Social Indicators Research Series

Volume 55

This series aims to provide a public forum for single treatises and collections of papers on social indicators research that are too long to be published in our journal Social Indicators Research. Like the journal, the book series deals with statistical assessments of the quality of life from a broad perspective. It welcomes research on a wide variety of substantive areas, including health, crime, housing, education, family life, leisure activities, transportation, mobility, economics, work, religion and environmental issues. These areas of research will focus on the impact of key issues such as health on the overall quality of life and vice versa. An international review board, consisting of Ruut Veenhoven, Joachim Vogel, Ed Diener, Torbjorn Moum and Wolfgang Glatzer, will ensure the high quality of the series as a whole. Available at 25% discount for International Society for Quality-of-Life Studies (ISQOLS). For membership details please contact: ISQOLS; e-mail: isqols@mail.vt.edu Editors: Ed Diener, University of Illinois, Champaign, USA; Wolfgang Glatzer, J.W. Goethe University, Frankfurt am Main, Germany; Torbjorn Moum, University of Oslo, Norway; Mirjam A.G. Sprangers, University of Amsterdam, The Netherlands; Joachim Vogel, Central Bureau of Statistics, Stockholm, Sweden; Ruut Veenhoven, Erasmus University, Rotterdam, The Netherlands.

For further volumes:
http://www.springer.com/series/6548

Qualitative Studies in Quality of Life

Graciela Tonon
Editor

Qualitative Studies in Quality of Life

Methodology and Practice

Springer

Editor
Graciela Tonon
Universidad Nacional de Lomas de Zamora
and Universidad de Palermo
Buenos Aires
Argentina

ISSN 1387-6570 ISSN 2215-0099 (electronic)
Social Indicators Research Series
ISBN 978-3-319-13778-0 ISBN 978-3-319-13779-7 (eBook)
DOI 10.1007/978-3-319-13779-7

Library of Congress Control Number: 2014956188

Springer Cham Heidelberg New York Dordrecht London

Printed on acid-free paper

Springer is part of Springer Science+Business Media (www.springer.com)

To my loving sons Pedro and Erica, and my dear husband Walter Who support my every day life and my work.

To my brother Gabriel
Who has been recently appointed Bishop.

Preface

The aim of this book is to show the importance of the development of qualitative studies in the field of quality of life. It is organized in two parts, and has been divided into ten chapters.

Part I, which comprises four chapters, deals with the theoretical-methodological reflection of qualitative studies; it examines the written production on the subject, the role of qualitative researchers, the role played by culture in qualitative studies and in the researchers'own lives, the follow-up of young researchers in their process of insertion in this field, and the challenge of integrating qualitative and quantitative methods for the study of quality of life, thus overcoming the traditional antagonism between them.

Part II contains six chapters that are concrete cases in which researchers have developed qualitative studies on quality of life in different disciplines and themes: Geography, Health, Communities, Youth, Childhood and Yoga in labor life, thus showing the possible new scenarios in the the history of quality of life studies.

Some of the chapters are the results of different research projects developed by the authors and/or myself and the other ones are the results of Doctoral Thesis that I directed in Argentina and Colombia. I am very grateful with the colleagues that work with me in this book.

Adopting a particular methodology implies a philosophical, theoretical and political decision and, in the case of qualitative methodology, it is an essential approach in understanding people's experiences of well-being and discovering new issues related to quality of life.

Qualitative Research Methodology Professor
Universidad Nacional de Lomas de Zamora
Universidad de Palermo, Argentina

Graciela Tonon

Acknowledgments

The authors wish to thank all the people who kindly accepted to be interviewed, without their collaboration, this book would not have been possible.

Contents

Part I Theory and Methodology

1 **Relevance of the Use of Qualitative Methods in the Study of Quality of Life** 3
Graciela Tonon

2 **The Qualitative Researcher in the Quality of Life Field** 23
Graciela Tonon

3 **The Role of Context and Culture in Quality of Life Studies** 37
Lia Rodriguez de la Vega

4 **Integration of Qualitative and Quantitative Methods in Quality of Life Studies** 53
Graciela Tonon

Part II Cases: Qualitative studies in quality of life in Geography, Health, Communities, Youth, Childhood and Yoga in Labor Life

5 **Qualitative Methodologies in Geography, Contributions to the Study of Quality of Life** 63
Claudia Mikkelsen and Josefina Di Nucci

6 **Qualitative Studies in Health-Related Quality of Life: The Case of Young People Living With HIV/AIDS** 97
Milton Décima

7 **Children's Quality of Life in the Caribbean: A Qualitative Study** 121
María Dilia Mieles-Barrera and Graciela Tonon

8 Qualitative Studies of Young People's Quality of Life in Urban and Rural Areas 149
Lucia Zanabria Ruiz

9 Young People's Rural Quality of Life in the Colombian Andes: A Qualitative Study Using Triangulation 179
Antonio José López López

10 A Qualitative Study on Yoga Practice in Quality of Labor Life 217
Lia Rodriguez de la Vega

Index 239

Contributors

Milton Décima Lord's Miracle Hospital, Salta, Argentina

Antonio José López López MEN, Colciencias, Bogotá, Colombia

María Dilia Mieles-Barrera Universidad del Magdalena, Santa Marta, Colombia

Claudia Mikkelsen Study Group on Population and Territory, Geography Department, Universidad Nacional de Mar del Plata, Buenos Aires, Argentina

Geographic Research Center, Geography, History and Social Sciences Institute, Universidad Nacional del Centro de la Provincia de Buenos Aires, Buenos Aires, Argentina

Josefina Di Nucci Geographic Research Center, Geography, History and Social Sciences Institute, Universidad Nacional del Centro de la Provincia de Buenos Aires. CONICET, Buenos Aires, Argentina

Lia Rodriguez de la Vega UNICOM, Faculty of Social Sciences, Universidad Nacional de Lomas de Zamora, Lomas de Zamora, Argentina

CICS, Faculty of Social Sciences, Universidad de Palermo, Ciudad Autónoma de Buenos Aires, Buenos Aires, Argentina

Graciela Tonon UNICOM, Faculty of Social Sciences, Universidad Nacional de Lomas de Zamora, Lomas de Zamora, Argentina

CICS, Faculty of Social Sciences, Universidad de Palermo, Ciudad Autónoma de Buenos Aires, Argentina

Lucia Zanabria Ruiz CICS Faculty of Social Sciences, Universidad de Palermo, Ciudad Autónoma de Buenos Aires, Argentina

Part I
Theory and Methodology

Chapter 1
Relevance of the Use of Qualitative Methods in the Study of Quality of Life

Graciela Tonon

This chapter is dedicated to the origin and evolution of qualitative studies in the quality of life field. At first it describes the characteristics and specificity of qualitative methods, considering that their main purpose is to understand meaning for participants in the study of the events, situations and actions in which they are involved, the context in which participants act and the influence these methods have on their actions, as well as the process in which the actions take place, which can enable the identification and generation of a new theory (Maxwell 1996).

Although not many studies have been developed through the use of qualitative methodologies in quality of life field, this chapter shows a summary of the studies that had been published in the Official Journal of ISQOLS, *Applied Research in Quality of Life*, since 2006 and the qualitative studies produced during the last decade through the Research Program on Quality of Life, Faculty of Social Sciences, Universidad Nacional de Lomas de Zamora, Argentina.

Finally, the chapter will point out that adopting a particular methodology implies a philosophic, theoretical and political decision and, in the case of qualitative methodology, it is an essential approach in understanding people's experiences of wellbeing and discovering new issues related to quality of life.

1.1 The Challenge of the Research

Strauss and Corbin (2002, p. 31) define investigation as a work flux that evolves through an entire investigation project, which implies a series of methodological decisions in each of its stages.

G. Tonon (✉)
UNICOM, Faculty of Social Sciences, Universidad Nacional de Lomas de Zamora, Lomas de Zamora, Argentina
e-mail: gracielatonon@hotmail.com

CICS, Faculty of Social Sciences, Universidad de Palermo, Ciudad Autónoma de Buenos Aires, Argentina

G. Tonon (ed.), *Qualitative Studies in Quality of Life*,
Social Indicators Research Series 55, DOI 10.1007/978-3-319-13779-7_1

The Word of science is more often considered as a creation of cognitive maps, molding and being molded by the actions and perceptions of the scientist, rather than an accumulation of knowledge (Bohm 1987 in May 2003, p. 21).

Research is a systematic rigorous activity carried out with the object of producing knowledge. It differs from other activities in the fact that it produces empirical evidence and uses clear and precise procedures to shed light on the way in which the results have been achieved, thus allowing for further argument. Its rigorousness is in keeping with the use of a specific language, an internal order (logical coherence) and a critical apparatus for reference, critical apparatus being understood as the entire set of bibliographical references that legitimize and support the research work (Vélez Restrepo 2003, p. 132).

In 2006, Greene identified four domains in social research:

a. The philosophical aspects derived from the consideration of the nature of the social world and that of social knowledge, the role of context, the researcher-researched relationship, and the question of subjectivity/objectivity.
b. The logics of research (methodology), which comprises the research questions, the construction of a design, and the proof, together with the methodological strategies, including the analysis, writing and interconnection of all these elements.
c. The research practice, which comprises the research methods and techniques, as well as the methods of analysis.
d. The socio-political aspects, which lead us to reflect upon the role of research in different societies, the interests behind research, and the possible relation it may have with governmental decisions.

Research is an intentional practice, with clear aims, which produces an acquisition of knowledge about the real world which differs from other activities such as common sense, art or religion.

1.2 The Quality of Life Field

The importance of the use of qualitative methodology in quality of life studies is related with the importance of considering people´s perceptions, opinions, feelings, ideas and interpretations. This kind of approach is essential to the understanding of people's experiences of wellbeing and to the discovery of new issues related with the quality of life field.

The study of the quality of life refers to the material conditions (social welfare) and to the psycho-social conditions (personal welfare); the latter, based on experience and on personal assessment, including positive and negative measures and a global view of a person's life. This is known as vital satisfaction, defined by Diener et al. (2006, p. 2) as the general assessment each individual makes of his own life, taking into consideration all the areas that constitute the life of a person at a given point in time.

Quality of life is the perception each person has of his/her own place in life, within a cultural context and the system of values he/she conforms to, as related to expectations, interests, and achievements.

In assessing quality of life people consider all the things that matter to them and judge the overall quality of their lives as a whole, while at the same time, people choose particular aspects in the domains of their lives and judge each of these domains separately (Inoguchi and Fujii 2013, p. 4).

Quality of life has, of late, generally referred to as the degree that determines a person's life to be desirable or undesirable in individual cases. Domains of satisfaction with life are to be understood as the people's judgment, when assessing different areas of their lives. However, in order to grasp a person's level of satisfaction in each area, it is necessary for the person in question to specify its importance, how much it is enjoyed, and how much of it should be subjected to change.

Although individual needs deriving in personal satisfaction vary in the different societies, it must be pointed out that the comparative measurements undertaken, so far, have traditionally presented a tendency towards correlation between economic status and satisfaction. Nevertheless, we coincide with Easterlin (1974) who believes that economic prosperity does not necessarily affect quality of life.

But quality of life is also conditioned by social structure, which may be considered in terms of demographic characteristics, cultural traits, psycho-social characteristics of the community, as well as the characteristics of its institutions, both official and private, which develop their action in this context (Ferris 2006). The author points out that the demographic foundation of a society and its institutional structure, provide the social environment for living conditions. In this sense, quality of life is elicited by two types of forces, endogenous and exogenous. The former include mental, emotional and psychological responses of the people towards their living conditions. The latter, on the other hand, include the social structure and the cultural influence of the community (Ferris 2006).

Casas (1999) states that, nowadays, quality of life is a concept which refers to the citizens' joint action in assessing what affects them, thus carrying political significance, contributing to the study of the people's well-being from the perspective of physical and psychological well-being, relating material needs to socio-emotional ones, and integrating psychological and social measurements of perception to the assessment of individual personal experiences.

1.3 The Use of Qualitative Methodology in the Study of Quality of Life

Even though the first attempts at applying qualitative methods in the field of Social Sciences were the ethnographic studies in the early twentieth century, we must point out that qualitative methods came into fashion once more in the 1980s, and that this tendency was extended all through the 1990s, with the increasing application of qualitative methodological texts in Europe and the USA together with its development in Latin American countries, especially regarding the use of participatory methods.

Qualitative methods have been generally applied to little known subjects, which explains why most of those studies are merely exploratory and are, likewise, used in circumstances that demand a revision of existing theories.

They have been traditionally conceived as a methodological resource for a first level approach to reality, which preceded a second instance in which the quantitative method was displayed.

The main purposes of using qualitative methods are to understand the meaning for participants in the study of the events, situations and actions in which they are involved, the context in which participants act and the influence of it on their actions and the process in which the actions take place, and at the same time enable the identification and generation of new theory (Maxwell 1996).

Understanding the meaning[1] for participants in the study of the events, situations and actions they are involved with and the accounts that they give for their life and experiences, as people perspectives conforms part of the reality the researchers try to understand in the study (Maxwell 1996, p. 17).

At present, there are a number of different proposals of qualitative methods applied to the field of social and human sciences: Phenomenology, Hermeneutics, Grounded Theory, Ethnography, Ethno-methodology, Content Analysis, Thematic Analysis, Discourse Analysis, Action Research, Participative Research, among others. Yet this chapter does not aim at presenting an abstract of every one of these proposals, since there is an extensive bibliography on each; the purpose is to reflect upon the peculiarities that qualitative methods have in common.

Qualitative studies are organized from generated ideas in relation with the importance of the analysis of the issue, with a core and keys of interpretation, not necessarily a hypothesis. The research purposes are focused on understanding something, gaining some insight into what is going on and why this is happening (Maxwell 1996, p. 16). The main feature of these studies is that they are holistic and inductive and that they require rigorous work over an extended span of time, their axes being discovery and comprehension.

Comprehension is a process that differs from information and scientific knowledge, and whose results are not definite. According to Arendt (1953–2005, pp. 32–33) comprehension precedes and prolongs knowledge and if a scholar wishes to transcend his own knowledge, he must be humble enough to become a careful listener of the populace in order to restore contact between knowledge and comprehension.

In this sense, Zemelman (2006, p. 33) points out the need to discuss a manner of comprehension of a historical moment in order to account for its diversity, which is quite different from the proof of a hypothesis. The researcher's capacity to articulate the diversities as they emerge, at a certain point in time, is what really matters.

[1] For the author "meaning" is used in a broad sense including cognition, affect, intentions and anything else that might conform the participant's perspectives.

Unlike the traditional theoretical background of quantitative studies, qualitative studies comprise a conceptual context formed by concepts, topics, beliefs and theories which support the project. Miles and Huberman (1994, p. 18) say that the contextual context explains either graphically or in a narrative form the main things to be studied, the key factors, concepts or variables and the presumed relationships among them.

The contextual context is not found, it is constructed by the researcher, hence, the importance of revising all the existing theories and previous researches (state of the art) in order to determine which of them may become a contribution to our project. In the construction of the conceptual context Maxwell (1996, p. 27) advises the consideration of the following: accumulated knowledge emerging from the researcher's experience, the theories and research already in existence in the thematic field, and the test research developed by the researcher.

Qualitative methods study inter-subjective meanings, situated and built by probing into the depths of social life in its natural development and exploring meaning for its actors. In this perspective, the world is built around meanings and symbols, the former being local, inherent to each individual and each group/culture and to their behavior within each historical moment. Furthermore, as is the case of every process of production of knowledge in social sciences, its results also affect the subjects. As Vélez Restrepo (2003, p. 143) says qualitative perspective is a social product whose production process is collective and transversally influenced by values, perceptions and meanings of the subjects in charge of their construction. An inter-subjective immersion into the desired knowledge of a particular reality is the condition which allows the comprehension of its internal logics and rationality.

The choice of qualitative methods implies a particular vision of the world which leads to a consideration of the essential meaning of the world (ontology), an idea of how it may be known (epistemology), and a way to guarantee the knowledge of the world (methodology) as well as a set of values to orient the task (axiology) (López et al. 2010, p. 132).

Studies of this kind offer two essential characteristics: *reflexibility* and *indexicality*.

The former originated in Garfinkel's ethno-methodology (1967). He states that ethno-methodology is the research of the methods people use to achieve and substantiate communication, decision making, rationality, and everyday life activity. It is, thus, an outlook on daily life and the rules that help the subjects (including the researcher himself) to understand and construct his own world. In this sense, *reflexibility* is the property which goes together with an activity when it presupposes something while making it observable, at the same time (Ruiz Olabuenaga and Ispizúa 1989, pp. 54–56). For Sotolongo Codina and Delgado Díaz (2006, p. 62) the *reflexibility* presumption considers that a system has been constituted in virtue of the reciprocal interference between the activity of the object system and the objectified activity of the subject.

Indexicality is the movement which reveals contextual meaning and shows the dependence of concrete acts on the situational context in which they occur; therefore, they can only be explained if the context has been understood. According to Ruiz Olabuenaga and Ispizúa (1989, p. 56) it aims at the double meaning every expression offers: a trans-situational meaning and a specific one, for individual situations.

Qualitative studies mostly work on description, defined by Strauss and Corbin (2002) as the use of words to express mental images of an occurrence, an aspect of the panorama, a scene, an experience, an emotion or sensation, where the narrative is made from the point of view of the person making the description. Every description includes a purpose, an audience, and a selective eye.

In qualitative studies, two kinds of description may be observed: fine descriptions and dense descriptions. The former are those which narrate an occurrence without attempting to show the intentions, motives, meanings or circumstances that surround it. Dense descriptions, on the other hand, reveal or lead to discover the subjacent knowledge, relationship structures which the persons under study may or may not understand, and act accordingly. They go beyond the act, probing into detail, context, emotion, and the affiliation network and micro-power (Ruiz Olabuénaga and Ispizúa 1989, p. 48).

Description may be the foundation for the interpretation and construction of a theory, though it is necessary to make clear that, while description incorporates concepts, it should be stressed that "describing does not equal theorizing", although description is basic to theorization.

Nevertheless, interpretation and theorization are not the same. Interpretation is related to the significance given to occurrences by the subjects under study. It is only when researchers take, both descriptions and interpretations, as sources of explanation that they can be said to be attempting to generate theory.

All interpretations are constructed inter-subjectively, and within a given context to which they belong, and which their constructions cannot avoid; this does not imply the validity of all interpretations, only that it is necessary that they should be contrasted to the daily practice of real and concrete subjects (Sotolongo Codina and Delgado Diaz 2006, p. 57).

Theorizing is a long and deep process which implies formulating ideas in a logical, systematic and explicative scheme. In the depths of theorization lies the interaction between making inductions, deriving concepts, their properties and dimensions, on the basis of given data and deductions. Thus, theory is more than mere findings, since it offers further explanation of the phenomena, which allow the development of a field of knowledge (Strauss and Corbin 2002, pp. 15–28).

Maxwell (1996, p. 33) pointed out that in qualitative studies it is possible to use a theory based on concepts and one emerged from inductive reasoning through the data of the study (grounded theory); likewise, theory can be used as a coat closer where you can find and hang anything in it or as a Spotlight in which case theory illuminates what you can see in your research.

Considering the abovementioned characteristics and specific aspects related to qualitative studies we may point out that, since this type of studies consider the person as a protagonist of the research processes, acknowledging the importance that context and meaning have to the actors, we conclude that qualitative methodology is a kind of approach essential in understanding people's experiences of wellbeing and discovering new issues related to quality of life.

1.4 Qualitative Studies in Quality of Life at the *Applied Research in Quality of Life*, Official Journal of the International Society for Quality of Life Studies (ISQOLS)

The *Applied Research in Quality of Life* (ARQOL) is the official journal of the International Society for Quality-of-Life Studies (ISQOLS), Richard Estes is his Editor in Chief, and it is published by Springer.

The Journal presents conceptual, methodological and empirical papers dealing with quality-of-life studies in the applied areas of the natural and social sciences. It aims at publishing papers that have direct implications for, or impact on practical applications of research on the quality of life. The articles are crafted from inter-disciplinary, inter-professional and international perspectives. ARQOL guides decision making in a variety of professions, industries, nonprofit, and government sectors, including healthcare, travel and tourism, marketing, corporate management, community planning, social work, public administration, and human resource management. It helps decision makers apply performance measures and apply assessment techniques based on such concepts as well-being, human satisfaction, human development, happiness, wellness and quality-of-life.

From its onset, in 2006, to August 2013, three specifically qualitative studies have been published in *Applied Research in Quality of Life*. Only these three articles are mentioned, since they are the ones which propose qualitative methodology as the only option used by researchers. It is worth mentioning that studies applying mixed methods have been published in this journal and they will be referred to, once more, in the eighth chapter of this book.

The first of those articles entitled *Revisiting the local impact of community indicators project: Sustainable Seattle as a prophet in its own land*, was written by Meg Holden. This article presented the results of a research on the policy impacts of community indicator projects in their localities and on manners of increasing the effectiveness of projects from the perspectives of different indicator organizations and policy actor groups. It was a case study in which data were gathered developing a historical analysis using archival and policy documents as well as newspapers, participant observations and deep interviews with people selected out of five groups: elected leaders, local government employees, nonprofit organizations, active citizens and businesses.

The second article was edited in 2009 and was entitled *Suerte (luck): spirituality and well-being in El Alto, Bolivia,* by Melania Calestani. It is a doctorate thesis which, years later, became one of the volumes of the Springerbriefs collection. This paper deals with the importance of faith and the consequent resort to supernatural forces in order to acquire a sense of well-being in a poor neighborhood in the city of El Alto, Bolivia. It was an ethnographic research carried out during twelve months where the researcher developed the participants' observations, informal conversations and informal interviews. The author concluded that

> Ethnography enables the analysis of the art of living, privileging a more unsystematic -yet rigorous- approach to accommodate different cultural contexts and the many perspectives that illustrate the scenarios of human life. Illustrating the value of such an approach and the complexities of social action can hopefully create space for further discussion on the importance of context and will highlight the malleability of concepts of well-being in everyday life, in opposition to universalist definitions based on material factors. (Calestani 2009, p. 73)

The third article, dating from 2010, is *Health related quality of life in Iranian breast cancer survivors: a qualitative study* de T. Harandy, F. Ghofranipour, A. Montazeri, M. Anoosheh, E. Mohammadi, F. Ahmadi, F. Shokravi and S. Niknami. This work analyses the role of cultural and social factors on quality of life, in relation to the state of health of women who have survived breasts cancer in Iran. The authors developed deep semi-structured interviews of 39 women diagnosed with breast cancer, at diverse stages, one year after diagnosis, and no longer on active invasive treatment. Two topics were discussed in the interviews: the effects of their illness in their QOL and cultural aspects affecting their QOL. Women agreed to be interviewed and authorized the interviews which were audio-taped and transcribed using members check. Results were analyzed using the words of the participants and organized in codes.

1.5 Qualitative Studies in Quality of Life at the Research Program on Quality of Life, Faculty of Social Sciences, Universidad Nacional de Lomas de Zamora, Argentina

Since the creation, in 2004, of the Research Program on Quality of Life of the Faculty of Social Sciences of Universidad Nacional de Lomas de Zamora, three research projects have taken place, developed with a qualitative focus and centered in the study of the relationship between quality of life and Access to university life.

The first project took place during 2005 and was entitled *A strategy in the improvement of the quality of life: the university as a space for the social integration of students.* Subsequently, and during the 2010–2011 period, the second project was developed under the name of *Images of the future and quality of life of young university students of the Faculty of Social Sciences of Universidad Nacional de Lomas de Zamora.* Both projects allowed the identification of the existing relationships between higher studies and level of satisfaction in the lives of the subjects under study. The report revealed a direct and positive relationship between the situation of studying at university and the perception of quality of life. These conclusions encouraged us to pursue this line of research, thus, advancing in the study of the quality of life of post graduate students, taking into consideration that, since 2009, the Faculty of Social Sciences of Universidad Nacional de Lomas de Zamora has been offering its graduates and teaching staff the opportunity to take up post-graduate studies, free of charge. Our latest Project, developed in the course of 2012–2013, is entitled *Quality of life and satisfaction with post-graduate studies: a study from the subjects' perspective.*

Presently, we shall very briefly introduce the most significant features and results of the first two projects, considering that they have already been published, and proceed to a deeper treatment of the third project one of whose central topics of study was, precisely, the definition of the concept of quality of life as expressed by the interviewed subjects.

First project: *A strategy in the improvement of the quality of life: the university as a space for the social integration of students.* Its aims were: to describe the role of university as a space for social integrating in the Departments of Greater Buenos Aires[2] in the early twenty-first century and identify the assessment the students made of their access to university, and the way it altered their quality of life. It was a descriptive study made through the qualitative method, the construction of meanings and the context in which the actors behave being part of the problem the research is about.

Semi-structured interviews were made to an intentional sample of students from Universidad Nacional de Lomas de Zamora, and two other national universities located in other Departments of Greater Buenos Aires, as well as three university professors from the abovementioned educational institutions who acted as key informers. This technique privileged the attainment of information pertaining the students' perception of their process of insertion in university life and the social role of university. The selected group of students was integrated by 10 subjects of both sexes, between 20 and 56 years old. The courses of study were the following: Advertising, Education, Social Work, Minors and Family, Law, Political Science and Mathematics.

The students greatly valued their access to university, whether to acquire knowledge, as an anticipatory mechanism of a possible future source of employment, or as a stage in the improvement of their quality of life; the latter being regarded in its broader sense rather than as a restrictive conception that relates the quality of life to material possessions.

In the students' discourse, the possibility of being inserted in the work-field was regarded as the final stage of development derived from previous ones such as: access to work spaces related to their courses of study, preceding their graduation, in order to become acquainted with the work-field; development of volunteer work; and the need to take up post-graduate studies. On account of the increasingly precarious working conditions, especially in the professions connected with social sciences, the expectations of working at the chosen profession began to take shape as a way of improving their personal quality of life and, in this sense, attending university has been a stage of improvement.

[2] The Departments of Greater Buenos Aires is the geographical region that surrounds the capital district. Its size is 3833 km^2 and it is organized in 24 departments. The most recent national census (2010) showed that its population is about 9.916.715 inhabitants, which is the equivalent to the fourth part of the total country population which amounts to 40.117.096 inhabitants. It is a region that presents polarized life conditions, ranging from settlements of extreme poverty to high-income gated neighborhoods.

Quality of life has been associated to vital satisfaction, to enjoyment, to "doing what I like" and, in doing so, with the possibility of personal fulfilment. Thus, quality of life has been recognized as an instance that confers entity to the experience people have of their own life styles and living conditions, conferring as much value to this experience, or even more, than to material conditions, historically considered "objective".

The second project was developed in the course of 2010–2011 and was entitled *Images of the future and quality of life of young university students of the Faculty of Social Sciences of Universidad Nacional de Lomas de Zamora*. Its aims were to describe the perception that young university students have of their quality of life, as related to the characteristics of their socio-political and economic context, and to identify their wishes and fears regarding their future insertion in the work field after their graduation. It was a descriptive study, with a qualitative perspective, which allowed a better understanding of the personal perceptions of the participants, giving way to the emergence of new categories, or to a new interpretation and significance of the same categories hitherto observed.

Ten university students were selected, males and females between 18 and 23 years old, newly incorporated to the Faculty of Social Sciences of Universidad Nacional de Lomas de Zamora. Each was selected for a different course of studies in that Faculty: Social Work, Psycho-pedagogy, Educational Sciences, Letters, Minors and Family, Social Communication, Journalism, Advertising, Public Relations, and Labor Relations.

A semi-structured interview was used as a technique, defined as *a gathering among subjects, and it is a technique that enables reading, comprehension and analysis of subjects, contexts, and social situations, also generating situations and acts of communication* (Tonon 2009, p. 5). The semi-structure was provided by thematic axes that responded to study oriented ideas, generated on the basis of a theoretical perspective, in coherence with the research design. Placing special attention on methodological rigorousness, the purpose of this kind of interview is, at the same time, to offer enough scope to avoid hindering the spontaneous emergence of new theoretical categories. The thematic axes were:

- Identification data: age, sex occupation, type and duration of job.
- Perception of present quality of life.
- Perception of the characteristics of the socio-political and economic context.
- Characteristics of the Departments of the Greater Buenos Aires.
- Expectations regarding a future insertion in the labor force: wishes and fears.
- Labor alternatives for the future.

For the data analysis we used Thematic Analysis, which is a method of qualitative analysis that allows for topics to be identified and codified within the dense descriptions obtained from the semi-structured interviews with the young students. The chosen phases for the thematic analysis were those of Braun and Clarke (2006).

The results demonstrate that all the subjects we interviewed lived with their families and were, in some cases, the first member of the family to enter university. Most of them were unemployed, but those who had a job considered it to be a contribution to the family economy. On the other hand, others considered that getting a job was an expectation related to certain relevant values at a personal level, such as the right to feel independent.

Thus, the expectations of making a living on their chosen professions, as an improvement in their quality of life, relates the young students' access to university studies to the empowerment of quality of life, on objective and subjective terms. Quality of life is related to satisfaction with life, with enjoying what they like doing. Quality of life is therefore acknowledged as something that makes their lives meaningful. The scenario is completed by their conception of education as an opportunity to become real citizens. The students' discourse further discloses the notion that obtaining a university degree implies having access to a job and, thus, to social prestige.

These young people describe their difficulties in obtaining jobs, which sheds light on the way they relate this issue to their quality of life. In this sense, it is important to point out that Sirgy et al. (2008, p. 88) have studied the effects of satisfactory employment on the quality of life of a community, and have concluded that a total satisfaction with one's community is partially affected by job availability which, in turn, has an impact on the financial as well as the labor and family fields.

The results show that the young students of both sexes are, in all cases, satisfied with their quality of life, even when this feeling is related to different aspects of the same: namely, job availability, healthy family relations, religious practice, the opportunity to carry on with their studies, and the achievement of an economic status.

Finally, we may add that the central role our research assigns to work, as a means of improving quality of life, came across as part of the process of interaction in the construction of citizenship. University studies (and the university as an institution) continue to be perceived as a distinctive value related to social mobility, in its broad sense, that is, not reduced to economic status but also regarded as an improvement of the "person", in other words, of quality of life in general. The expectation of making a living on the chosen professions came up as an improvement of the quality of life, relating access to university to the empowerment of the quality of life, both in objective and subjective terms. The feeling of satisfaction with one's life and the enjoyment derived from doing what one likes, lead quality of life to be recognized as a state which makes one's life meaningful.

The third project was *Quality of life and satisfaction with post graduate studies: a study from the subjects' perspective*. Its aims were: to identify the situations which led the post graduate students in question to take up their studies; to interpret the descriptions of their quality of life made by the participants; to determine their alleged level of satisfaction with their present studies; and to identify whether the initiation of post graduate studies has, in fact produced a change in their quality of life, particularly in their work field.

The abovementioned was a descriptive study which proposed a qualitative perspective. The sample was integrated by students of post graduate courses from the Faculty of Social Sciences of Universidad Nacional de Lomas de Zamora (Specialization in Didactics and Curriculum, Masters in Curriculum, Specialization in Labor Relations, Masters in Labor Relations, Specialization in Social Communications, Masters in Social Communications). The mode adopted was that of the plain simple for qualitative studies which requires the researcher to make a list of the essential features each selected unit should possess; 18 subjects were interviewed to that effect. The selection was made taking into account the parameters of sex, age, and whether or not the subject was a student and/or ex-student of Universidad Nacional de Lomas de Zamora.

The semi-structured research interview was used from a perspective that sets aside the traditional reductionist outlook which has so far been attributed to the semi-structured research, i.e., as a simple tool to gather information (Tonon 2009, p. 71). Like in the previous researches, the interviews had a script based on the following axes:

- Identification data: age, sex, occupation, time and duration of job.
- Description of the decisive factors leading to post-graduate studies.
- Description of the subjects' family reactions regarding the subjects' decisions.
- Description of the subjects' quality of life.
- Degree of satisfaction with post-graduate studies: pedagogical, administrative, and education.
- Opinion about the university as an institution.
- Description of the possible relationship between post-graduate education and quality of life.
- Future perspectives regarding the possible changes in their lives, in general, and particularly as regards the job offer that a post-graduate degree is likely to generate.

In this research, the thematic analysis proposed by Braun and Clarke (2006) was used in order to identify, analyze, and inform about topics and structures thus revealing, not only the experiences but also the meanings and realities of the subjects, as well as examining the ways in which events, realities, meanings, and experiences are dictated by society. Thus, thematic analysis becomes a strategy of qualitative data analysis through which results are systematized and inferred.

The interviewed subjects were between 27 and 53 years old, ten of them were females and eight of them males, most of them residing in the Departments of Greater Buenos Aires and have obtained their degrees at the Universidad Nacional de Lomas de Zamora, some have graduated recently, while others are re-commencing their studies after several years. In some cases, they have alleged not being the only university students in their families but, in most cases, they were taking up post-graduate studies for the first time.

The subjects' interview discourse reveals their acknowledgement of a good or very good quality of life and, only one of them did not show complete satisfaction with the life he had.

The definition of quality of life appears in the subjects' discourse as associated to family life, housing and environment, leisure time, health, job, education and politics; but it is mainly defined as good living, satisfaction with their activities, personal fulfillment, happiness, and harmony. One significant fact is that the definition of quality of life is not preeminently associated to money or economic welfare, it is only related to the money earned at work, but only as a contribution to personal and family welfare.

> Look, I believe quality of life is not a synonym of salary raise, in my specific case it would be the opposite; I think quality of life has to do with feeling useful and satisfied with the profession one has chosen, with one's family circle, as persons, which is not the same as just one's income. (female, 40 years old)
> It's difficult to define quality of life but, let's say, if I had to use classical parameters and common sense, I'd say, well, I own a house, I have a job, my work enables me to be in a fairly good position, I go on holiday in Summer, in Winter I can also go on holiday, if I have the time; I can pay for my daughter's kindergarten, she's taking swimming lessons, gym lessons, I'm also taking swimming lessons. Let's say, I can indulge in certain things I like, nothing showy. I have my own car; I'm still paying for it in installments. (male, 34 years old)
> Well, er…, I'm lucky to have an income that allows me to have a quality of life, doing what I like, not everything but, well, a few whims… (female, 30)

Family is a core determinant of life satisfaction and personal development. Mattew (1986) found that people with spouses and friends are more likely to be physically and mentally healthier than people living alone. The roles of the spouse and of the friend provide emotional support and well being (Requena 1995).

> I've got my husband, so I consider my quality of life to be good. (Female, 27 years old)
> I'm fulfilled… I've got my loved ones, which is what contributes quality of life, to a greater degree. (Female, 50 years old)
> Being able to exploit and develop my abilities for the benefit of others and, obviously… my quality of life, I think I'm going to be alright if the people around me are alright, that's what comes to mind, that those who are with me should be well. My surroundings, my context; obviously, I prioritize my family, friends, my surroundings, my work, my studies. I'll feel well if those who are dear to me are well, this is my conception in this matter. (Male, 29 years old)
> As to emotions, which also influence my life, I'm in a stable relationship. I have a good quality of life. (Female, 30 years old)

In their discourse there is a preeminence of the connection between having a job and pursuing post-graduate studies with an improvement of the quality of life in terms of personal achievement; and the pursuit of post-graduate studies as a form of improvement of their labor conditions.

Employment plays an important role on people's social lives and also confirms their conformity with social norms (Marks et al. 2004, p. 14). Various authors have observed a positive correlation between having a job and life satisfaction. Such is the case of the studies made by Jackson (1993, 1994, and 1998) y Rodgers (1977) involving women and quoted by Mammen, Bower and Lass (2009). Personal development captures curiosity, enthusiasm, absorption, flow, exploration, commitment, creative challenge and also potential meaningfulness (Marks et al. 2004, p. 4).

> Post-graduate studies have a lot to do with quality of life, they offer the chance to gain access to a place of learning, and that place of learning gives you personal satisfaction; because my presence here is a question of personal growth. (Female, 50)
> I attend a post-graduate course for personal satisfaction, one gets ahead, comes into contact with people who want to make progress and with whom you can hold conversations at a totally different level from the ones on the streets, or habitually at work. (Female, 33)

> Post-graduate courses offer this possibility … and the quality of life … not only by associating work to economic welfare, but also regarding work as a generator of other activities which broaden your personal spectrum, as when you open up to doing awesome things, surprising things. And you say, "Wow, this can actually be done!" Not always the same routine... (Female, 53)
> Well, I have my work, my husband's got his, we both study, he attends a private university but I've always studied at public university; in this sense, I consider my quality of life to be good. (Female, 27 years old)
> Many relationships …, not only can I improve my quality of life regarding my work field by taking a post graduate course, but it also helps you acquire another train of thought, it opens your mind. Attending a post-graduate course changes your mentality; with the influence of TV, the radio, your family, it gives you another outlook on things … I don't know what else to say. (Female, 30 years old)

The relationship of quality of life with the environment and habitation is one of the most popular options offered by the interviewed subjects. Some authors (Veenhoven 2009; Inoguchi and Fujii 2013) point out that the livability of the environment refers explicitly to the characteristics of the environment and is not limited by material conditions. The habitability of an environment is a term used for the quality of housing in particular (Veenhoven 2009, p. 8).

> The places and environment where people live and the resources and activities available to them affect quality of life directly, but such objective conditions of life also affect quality indirectly through a set of values held by the same people (Inoguchi and Fujii 2013, p. 4)
> What the interviewed subjects say:
> Quality of life; I associate it more and more to the preservation of our space, looking after ourselves, posing whether we can really generate environments- fair, loving spaces…And, in looking after each other and, in the environment, in the field I cover, there is a definition of quality of life. (Female, 53 years old)
> As to the place I live in, though there are no sewers where I live, it's something that is beyond me; but regarding my quality of life, I consider it good, in general lines. My environment has no specific needs …this, at times, has got a bearing on it but, it's good, I should say it's good. (Male, 34 years old)
> It's obvious that one would always wish to have more, for instance, in my case, I'm renting. Owning a house, obviously… but the general context is good. (Male, 29 years old)
> Good; the house is rather small, very small, especially taking into account our kid. My immediate aim is to enlarge the house, but everything else is excellent; we're in good health, we have a job, our boy can even go to nursery school, has already got his education project; we have leisure time, we don't need anything else. (Female, 38 years old)

Three subjects have related quality of life to activities they carry out for leisure or for pleasure. In relation with the effects of leisure activities on people's quality of life, Cini et al. (2013) reported positive effects. The authors point out that leisure activities provide opportunities for self determined behaviors that exist when people freely choose to engage in activity out of a sense of interest, out of mere enjoyment of the activity itself, which is important in coping with stress and enhancing well-being (Cini et al. 2013, p. 46).

> I relate my quality of life with leisure time. (Male, 28 years old)
> Full, very good, my quality of life; I was able to go swimming again, because I had always had this activity, always. And, well, now I've gone back to this activity I had abandoned. (Female, 50 years old)
> I love dancing, I really like dancing the tango and "salsa". (Female, 33 years old)

One of the interviewed subjects relates quality of life with good health. Good health is widely considered to be a key to living a happy life but causality can work the other way around. Well-being is also a key to good health as there is strong evidence that happy people are healthier and live longer (Marks et al. 2004, p. 16). In his book Etica a Nicómaco, Aristotle admitted the importance of good health in his definition of happiness. Health related QOL concentrates on an accurate depiction of the way health influences and is influenced by the experience of the body and the mind within a social and cultural context (Patrick 2006, p. 399).

> If quality of life is also related, or so I think, to one's environment, to the environment, to the wholesome feeling of being involved with one's family, friends, and such, I could say that my quality of life is good, healthy. And if it were to be about, say, personal projects one has been able to achieve, I'd say that I'm in good health. (Male, 36 years old)

One of the subjects also related quality of life with his political activity, pointing out the flexibility this generates in him. In this sense, there is a coincidence with Martinez Manzano (2008, p. 10) who refers to Aristotle when he expresses that political life seeks honors, though its real nature consists in the exercise of virtue in the context of the citizens' coexistence.

> I'm interested in politics ... one has a kind of social flexibility, different from other people's. Yes, I think I know... what I want. Well, my quality of life is very good. (Male, 27 years old)

But the interviewed subjects, essentially, define quality of life in terms of satisfaction, personal enrichment, transcendence, happiness and harmony.

According to Veenhoven (1996), life satisfaction or vital satisfaction, is the degree of positive assessment of global quality of life, i.e., how much a person enjoys the life he/she leads. The relevant dimension for the measurement of life satisfaction is the degree at which a measure is relevant to oneself. Life satisfaction captures satisfaction, pleasure, enjoyment and contentment (Marks et al. 2004, p. 4).

> I believe that quality of life is related to satisfaction and a post-graduate course; personally, I believe this brings deep satisfaction. Beyond the fact that it allows for subsidiary jobs, even if that were not the case, I believe it has to do with a question of inner satisfaction, self improvement, other bonds, other outlooks, to other ways of listening; intangible satisfactions which are related to quality of life. Experiencing the satisfaction of doing the things I'm interested in and being interested in what I do, this is quality of life to me; being satisfied with the things I do gives me moral well-being and ease of mind. (Female, 38)
>
> There's a relation with the term personal development but, in my conception of quality of life development, when I define it, I take it as a question of personal development as a professional and, well, obviously, the post-graduate course will afford me all that, and has already done so, to a greater or lesser extent, through the curricular subjects, the different experiences and class mates, and a lot of other things that are reflected professionally through many of the things I've learnt. And, well, this is also reflected in my quality of life. (Male, 29)
>
> From the personal satisfaction of knowing, learning... (Female, 40 years old)

Smith (1980, pp. 21–27 in Sirgy 2006, p. 356) sketched six views of the good life: maximum gratification of desire, dominant end view, purpose in life, living up to one's major expectations, human flourishing and satisfaction of need. The author said that the first four views posit the good life as an end or product, while the two final ones posit it as a process.

A good life must be good for something more than itself. This presumes some higher values (Veenhoven 2009, p. 8). Gerson (1976, p. 795 in Veenhoven 2009, p.) referred to the latter as transcendental conceptions of quality of life.

> I relate quality of life, more and more, with a good life, I mean, the things we are generating in order to have a better coexistence with ourselves and with others. (Female, 53 years old)
> Quality of life is the chance we have to, intelligently, select the things that are going to enrich us, improve us, and make us grow up. I understand that quality of life is not only about material things, it also relates to emotions, thoughts, and transcendent things, because I believe in transcendence, and I believe that is also quality of life. (Female, 47 years old)

Things can be intrinsically valuable or instrumentally valuable. The things that are intrinsically valuable are those regarded as good, for what they are, or good as ends, themselves. The things that are instrumentally valuable are the ones regarded as good for obtaining other things, or good as a means of obtaining things that are regarded as intrinsically valuable (Michalos 2006, p. 353).

Reflecting on that old model of harmony, today one might say that people are happy when their heads and hearts are together, such people can be said to be happy (Michalos 2006, p. 355). Aristotle said that the proper, intrinsically valuable aim of human beings is happiness "to be happy is to live well and to do well". Happiness should be placed among the things that are themselves pleasurable, not for any other reason, for happiness does not need anything other than itself; and the activities selected for what they are, are those which do not seek anything beyond the activity itself (Aristotle 1176b, p. 281). The happy life is the life of virtue and effort (Aristotle 1177b, p. 283). Happiness is the major possession sought by the nature of human beings. For Aristotle, happiness is the ultimate end, since it is always sought for itself, while making the subject independent and self-sufficient; for whoever reaches it is content with it and needs nothing more.

> Perhaps we should review our concepts of quality of life to check whether we are referring to the same thing. To me, quality of life is related to a state of harmony; it's rather utopian to think of a state of harmony, but being somehow firm in one's position, balanced, happy, is not a utopian state. I regard quality of life, not so related to financial gain … with welfare, but with the satisfaction of basic needs, of course. (Female, 50 years old)
> Quality of life……………………it's very subjective, isn't it? (Female, 30 years old)

To conclude, we may say that the definition of quality of life extracted from the discourse of the interviewed subjects is essentially considered in terms of satisfaction, personal enrichment, transcendence, happiness, and harmony. A significant finding is the fact that quality of life is not essentially associated to money or economic welfare, for money has only been associated to work, and in terms of personal and family welfare. It is identified as a positive relationship between having a job and taking up post-graduate studies, in terms of personal development and the chance/opportunity of improving working conditions. The environment and habitation, the most often mentioned, appear integrated with personal and community life development. Lastly, the access to leisure activities that generate pleasure, good health, and political activity complete the definition.

1.6 Conclusions

If we agree to the fact that quality of life offers us the possibility of a new theoretical outlook—which aims at working on potentialities rather than deficiencies, and on a community anchorage which includes the analysis of the socio-political context where a person is considered as subject and protagonist—we may then state that quality of life poses a social and political reality necessarily based on an integrated respect for human rights (Tonon 2003).

This chapter has led us to consider that deciding on a particular methodology implies a philosophic, theoretical and political decision. In this sense qualitative research constructs and interprets meanings within specific social and cultural contexts, thus, becoming a sense generator (Torres Carrillo 2006, p. 100).

The use of the qualitative methods in the study of the quality of life of persons, groups, communities and nations, is suitable and important, though researches made through qualitative methods have not yet been highly developed.

Likewise, it would be interesting to understand what Schultz and Meleis expressed two decades ago:

> If we admit that there are different forms of knowledge, different unknown things to be discovered, different inclinations of the knowledgeable to discover, and different aspects which can be found out about the same phenomenon, we will then, perhaps, develop more appropriate criteria to learn from what we already know, and then to know what we wish to know (Schultz and Meleis 1988. p. 221 in May 2003, p. 15)

References

Arendt, H. (2005). *De la historia a la acción*. Buenos Aires: Editorial Paidós.

Braun, V., & Clarke, V. (2006). Using thematic analysis in psychology. *Qualitative research in Psychology, 3,* 77–10. (Edward Arnold Publishers).

Casas, F. (1999). Calidad de vida y calidad humana. En *Revista Papeles del Psicólogo N° 74.* Madrid. pp 46–54

Calestani, M. (2009). "SUERTE" (Luck): Spirituality and well-being in El Alto Bolivia. *Applied Research in Quality of Life, 4,* 47–75.

Cini, F., Kruger, S., & Ellis, S. A. (2013). Model of intrinsic and extrinsic motivations on subjective well-being: the experience of overnight visitors to a national park. *Applied Research in Quality of Life, 8,* 45–61.

Diener, E. (2006). Guidelines for national indicators of subjective well-being and ill-being. *Applied Research in Quality of Life, 1,* 151–157.

Easterlin, R. (1974). Does economic growth improve the human lot?. Some empirical evidence. http://graphics8.nytimes.com/images/2008/04/16/business/Easterlin1974.pdf. Accessed 3 Dec 2013.

Ferris, A. (2006). A theory of social structure and the quality of life. *Applied Research in Quality of Life, 1,* 117–123.

Garfinkel, H. (1967). *Studies in ethnomethodology*. Englewood Cliffs: Prentice-Hall.

Greene, J. (2006). Toward a Methodology of Mixed Methods Social Inquiry. *RESEARCH IN THE SCHOOLS. Mid-South Educational Research Association Vol. 13. No, 1,* 93–98.

Inoguchi, T., & Fujii, S. (2013). *The quality of life in Asia. A comparison of quality of life in Asia.* Dordretch, Heilderberg, New York, London: Springer.

Jackson, A. P. (1993). Black, single, working mothers in poverty: preferences for employment, well-being and perceptions of preschool-age children. *Social Work, 38*(1), 26–34.
Jackson, A. P. (1994). Psychological distress among single, employed, black mothers and their perceptions of their young children. *Journal of Social Service Research, 19*(3–4), 87–101.
Jackson, A. P. (1998). The role of social support in parenting for low-income single, black mothers. *Social Service Review, 72*(3), 365–378.
López, Jorge S., Blanco, F., Scandroglio, B. (2010). Rasskin Gutman, Irina. Una aproximación a las prácticas cualitativas en psicología desde una perspectiva integradora. *Papeles del Psicólogo, Vol. 31, Núm. 1*, enero-abril, pp. 131–142. Consejo General de Colegios Oficiales de Psicólogos. España. Retrieved from: http://redalyc.uaemex.mx/src/inicio/ArtPdfRed.jsp?iCve=77812441013. Accessed 28 Oct 2013.
Mammen, S., Bauer, J., & Lass, D. (2009). Life satisfaction among rural low-income members: the influence of health, human personal and social capital. *Applied Research in Quality of Life, 4*, 365–386.
Marks, N., Shah, H., & Westall, A. (2004). The power and potential of well-being indicators. Measuring young people's well-being in Nottingham. Nef. Retrieved from http://s.bsd.net/nefoundation/default/page/file/fc446058e067754539_xwm6vurfq.pdf. Accessed 5 Feb 2014.
Martinez Manzano, T. (2008). Introducción en Aristóteles, *Etica Nicomáquea,* Bs. As. Biblioteca Clasica Gredos (pp. 7–17).
Maxwell, J. (1996). *Qualitative research design. An interactive Approach.* New York: Sage publications.
May, K. (2003). Conocimiento abstracto: un caso a favor de la magia en el método. En J. Morse (comp.), *Asuntos críticos en los métodos de investigación cualitativa* (pp. 14–27). Medellin: Universidad de Antioquia.
Miles, M., & Huberman, M. (1994). *Qualitative data analysis: An expanded sourcebook.* Thousand Oaks: Sage.
Michalos, A. (2006). Conceptual and philosophical foundations. Sirgy, J., Michalos, A., Ferris, A., Esaterlin, R., Patrick, D., Pavot, W. The quality of life (QOL) Research movement: Past, present and future. *SIR 76* (343–466). pp. 351–383.
Patrick, D. (2006). Short history of health realted quality of life research. Sirgy, J., Michalos, A., Ferris, A., Esaterlin, R., Patrick, D., Pavot, W. The quality of life (QOL) Research movement: Past, present and future. *SIR 76* (343–466). pp. 399–408.
Requena, F. (1995). Determinantes estructurales de las redes sociales en 10s hombres y las mujeres. P*apers, 45,* 33–41.
Ruiz Olabuenaga, J., & e Ispizúa, M. (1989). *La descodificación de la vida cotidiana.* Bilbao: Universidad de Deusto.
Schultz, P., & Meleis, A. (1988). Nursing epistemology: tradition, insights, questions. Image: *Journal of Nursing Scholarship, 20*(4), 217–221.
Sirgy, M. J., Michalos, A. C., Ferriss, A. L., Easterlin, R. A., Patrick, D., & Pavot, W. (2006). The quality-of-life (QOL) research movement: Past, present, and future. *Social Indicators Research, 76*(3), 343–466.
Sirgy, M. J., Gao, T., & Young, R. (2008). How does residents' satisfaction with community services influence quality of life outcomes? *ARQOL, 3*(2), 81–105.
Smith, M. L. (1980). *Solving for some unknowns in the personal equation (CIRCE Occasional Paper).* Urbana: University of Illinois.
Sotolongo Codina, P., & Delgado Díaz, C. (2006). *La revolución contemporánea del saber y la complejidad social.* Bs. As: CLACSO Libros.
Strauss, A., & Corbin, J. (2002). *Bases de la investigación cualitativa. Técnicas y procedimientos para desarrollar la teoría fundamentada.* Colombia: Universidad de Antioquía.
Tonon, G. (2003). *Calidad de vida y desgaste profesional. Una mirada del sindrome de burnout.* Bs. As: Espacio Editorial.
Tonon, G. (2005). Un lugar en el mundo: la universidad como espacio de integración social para los estudiantes. Revista Hologramàtica. Edición N° 3. Diciembre. Facultad de Ciencias Sociales.

Universidad Nacional de Lomas de Zamora. pp 41–49. Retrieved from www.cienciared.com.ar/ra/doc.php?n=134, September 22, 2013.

Tonon, G. (2009). La entrevista semi-estructurada como técnica de investigación. En G. Tonon (comp.), *Reflexiones latinoamericanas sobre investigación cualitativa* (pp. 46–68). San Justo: Prometeo-UNLAM.

Tonon, G., & Aragón, S. (compiladores-editores) (2012). Jóvenes ciudadanos: experiencias de participación en América Latina. Llavallol, UNI-COM, Facultad de Ciencias Sociales, Universidad Nacional de Lomas de Zamora.

Torres Carrillo, A. (2006). *Subjetividad y sujeto: perspectivas para abordar lo social y lo educativo. Revista Colombiana de Educación* (N° 50) (pp. 87–103). Bogota: Universidad Pedagógica Nacional.

Veenhoven, R. (1996). *Developments in satisfaction research. Social Indicators Research 37: 1–46*. The Netherlands: Kluwer Academic Publishers.

Veenhoven, R. (2009). *Well-being in nations and well-being of nations Is there a conflict between individual and society? Social Indicators Research 91:5–21*. The Netherlands: Springer.

Vélez Restrepo, O. (2003). *Reconfigurando el Trabajo Social.* Buenos Aires. Espacio Editorial.

Zemelman Merino, H. (2006) *Pensar la sociedad y a los sujetos sociales. Revista Colombiana de Educación. N° 50* (pp. 15–33). Bogota: Universidad Pedagógica Nacional.

Chapter 2
The Qualitative Researcher in the Quality of Life Field

Graciela Tonon

2.1 Subjectivity and Persons

In qualitative studies the emphasis placed on the existential thing, makes an impact on the process of production of knowledge, recognizing the word as the place where the meaning is constructed and the research practice is understood, that is, as a dialogic process between the researcher and the interviewed subject, opening a space for coproduced knowledge.

Considering that this is not a book on philosophy, we shall abstain from making a deep analysis of the concept of subjectivity. Nevertheless, and taking into account that subjectivity is inherent to qualitative studies, we coincide with Lechner (2002, p. 43) in that subjectivity is a complex phenomenon which embraces values and beliefs, mental dispositions and practical knowledge, norms and passions, experiences and expectations.

Torres Carrillo (2006, p. 94) believes that subjectivity is transversal to social life and is present in all social dynamics of daily life, both in micro-social and macro-social spaces, as well as in the daily inter-subjective experience and in the institutions that constitute the structure of an age.

If we consider that the human phenomena are subjective, due to their specific quality, then subjectivity is not opposed to objectivity. The qualitative researcher works on the subjective productions of each of the persons he/she studies and, in the quality of life field in particular, that subjectivity acquires special importance, since quality of life is a concept composed of two dimensions, objective and subjective, the same as social reality.

G. Tonon (✉)
UNICOM, Faculty of Social Sciences, Universidad Nacional de Lomas de Zamora, Lomas de Zamora, Argentina
e-mail: gracielatonon@hotmail.com

CICS, Faculty of Social Sciences, Universidad de Palermo, Ciudad Autónoma de Buenos Aires, Argentina

G. Tonon (ed.), *Qualitative Studies in Quality of Life*,
Social Indicators Research Series 55, DOI 10.1007/978-3-319-13779-7_2

Natanson (1974, p. 23), commenting on Schutz, points out that, for the social researcher, his objects are not only objects of observation but also beings possessing their own pre-interpreted world and carrying out their own observation, i.e., they are fellow creatures inserted in a social reality. The world we live in is intersubjective because we live in it, relating with others, it is a world of culture and "a universe of meaning, a texture of reason we must interpret in order to orient and conduct ourselves within it". (Schutz 1974, p. 41).

The qualitative researcher is expected to feel personally involved in every step of the research process, because every consideration and decision will have to be based on entirely personal grounds (Fink 2000). According to Jaramillo Echeverri (2006, p. 112) being a subject in the research is the chance of sharing and relating reflective experiences with the subjects of research and placing oneself, intentionally, in their circumstances.

The manner in which we feel and experience a certain society is not only determined by the objective connotation of the problems we are affected by, but also by the ways in which those problems become subjective (Gonzalez Rey 2006, p. 241 quoted in Diaz Gomez 2006b). In this sense, the reconstruction of reality, a major task in qualitative research, is achieved when it stems from the actors and situations proposed by the researcher's presence (Vélez Restrepo 2003, p. 148).

Likewise, it is important to remember the place of sensitivity in this process. Being sensitive means being able to penetrate and give significance to incidents and events shown by the data (Strauss and Corbin 2002, p. 52). Thus, personal/professional experience may increase that sensitivity if used appropriately. In this sense, Boyatzis (1998) points out the need to apply creativity to the direct study of the phenomena.

Qualitative research requires the researcher to distinguish between his own world and the world of others so that they may both be analyzed. It requires the researcher to be able to conceptualize, write and communicate. According to Morse and Field (1995, p. 1) "doing qualitative research is an intense experience, it enriches one's life, it captures one's soul and intellect".

2.2 Participation of the Researcher in Every Stage of the Research: The Importance of Transcription and Quoting

An important issue to consider is, precisely, the participation of the researcher in each of the tasks required in the development of a research process.

In the role distribution within a research team, we traditionally observe a watershed dividing two groups: those who carry out the field work and the ones who collect the data and analyze it.

Though it is understood that the stages in the professional lives and development of the members requires that each of the researchers should train in different activities and carry them out, the task of transcribing and quoting the interviews or team meetings is a question that requires special attention, since it has been observed that, in a great number of cases, the researchers who carry out the interview and/or coordinate a group, are not the same persons who will later transcribe and quote the data derived from those situations.

It is necessary to remember that the use of the interviewing technique in the research field is not reduced to an encounter between the researcher and the subject of the research. Once this encounter has taken place, it is the researcher's task to devote to the transcription of the said material and to its quoting, as soon as possible.

Mero-Jaffe (2011, p. 232) quoted Kvale (1996) who defines transcription as the transference of spoken language with its particular set of rules to the written word with a different set of rules and, at the same time, quoting Lapadat (2000), the author considers that this process of transforming uninterrupted dynamic oral language spoken in a particular context to a static form of representation (written language) is necessary for the management and organization of data, since only written language can be managed; in other words, sorted, copied, examined, evaluated and quoted.

The task of transcribing and quoting will allow the researcher to remember gestures and peculiarities of the experienced scene which may turn into clues to the analysis of the collected material. By placing, on the right hand column of the transcription page, the significant terms that may help record peculiarities of the situation in which the person answered the questions, the researcher will be able to, simultaneously, associate those details to the key concepts that will guide the definite process of analysis. This is so, because the qualitative methods attempt to clarify the meanings of society life, thus, they cannot simply examine the mere content or surface of what was said, but it is vital that it should also analyze the way in which it was said, and in what context in order to recover the meaning or possible meaning of the words (Farías and Montero 2005, p. 5).

If, on the other hand, the transcription and quoting had been made by another member of the team, it is clear that the latter would be unable to recover those details, basically, due to the fact that he/she has not experienced the scene; therefore, the researcher who made the interview would be required to read the transcription immediately and place those meaningful concepts in the aforementioned column. If this process were not carried out a short time after the interview, part of that information would be irremediably lot and, with it, the possibility to advance in the analysis of concepts which are significant to the achievement of the final product of the research.

In this respect, let us consider the comment made by a vastly experienced researcher, on the impressions she obtained while using qualitative methods and semi-structured interviews in the development of her studies in the quality of life field:

> In my personal experience in qualitative studies, the researcher's task is crucial, for there is a mutual influence between the researcher and the approached social actors. As we know, qualitative research is an interpretive process concerned with the way in which the social actors produce and interpret the social world, assuming that reality is multiple and subjective.
> In the case of the semi-structured interview, conceived as an encounter between persons, the ethics present in the communicative situation becomes fundamental; it should create a space for interchange in which the main concern should be to listen to the person interviewed, to the meanings he conveys, which emerge from his own context of significance generated in the dialogic space.

> On the researcher's part, it requires generating confidence, an initial clarification of the job to be carried out, and the guarantee that the name of the person interviewed will be kept anonymous and the interest aroused by his/her expressions, confidential. All of which implies the researcher's acknowledgement of his/her historical position which, in turn, makes his interview unlike a similar one made by another researcher, fundamentally acknowledging the fact that we are dealing with subjects, not objects.
> It is ideal, I believe, that the person carrying out the interviews should be the one to read them, transcribe them, and quote them, in order to increase familiarity with the data and whatever field notes might have been taken, thus recovering images and even tones and voice inflexions; all these codes of communication make it more significant.
> I mention the specific case of transcriptions because, if made by someone other than the interviewer, however conscientiously made, it will fail to reflect tones of voice, associated images, and intention, which will indeed be captured in the "reading" of the person who has actually experienced it and quoted it in the transcription. So important is this that it might be determinant to the questions posed on a re-interview, and of the utmost importance to its analysis.
> In my humble experience, participating in the whole process is the way to contribute some real understanding of the study in question. I find it useful to associate everything; images, voices, my various listening sessions, note-taking; that is why I am so insistent on step-by-step participation. (Female, 47 years old, expert in quality of life and diversity studies).

If, on the other hand, the interviews had been developed for a Doctorate or Master's Thesis, the importance of the transcription and quoting being made by the authors, would not be arguable. If that work were done by another person, the author of the thesis would, clearly, miss the opportunity to obtain a profound knowledge of the results of the research in process.

2.3 Three Dimensions for Analyzing the Qualitative Researcher's Role

We will propose three dimensions for the analysis of the role of the qualitative researcher: personal dimension, professional dimension and political dimension (Tonon 2013).

- Personal dimension: is centered in the researcher's perceptions and experiences.
- Professional dimension: considers the role of the original-traditional professions and the emergence and inclusion of new professions in the research field.
- Political dimension: analyses the decision process in the academic research field; this implies the analysis of the power systems and their different forms of expression.

2.3.1 Personal Dimension

It is centered round the perceptions and personal experiences of the subjects, at an initial stage; and though it is the essential and structuring dimension of every research process, it is also the least considered in the academic scope, maybe, because in that field, research is a "natural activity" to a university professor, a university student and/or an acting professional.

In qualitative studies, the process begins with the researcher's recognition of his/her own socio-cultural and historical position, which implies ethics and politics in connection with the research (Gianturco 2005). Doing qualitative research requires the researcher to be methodologically versatile, to have extensive knowledge of theory, to be persistent and focused in the research and to be able to conceptualize, write and communicate (Morse and Field 1995).

This scenario requires the trust that stimulates the collaboration and allows the subject interviewed to reduce the uncertainty in the circumstances. At the same time confidentiality is necessary to preserve the intimate and secret information conveyed by the person (Tonon 2009).

In my personal practice as a researcher and professor of research methodology in various courses of study and post-graduate courses within the field of Social Sciences and Humanities, I have been able to observe that, in order to be initiated in the role of researcher, certain conditions are previously required and, if that were not the case, a firm decision to achieve them would be necessary.

When I refer to conditions, I do not mean the storage of a certain amount of information in the brain, or having a certain IQ; in fact, I have had brilliant students, academically speaking, who have not been successful in the research field. What I allude to refers to certain attitudes such as being open to discovery, the need to go on learning, not being afraid to revise the history of one's own learning; all of which confront each of the subjects with the risk of verifying or, failing to verify what they have, in fact, incorporated.

In the case of professionals of long standing, it is not easy to notice whether they have submitted their practices to enough reflection. It is not easy, either, to become aware that, thinking out a research problem and carrying out a research project, is a task that differs from participating in a case of assistance to a subject or family, or carrying out a pedagogical proposition, or again conducting a social project or generating a public policy. It is the same as the difference between writing a report, a project of a professional intervention, or a professional book; between writing a scientific article, a scientific research report or a Doctorate or Master's Thesis. Thus, at the first sign that the research problem must be re-formulated, and/or the text must be amended because it is not argumentative enough, the persons show attitudes of frustration, anger, or the intention to abandon the research.

The following expressions were uttered by post-graduate students undergoing their first experience in qualitative research.

> When I began this research process, I thought it was not unknown to me. I took for granted that I knew something about it; little by little, this sensation vanished. Doubts began to arise, uncertainty, anguish and, somehow, the decision to accept the challenge. (Female, 46 years old, post-graduate student).
>
> Life, at university and outside, personal and professional, has taught me and is actually teaching me that, if I don't enjoy it, I'm not living it, only passing; that's why what I like the most about this path "towards research" is, above all,my inner search. If I weren't at ease with the people I'm with, week after week, I wouldn't be able to go on… The path leading to research isn't at all easy; many sleepless nights, many comings and goings, often, the feeling that what has been accomplished is not enough, that I'm behind, that I won't make it, that I'm about to give up; yet, I'm still here, trying hard every day… which is far more than it seems to be. (Female, 48 years old, post-graduate student).

> I'm going through a stage when I think the following: "With practice we can construct what we really want". Learning how to do research by using the right method; this demands great perseverance, order, patience, intelligence, etc. But, above all, there must be passion for the subject of our research for, only that passion will encourage us to train in order to become good researchers, because we can't do anything properly if we don't get to like it, first. (Male, 32 years old, post-graduate student).
> In the first place, focusing on this research process is something new to me. It's taking a new path full of doubts, curiosity, the will to search more and more, to read and re-read; a path of self-questioning, of deciding what I want to do, of thinking a lot. A path which, on the one hand, arouses uncertainties, generates nervousness, anxiety, restlessness, but which, at the same time, allures me, attracts me. Accepting this challenge also has a positive effect for I want to learn and feel like doing so, and doing it well, becoming committed. One often has mixed feelings; at times, we feel that we're stuck, that we can't move on. But the moment one finds or discovers something, one pushes forward, and new doubts arise, or tentative answers; and that's the way we come and go. This is a great challenge to me; it draws me on, and I'm determined to face it. I know it's not easy, but it's not impossible, either. (Female, 39 years old, post-graduate student).
> I've never thought of doing research and it's one of the difficulties I've found in the post-graduate course. I feel that I know nothing and, suddenly, I construct something meaningful out of something that arises… I believe myself to be strongly committed to the task, which is not easy. (Male, 55 years old, post-graduate student).

The abovementioned discourses show how post-graduate students, initiated in research work, share mixed feelings; on the one hand, eagerness to learn and make progress in the project development; and, on the other, the difficulties they find in reviewing their own learning histories, in paving a new way which requires them to go on with their studies and which, in their own words, implies a great challenge.

Thus, the decision to become qualitative researchers, above all, leads them straight away to a revision of their own histories and to introspection. It is necessary for them to keep up an open and humble attitude for, if the subjects possessed knowledge of everything, they would be unlikely to be able to learn.

2.3.2 Professional Dimension

This dimension considers the possibility of including in the scientific field, subjects whose professions have emerged only in the last decades.

The professional peculiarities of each of the researchers designate and condition the development of their future careers. There are professions traditionally devoted to research work, while others have come to emerge in this field, in the course of the last two decades.

Thus, those whose professions have, historically, produced theory and who impose them through traditions, can be distinguished from those whose stereotype has been, historically, focused on practice rather than theory, and are beginning to be sequentially included in the scientific field.

This is a complex and contradictory process, and it is a source of opposition and confrontation. The re-location of points of power, formerly typical of generational changes, is also occurring nowadays among traditional and emerging professions.

The challenge consists in allowing them all to develop and move forward, according to their specific knowledge and interests, with a vision of the future which envisages integration rather than separation. It should be understood that new professions and new proposals should not be considered as a peril, that the professionals incorporated in the new scenario are to be regarded as a contribution to the field and, therefore, as new colleagues rather than new competitors.

2.3.3 Political Dimension

It refers to the analysis of the decision-making processes in the scientific-academic field, which implies the consideration of the systems of power and their different expressions.

Diaz Gómez (2006a, p. 225) has expressed that the production of knowledge goes hand in hand with institutionalization processes and with the generation of power mechanisms that privilege certain kinds of research and allow the spreading of specific knowledge and perspectives of theory, as well as the preeminence of a kind of discourse which is becoming natural and, therefore, widespread in university classrooms and research scenarios.

Bourdieu (2000, p. 89) acknowledges two forms of power in scientific fields: an institutional political power held by those who formally stand in "decisive positions", and a specific power, based on personal prestige, therefore less institutionalized, and born of invisible colleges of scientists united by mutual recognition. Moreover, the author considers that the former type of power is obtained through political strategies which respond to the rules of bureaucratic capital and constitute what is known as *institution science* which establishes routine practice as a model of scientific activity (Bourdieu 2008, p. 47); whereas the latter is achieved by accumulating purely scientific capital, solely derived from effort and scientific work. This explains why prestige is not necessarily a synonym of power. (Bourdieu 2000, p. 90). Thus, if the assessors and those assessed end up being colleagues and competitors, due to the conflict of interests among the members of the scientific field, the aforementioned situation is aggravated, the fields may be turned into "machines", generating a pathological situation (Bourdieu 1990). The author (1990, pp. 157–158) expressed the difference between the two concepts by identifying the field as the place where the agents and institutions struggle with different forces and according to the constituent rules of this space; and though the ones who predominate, are well equipped, they also experience the resistance of the rest; whereas, when the dominators of the field possess the means to neutralize the resistance, the latter becomes a "machine".

Thus, the communication of knowledge in academic discourse is imposed, responding to position, the market flow and/or the prevailing fashion. Bourdieu (2008, p. 44) sustains that there is a socially acknowledged scientific rank, generally considered valid, which bestows on those who represent it or appear to, the monopoly of the scientific point of view.

It has been observed that, in different periods, the same text books have been used for different subjects, belonging to the same course of studies, without arousing concern in the external analyst. Something similar occurs with research topics, there being a recurrence in the study of certain theses, prompted by the market and/or the prevailing fashion.

This generates a subtly dangerous situation for it conceals new horizons of development, especially from young teachers and researchers.

Breaking with the establishment is a great challenge and, in this sense, the use of qualitative methods in the scenario of social research enables the acknowledgement of the leading role of subjects in the research processes of the social and humanistic sciences field, while attempting to make progress in the quest to overcome the dichotomy between qualitative and quantitative methods, with the object of integrating both, an issue which will be developed in the last chapter of this book.

Coinciding with Torres Carrillo (2006, p. 100) we shall state that qualitative research allows us to detect the degree of political and cultural determination in the researcher and in his/her research work.

2.4 Following up the Initiation in Research of Young Graduate and Post-Graduate Students

A decade ago, I began my work as tutors to young researchers, a task we have developed within various research programs and curricular spaces in diverse academic institutions in Argentina. This work was developed in the Quality of Life Research Program of the Faculty of Social Sciences of Universidad Nacional de Lomas de Zamora, the tutorial of Theses for the Doctorate in Psychology, and of research papers for students reading for the Degree in Psychology at Universidad de Palermo; also, the tutoring of graduate students in the Scholarship Program to stimulate scientific research by the National Inter-university Council.

I have worked with young people between 23 and 30 years old, males and females, in their initial experience as researchers; graduated in Political Science, Psychology, Social Work, Educational Sciences.

This section comprises there axes for reflection: the university-research-quality of life relationship; the insertion of the young student/reseracher in the scenario of research; and the tutor's role (Tonon and Toscano 2013).

2.4.1 The University-Research-Quality of Life Relationship

From a traditional outlook, the university structure is conceived as historically founded on scientific knowledge and stems from the consideration that the science system is formulated through basic research founded on the advance of knowledge and the re-affirmation of its concepts; as well as on applied science, which has an outstanding social application (Plascencia Castellanos 2006, p. 31). Likewise, university has been, traditionally, ascribed four functions: formal education in academic disciplines and professional areas, research, extension- society service, and the production of national figures.

Nevertheless some authors, like Duderstadt (2010, p. 82), consider that university should not be considered as a mere knowledge factory, for teaching and discovering further defy the existing order and lead to change, by attempting to transform knowledge into wisdom.

And it is, precisely, in the history of higher education in Latin-America that a new era has begun; an era in which knowledge is not only necessary to achieve social welfare but is also instrumental in the improvement of every person's quality of life (Duderstadt (2010, p. 413).

The new trend propounds a switch from the formal university degrees, mainly aimed at young students, to a mode of learning which aims at ensuring the continuity of education for a life-time. Thus, continuous learning has become necessary to guarantee working stability and relevance, as shown in former researches (Tonon 2005, 2010) mentioned in Chapter 1 of this same text-book, illustrating the importance of work in the increasing improvement of people's quality of life.

Duderstadt (2010, p. 425) sustains that "education is regarded, today, as the hope for a significant and satisfactory life", he adds that, in that respect, both education and each subject's abilities, are increasingly being regarded as the keys to a personal quality of life and to the quality of life of society as a whole. (Duderstadt 2010, p. 425).

Unfortunately, the traditional concept of university campus, and the high costs that its organization involves, can no longer meet the current demand—which is impossible to foresee. This situation necessarily leads to the gradual yielding of the reductionist model still in force as certifier of knowledge, to the model of university as a space for the construction of citizenship and democratization of knowledge, as well as for the improvement of personal quality of life.

In the abovementioned university scenario, research becomes a social opportunity to young people for, according to Sen (2000), it increases the persons' potential. Moreover, in the words of Castillo Garcia (2007, p. 799), society and education are the scenarios in which young people are able to evolve as subjects in a certain social reality. Learning to do research and being initiated in the research profession, represents an opening, to young men and women, for the development of knowledge and future labor prospects—both of which are necessary to improve their quality of life.

Nevertheless, this process is not viable if pursued in isolation; it requires experienced teacher-researchers to guide the insertion of the young researchers in order to enable them to achieve their aims and avoid frustration.

2.4.2 *Insertion of the Young Students in the Scenario of Research*

In order to describe the process of insertion of the young students in research work, it is, above all, necessary to explain that we regard research as a process of discovery which, though responding to logical and organized guidelines, also involves creativity and reflexibility. This is, perhaps, the most arguable and difficult point to understand: the integration of structured and serious (non rigid) logics with the possibility of creativity and innovation.

The reception of young people who have been selected from different scholarship programs and need to comply with specific curricular demands in order to gain credits for the completion of their courses of studies (as in the case of papers for an university degree), requires the tutor's primary analysis of the subject's background and biographical details. Schutz (1974, p. 17) defines it as the acknowledgement of the fact that the actor's present situation stems from the sediment of all his/her previous subjective experiences, which he/ she does not experience as anonymous, but as subjective and exclusive.

The young researchers will arrive, equipped with background knowledge (Schutz 1974, p. 17), that is, with accumulated experience that will determine their capacity to resolve any new situation they might be confronted with. They may even possess systematized knowledge about the significance of research or, on the other hand, maybe none at all—which explains these young researchers' need to adopt a misleading attitude regarding their present situation in this field.

The first resarcher-tutor encounter is a significant human encounter to both, and it cannot be reduced to a mere administrative formality. By interacting, they will both perceive a change within themselves and this new bond will generate commitment in the development of that shared process, in which plays a role; one being the "teacher", and the other, the "apprentice". This brings to mind the words of Wainerman (2001, p. 21) who pointed out that a researcher can only learn through a teacher as in the medieval guilds, for there is something in the researcher's role that cannot be coded and which is difficult to transmit. Research is a craft and, as such, it involves personal experience as well as intellectual-professional activity.

The young researcher and his tutor will then share the research adventure, implying by adventure, quoting Diaz Gomez (2006a, p. 228) a process in which there is a reference of the path to be followed (even when the details may be unknown), accompanied by an element of surprise, questioning and expectation; a situation which clearly differs from a package-tour whose itinerary has been prepared by somebody else and which does not contemplate the freedom of the actors.

This adventure route requires care and organization, which brings up a question: What should the young researcher be taught? In order to deal with this question, we shall organize it in two dimensions: learning acquired within the human and social dimension, and learning within the intellectual and operative dimension.

Learning acquired in the human and social dimension triggers attitudes of commitment with one's work and with other people; learning how to apply life experience to intellectual work, examining and interpreting it (for having experience means that our past has a bearing on our present), affects our capacities for future experience (Wright Mills 1961, p. 207); thus, understanding the acting context; overcoming adversity without resigning our dreams.

Learning acquired in the intellectual and operative dimensions involve the following:

a. devoting oneself to reading, taking into account that this activity implies the reconstruction of meaning in a text by relating the informative clues it contains with the reader's own knowledge (Carlino 2006). The young researchers will endeavor to obtain books, scientific articles and written productions referred to their research theme, as well as any other material that will allow them to broaden their field of study and go beyond the mere objectives; for, taking down notes on a book, invites reflection (Wright Mills 1961, p. 210);
b. training in writing skills, on the basis that writing is recovering the recollections of one's accumulated knowledge on the topic by expressing it on paper (Carlino 2006) producing summaries of the texts, files, charts, diagrams, that is, constructing an archive in which professional activities coexist with personal experience. (Wright Mills 1961, p. 208);
c. avoid neglecting the, so called, (Wright Mills 1961, p. 207) i.e., those ideas that cross our minds in a disorderly way, as well as the ones that arise from conversations overheard along the corridors of an institution or on the street, and which come across as causal associations which may be considered irrelevant at the moment, while becoming meaningful in the future.
d. Work steadily and systematically until the task is concluded.

2.4.3 *Role of a Tutor*

In previous papers we have already pointed out that, the path from practice to theory, and from theory to practice, has traditionally been the least chosen and valued, especially in university studies (Tonon 2005). Fortunately, we have concluded that, both practice and theory, conform an integrated unit; that they need and nurture each other, which implies that their relationship is based on mutual assistance rather than confrontation.

The follow-up of a young student's graduate and/or post-graduate studies, in a process of insertion into research, requires a tutor to construct a work mechanism based on task supervision. From our point of view supervision is:

> A theoretical-methodological process displayed in two spaces: professional activity and academic formation. Its objective is the acquisition of new information and new skills, required in everyday professional performance, as well as reflection on the emotional and affect impact that every situation would have had on the tutored student if he/she had been acting professionally. It is based on a holistic conception of reality in which theoretical knowledge interacts with practical experience (Tonon 2004, p. 11)

Becoming a tutor to young researchers firstly requires a certain attitude towards life and then, a store of knowledge and experience in the thematic field; it should be noticed that, in this case, the order of the factors does modify the result. There are eminent researchers, prize winners, and authors of famous scientific production, but none of these turn them into better tutors.

The tutor's job demands from whoever undertakes the task, a certain human attitude which implies a series of requirements:

a. commitment with the young researcher and his task.
b. generosity in transmitting knowledge.
c. love teaching as much as he/she loves research.
d. being a good listener.
e. not being prejudicial.
f. knowing when to draw the line.
g. Enjoying and sharing the young researcher's achievements, that is, not being fearful that the apprentice might, someday, surpass the teacher.

The process of standing by someone doing research requires that each of the subjects acting in it should first make an introspection and assess their possibilities and their limitations. Thus, the task of training and supervising a young researcher cannot be reduced to certifying the case history in the tutor's curriculum. It is, in fact, much more; it is an encounter between subjects, with all the complexities and seriousness that human relations imply, and which has an impact on the quality of life of those involved in the relationship.

Just as the apprentice in the Middle-Ages learnt from his master, today, in the XXI century, the young researcher will learn from his tutor, not only theory and/or research methods and techniques, but also attitudes and values. Something similar will happen to the tutor, for he will have much to learn from the young researcher. For both share the love of discovery and knowledge, as well as the inclination to transmit them and put them at the society's service, quoting Aristotle (1144a5–2008) "knowledge produces happiness for, being a part of total virtue, its possession and practice produce happiness".

2.5 Conclusions

Strauss and Corbin (2002, p. 36) have pointed out that every researcher has personal preferences, since he/she is familiarized with, and better able to conduct a certain type of research, and this situation prevails when the moment comes to decide which method to use, even when the aim of the research and the nature of the questions that arise may influence the decision.

Subjectivity is a system constituted in the history of a person, stemming from the multiple consequences of a subject's social trajectory, and which cannot be separated from that subject's production of subjective senses (González Rey 2006, p. 245 quoted in Diaz Gomez 2006b)

> Qualitative research produces important impacts on the setting of the subjectivities engaged in, in the act of research. His/her questions, acts, and cultural heritage, turn the researcher into an instrument through which another subject's expression and discourse are potentiated and shaped in the analysis and interpretation. Understanding another (others) implies triggering the question, "Who am I?", and that situation arouses countless feelings anchored

in our memories, sensations, and experiences which constitute the soul of research (Vélez Restrepo 2003, p. 147)

Accompanying a young researcher at the stage in which he/she is inserted in the research field is a noble task which implies true commitment from whoever decides to undertake it. And, since it is an encounter between subjects who will share their work in their different roles, far from being a simple task, it implies complexities.

Qualitative research is an extraordinarily absorbing intellectual exercise; and the good qualitative researcher has a vast knowledge of social science theory, is persistent in fitting the emerging model both the setting and to the literature, and never hesitates to redo the analyses (Morse 1995, p. 17).

In the light of what we have explained above, on approaching research in the quality of life field, from the perspective of qualitative methods in particular, it is necessary to remember that the researcher is a subject who relates to other subjects, and that the product resulting from those research processes will have been socially and historically constructed.

References

Aristóteles. (2008). *Ética Nicomáquea*. Buenos Aires: Biblioteca Gredos Clásicos.

Bourdieu, P. (1990). *Sociología y cultura*. México: Editorial Grijalbo.

Bourdieu, P. (2000). *Los usos sociales de la ciencia*. Buenos Aires: Ediciones Nueva Visión.

Bourdieu, P. (2008). *Homo Academicus*. Buenos Aires: Siglo XXI Editores.

Boyatzis, R. (1998). *Transforming qualitative information*. Thousand Oaks: Sage Publications.

Carlino, P. (2006). *Escribir, leer y aprender en la universidad: una introducción a la alfabetización académica*. Buenos Aires: Fondo de Cultura Económica.

Castillo García, J. (2007). La configuración de ciudadanías en estudiantes universitarios de pregrado. *Revista Latinoamericana de Ciencias Sociales, Niñez y Juventud, 5*(2), 755–809. (Universidad de Manizales- CINDE. Colombia).

Díaz Gómez, A. (2006a). Formación compleja en humanidades en el ámbito de la educación superior. In P. Sotolongo Codina y C. Delgado Díaz (Eds.), *La revolución contemporánea del saber y la complejidad social* (pp. 223–232). Buenos Aires: CLACSO.

Diaz Gomez, A. (2006b). Subjetividad y subjetividad política. Entrevista con el psicólogo cubano Fernando González Rey. En *Revista Colombiana de Educación N° 50*. Primer semestre 2006. Universidad Pedagógica Nacional. Colombia. pp. 239–252.

Duderstadt, J. (2010). *Una universidad para el siglo XXI. Tomo 2*. Colección Educación Superior. Fac. Ciencias Sociales. Universidad de Palermo. Buenos Aires.

Farías, L & Montero, M. (2005). De la transcripción y otros aspectos artesanales de la investigación cualitativa. *International Journal of Qualitative Methods 4*(1), pp. 1–14.

Fink, A. (2000). The role of the researcher in the qualitative research process. A potential barrier to archiving qualitative data *forum qualitative social research. Volume 1, No. 3, Art. 4*—December 2000.

Gianturco, G. (2005). *L'intervista cualitativa*. Facoltá di Psicología. Universita degli studi di Roma La Sapiencia. Roma.

Jaramillo Echeverri, L. (2006). Ser sujeto en la investigación: investigando desde nuestra subjetividad. En *Revista Colombiana de Educación N° 50*. Primer semestre 2006. Universidad Pedagógica Nacional. Colombia pp 105–120

Kvale, S. (1996). *Interviews: An introduction to qualitative research interviewing*. London: Sage.

Lapadat, J. (2000). Problematizing transcription: Purpose, paradigm and quality. *International Journal of Social Research Methodology, 3,* 203–219

Lechner, N. (2002). *Las sombras del mañana. La dimensión subjetiva de la política.* Santiago de Chile: Lom Ediciones.

Mero-Jaffe, I. (2011). 'Is that what I said?' Interview transcript approval by participants: An aspect of ethics in qualitative research. *International Journal of Qualitative Methods 2011, 10*(3), pp 231–247.

Morse, J. & Field, P (1995). *Qualitative research methods for health professionals.* Thousand Oaks: Sage.

Natanson, M. (1974). Introducción. En Schutz, A. *El problema de la realidad social* (pp. 15–32). Barcelona: Amorrortu.

Plascencia Castellanos, G. (2006). *Palabra libre. Condición de la universidad.* México: Universidad Iberoamericana.

Schutz, A. (1974). *El problema de la realidad social.* Barcelona: Amorrortu.

Sen, A. (2000). *Desarrollo y libertad.* Colombia: Siglo XXI Editores.

Strauss, A. & Corbin, J. (2002). *Bases de la investigación cualitativa. Técnicas y procedimientos para desarrollar la teoría fundamentada.* Colombia: Universidad de Antioquía.

Tonon, G. (2004). La supervisión como cuestión profesional y académica. En G. Tonon et al *La supervisión en Trabajo social: cuestión académica y cuestión profesional* (pp. 13–49). Buenos Aires: Espacio Editorial.

Tonon, G. (2005). *Una estrategia de mejoramiento de la calidad de vida: la universidad como espacio de integración social para los estudiantes.* Programa de Investigación en Calidad de Vida. Facultad de Ciencias Sociales. Universidad Nacional de Lomas de Zamora.

Tonon, G. (Ed.). (2009). *Reflexiones latinoamericanas sobre investigación cualitativa.* San Justo: UNLAM/Prometeo Libros.

Tonon, G. (2010–2011). *Calidad de vida e imágenes de futuro de jóvenes estudiantes universitarios.* Programa de Investigación en Calidad de Vida. Facultad de Ciencias Sociales. Universidad Nacional de Lomas de Zamora. Programa Nacional de Incentivos para docentes investigadores, Ministerio de Educación.

Tonon, G. (2013). *La integración de métodos de investigación en Ciencias Sociales: la triangulación y los métodos mixtos.* Documento de investigación número 135. Serie Documentos de investigación del Colegio Mexiquense. Toluca México. Mayo 2013.

Tonon, G. & Toscano, W. (2013) Acompañar el proceso de iniciación en investigación de jóvenes estudiantes de grado y posgrado. *Revista Kairos Año 17. Número 31.* Universidad Nacional de San Luis. San Luis, pp 1–9.

Torres Carrillo, A. (2006). Subjetividad y sujeto: Perspectivas para abordar lo social y lo educativo. En Revista *Colombiana de Educación N° 50.* Primer semestre. Universidad Pedagógica Nacional. Colombia pp. 87–103.

Vélez Restrepo, O. (2003). *Reconfigurando el Trabajo Social. Perspectivas y tendencias contemporáneas.* Buenos Aires: espacio Editorial.

Wainerman, C. (2001). Acerca de la formación de investigadores en ciencias sociales. En Wainerman, C. & Sautu, R. (Eds.), *La trastienda de la investigación.* Tercera edición ampliada. Buenos Aires: Lumiere. pp. 15–43.

Wright Mills, Ch. (1961). La imaginación sociológica. Buenos Aires: Fondo de Cultura Económica.

Chapter 3
The Role of Context and Culture in Quality of Life Studies

Lia Rodriguez de la Vega

Dube (1999) points out that culture should be understood as an essential element in the production and reproduction of daily social life, that is to say, as the attitudes, norms and symbolic and structured practices by which social relations are perceived, articulated and experimented thus, defining this way culture in and by those relations, which are predicated to its power.

Culture endures forms in which practices and specific belief systems are implied in social relations and experienced within them.

The inclusion of culture by the social actors, leads to the question of identity, regarded as a set of internalized cultural repertoires through which social actors symbolically outline their borders, thus differentiating themselves from the rest of the social actors, in socially structured and historically specific contexts (Giménez 2000).

On the other hand we presume, like Shin et al. (2003), that quality of life is a multidimensional phenomenon which involves a variety of elements that refer to human needs whose satisfaction requires material and immaterial elements.

Likewise, we believe that the objective and subjective dimensions of life are distinct entities and that people carry out a positive or negative assessment of their life experiences according to what they consider to be good, their conception of it, and of everything that occurs in a specific cultural background, in space and time. Quoting Christopher (1999), the notions of well-being have cultural roots.

Considering the above mentioned, this chapter focuses on the notion of culture, the research on the relationship between culture and quality of life, and the impact of culture on the qualitative researcher.

L. Rodriguez de la Vega (✉)
UNICOM, Faculty of Social Sciences, Universidad Nacional de Lomas de Zamora, Lomas de Zamora, Argentina
e-mail: liadelavega@yahoo.com

CICS, Faculty of Social Sciences, Universidad de Palermo, Ciudad Autónoma de Buenos Aires, Buenos Aires, Argentina

G. Tonon (ed.), *Qualitative Studies in Quality of Life*,
Social Indicators Research Series 55, DOI 10.1007/978-3-319-13779-7_3

3.1 Culture

Giménez (2005), refers to the force of the symbolic conception of culture, and the impact deconstructivist criticism of Geertz's original position has had on it; ergo, being considered as "a set of disperse and off-centered symbolic practices", "as a symbolic repertoire of action strategies" (p. 3).

He further sustains that defining culture through a reference to the symbolic processes of society, confers the latter a specific and autonomous field, as a dimension of life in society. This conception leads to the fact that culture is particularized and pluralized in what Sewel calls "concrete cultural worlds" (Socially structured historical contexts) (1999, p. 52), thus allowing the use of the term "cultures".

Thompson (1998) on the other hand, considers that culture may be understood as a set of historically transmitted guidelines on meaning, embodied in symbolic forms through which individuals communicate and share their beliefs, experiences, etc.

Closely related to the idea of culture is the question of identity, the conception of the former having consequences on the latter.

Giménez (2005) distinguishes interiorized forms from objectivized forms of culture and considers that the semiotic conception of culture requires the symbolic models, to be related to the actors, who incorporate them subjectively and express them in practice; the underlying concept being that there are no actors without culture, and viceversa. In other words, culture is "habitus" (Bourdieu 1980), it is experienced from the point of view of the social actors and their practices, this being the really existent culture, the one found in social experiences and the "worlds of life" of the interacting actors.

In this sense, Giménez (2004) points out that the theory of identity is part of the broadest background of the social theories, whereas identity is an essential parameter which defines the social actors, conceived, according to Bassand and Hainard (1985), as having the following characteristics: (a) it occupies one or various positions in the social structure, (b) it permanently interacts with other social actors, in a permanent process of socialization and learning, (c) it possesses a certain form of power and a self-image with relation to others, and d) it generally has a project, and the means to carry it out. There is no sense in action without social actors which are, in turn, defined (among other elements) by their identities.

Grimson (2012), on the other hand, marks a distinction between culture and identity by pointing out that, while the cultural aspect refers to practices, beliefs, and routine and sedimentary meanings, the aspect of identity alludes to the feeling of collective ownership. He considers that being aware of this distinction allows an understanding of the shifting of the cultural and identity borders, taking into account that they do not always coincide.

Restrepo (2010) considers that identities are relational, that they are expressed by marking differences hence they are not marginal and, therefore emit practices to delineate "us" as an alternative to "others", thus identity and difference become mutually constitutive. In that respect, Grossber (2003) points out the need to develop relational methodological frames for the study of identity and differences in their mutual constitution.

He, furthermore, adds a relevant observation regarding the fact that identities do not only make allusion to differences but also to inequality and domination, i.e. that the abovementioned border marking is related to preservation or confrontation of different hierarchies (social, political, etc.). Thus, identities acquire sense both for those who assign them and for those who assume them.

He believes that identities (individual and/or collective) are not defined forever; their denotative and connotative elements derive from concrete practices of meaning and from a specific interaction among different subjects, thus evidencing a multiplicity of meanings.

Regarding interactive construction, social identities require, as a condition of plausibility, stable interaction contexts constituted as "familiar worlds" related to everyday life, which the social actors are acquainted with from within, for practical purposes.

In connection with this, Schütz (1974) points out that the experiencing of common sense in everyday life is a reference of signification which "constitutes the result of the selective and interpretive activity that men carry out as a part of nature, or in the act of observing it" (p. 37).

This intersubjective world of everyday life which existed before we were born and has already been experienced by others (as predecessors) as an organized world is now subject to our experience and interpretation. Moreover, this world possesses types of experience which are common to all men, and such typifications are everyday life structures that regulate both their comprehension as well as their personal experiences. Thus, man is immersed in a biographically determined situation, is defined by a physical-socio-cultural environment, which furthermore includes a moral and ideological position. In other words, society is also equivalent to a social space constituted by differentiated fields (Bourdieu 1987) all of which constitute the exogenous social context of social identities.

3.2 Identity Regarded as a Value and Values Regarded as Components of Identity

Identity is valuable to the subjects because it is the central value around which subjects organize their relationship with the world and with the other subjects, and also because all differentiations/distinctions inherent in such identity imply a search for self-value in relation with others (Lipiansky 1992).

In the development of men's social lives, we will find the foundation values they are regulated by, and the substance of their knowledge and beliefs. These norms affect the social order and, quoting Goodenough (1975), those values, with overlapping beliefs and feelings, acquire their own logic within which they not only understand but also make life meaningful.

This diversity of values is reflected in the perception of the quality of life of the subjects and of the groups they belong to. In this connection, Hofstede (1984), probing into the cultural relativity of the concept of Quality of Life, points out that "quality" is a question of values and is related to the "good" and "bad" standards; moreover, that those values partly depend on personal choices and, to a great extent, to the cultural context.

3.3 Quality of Life and Culture

Christopher (1999) argued that definitions of well-being are culturally rooted and in the same direction, Kawana-Singer et al. (2010) consider that quality of life is a multidimensional and subjective experience of well-being that is culturally constructed. Diener and Diener (1995), for example, found, at the individual level of analysis, that self-esteem was correlated with subjective well-being, but the correlation between subjective well-being and satisfaction with different aspects of life, varied according to the country (individualist or collectivist nation).

Regarding subjective well-being, which according to Diener and Fujita (1994), comprises the assessment people make of their lives, both in the affective and cognitive areas, Triandis (2000) adds that an adequate way of understanding the significance of the construct is by considering the factors related to it, and that the factor that predict subjective well-being may differ according to the different cultures. In this regard, he highlights that Diener and Suh (1997, quoted in Triandis 2000) found that emotions predicted people's subjective well-being in individualistic cultures, while in collectivist societies this was achieved by emotions and behavior in compliance with norms.

On the other hand, Oishi et al. (1999) pointed out that values mediate subjective well-being while, according to Triandis (2000), literature shows that, at cultural level, individualism is correlated with subjective well-being, and collectivism with tightness. He explains that in the latter societies (collectivist), people experience high levels of anxiety, fear of not being "correct" or "appropriate" in their behavior, which might cause them to be criticized, rejected or excluded.

Diener and Diener (1995) pointed out that satisfaction was more strongly predicted by self-esteem in individualistic cultures than in collectivist ones.

Another example is given by the social and interpersonal natures of the processes that underlie the effects of marital status on subjective well-being, which suggest that the relation between them (subjective well-being and marital status) may be different across different cultural contexts, considering cultural variables that may influence the negative effects of divorce. Related to this, because collectivist cultures give more importance to norms and individualist cultures to emotions (Triandis 1995, 1996), the subjective well-being of persons who live with a significant other in an individualist culture, may be just as high as that of married persons while in a collectivist culture, it may be not as high as that of married ones (Diener et al. 2000).

Forougui (1995) investigated the quality of life cross-cultural differences amongst Persian immigrants to Australia, Australians and Persians residing in Iran, and examined the mediating role of social support on life quality. Considering these three samples, the most important result was that, despite the fact that objective quality of life was significantly different across the three groups, no such differences were observed for the subjective quality of life and no relation was found between years of residence in Australia and social integration with subjective well-being. Considering the impact of social support and life quality, it was found a positive relation between subjective support for the Persian and Australian sample, but it was not found for the Persian-Australians.

Schumaker et al. (1993), examined the relationship between loneliness and life satisfaction in residents of Fukoku, Japan, and Melbourne, Australia, using the Revised UCLA Loneliess Scale (Russell et al. 1980) and the Satisfaction with Life Scale (Diener et al. 1985). Australian subjects showed significantly greater life satisfaction and less loneliness than Japanese subjects, and results suggest that loneliness in Japanese subjects did not emotionally translate into life dissatisfaction as it did in Australian subjects.

Gokdemir and Dumludag (2011) focused on the role of socio-economic factors (income, unemployment levels), and non-economic factors (identity, religion and culture), to explain the reasons for disparity of happiness levels among Moroccan and Turkish immigrants in the Netherlands (Amsterdam, Arnhem, Den Haag, Rotterdam and Utrecht). The results showed that Turkish immigrants report much lower levels of life satisfaction than Moroccan immigrants, while the socio-economic factors considered failed to explain why this happens. The findings showed that the effect of absolute income for Turkish immigrants was insignificant and the effect of relative income, matters to them. The authors studied the role of identity, language, religion, media, and discrimination to explain the different levels of life satisfaction for immigrant groups and found that a strong sense of "Dutch" identity has a positive effect on life satisfaction (although Moroccans with a strong sense of Dutch identity are more satisfied with their lives than Turks with a strong sense of Dutch identity). Finally, results showed that immigrants who identify themselves as Muslims are far more satisfied than the other immigrants identified as Turkish or Moroccan.

Skevington (2002) explains the reasons for the need of cross-cultural measures and points out that the pragmatic studies by which they are enforced provide theoretical evidence of the universality or relativity of the very concept of quality of life. She mentions that The World Health Organization Quality of Life Assessment group (WHOQOL) defines quality of life as "the individuals' perceptions of their position in life, in the cultural context and value system he lives in, and in relation with his aims, expectations, standards, and worries" (p. 136). Furthermore, the group has put forth that perceptions and interpretations are rooted in people's culture and that they should be regarded as the first definition of quality of life which has, directly and formally, incorporated cultural components to the body of the definition rather than recognize cultural influence as an external variable.

Verkuyten and Kwa (1994) studied whether, among minority young peoples, alternative forms of ethnic self-identification are equally healthy in terms of psychological well-being, considering Chinese and Turkish young peoples living in the Netherlends. They distinguished four different types of self-identification, following Berry et al. (1986): acculturative, assimilative, dissociative and marginal.

All types were found among Chinese and Turkish young peoples, but the Turkish subjects showed a stronger dissociative self-identification than the Chinese. Among the Chinese, an acculturative and especially a marginal orientation were associated with less happiness, decreasing self-concept stability, and decreasing collectivistic orientation, while among the Turkish subjects both of these orientations were associated with lower self-esteem.

In the scope of an exploratory research of the individualist-collectivist construct and well-being, Owusu-Ansah (2004), examines the relationship between cultural orientation and subjective well-being in Ghana, confirming that in such a collectivist cultural context, high levels of collectivism might be associated to high levels of subjective well-being. Nevertheless, individualism has also been positively associated to subjective well-being.

Theuns et al. (2012) pointed out that, in cross-cultural research on quality of life, researchers deal with the impossibility to compare subjective wellbeing assessments across cultural groups and they sustain that the Information Integration Theory provides a framework that allows a better understanding of the composition of the concept of "satisfaction with life as a whole", across different cultural groups. In this context, they studied the way students in Algeria, Belgium and Poland integrate information on a variety of life domains into an appraisal of "satisfaction with life as a whole" and found that different integration models coexist in all the studied groups, and that the prevalence of these strategies differs across groups, concluding that cultural differences in the conceptualization of overall satisfaction with life exist, and that differences between cultures result from different distributions of these conceptualizations.

3.4 The Impact of Culture in the Work of a Qualitative Researcher

From the researchers' stand-point, it is necessary to point out the impact of culture on their personal, professional and political dimensions (Tonon 2013).

Regarding the personal dimension, two fellow historians describe their personal attitudes towards diversity, in close connection with the plurality which characterizes their original contexts, highlighting imagination, open-mindedness, the attitude of trying to stand in the other's place, etc.:

A fellow historian, 47 year old female, explains:

> Originally belonging to an urban and foreign family circle crossed by long preserved narratives, previous to relocalization, allowed an early training in cultural diversity. Melodies evoking far-off lands, like Egypt in Aída; descriptive literature of fascinating scenarios imagined by Salgari; family stories about general and particular events that took place during the European World Wars in East Africa, and the very spirit of those times, became a challenge to imagination and knowledge.

Another fellow historian, 44 years old, narrates:

> My genes are, somehow foreign; a Paraguayan mother of Spanish and Italian descent, has made me broad-minded which, I think, is what helps me regard things without prejudice, think twice before giving my opinion, because I try to stand in the other's shoes…

In that respect, Scott (2008) sustains that research is not an area free from values and subjectivity the researcher is always present. Frost et al. (2010) point out the habitual use of that term "subjectivity" makes allusion to a representation of the individuals' inner world, which makes them uncognizable to a stranger and only partly cognizable to its owner.

Hence, the research process affects the researcher which is, in turn, affected by the researcher. This requires the researcher to be reflective and self-critical regarding his subjectivity in the research, and also the effect of the latter on his own.

Finlay (2005) makes allusion to a research process which implies a reflective commitment with the "embodied intersubjective relationship" we have with the participants in the research. He describes three impenetrable levels of reflexibility which culminate in a reciprocal and an interconnecting insertion of others in our selves, and of ourselves in others, in which the understanding of others and our self-understanding are merged in a mutual transformation. Subsequently, Finlay (2009) gives further details on two processes related to subjectivity and the researcher, namely, epoché and reflexibility.

As to the professional dimension, some specific aspects of the original profession and up-bringing become evident in a 47 year old fellow historian, in her allusions to the closeness to diversities and the production of knowledge she has found in different institutional environments. These are her views:

> Once I had found my way, academic contents enhanced my knowledge, paradigms, and methodologies, but did not always succeed in paving the way: omitted spatiality, stigmatized cultures, controversial values, and prejudiced looks, produce alert signs. In that sense: How could multicultural boundaries be bridged if knowledge seemed to be limited to a dominating center which alienated the whole? The wish to exceed that Eurocentric structure and plunge into a qualitative research on historical-cultural issues, on topics that had never been embraced or deemed to be subject to revision/up-dating, gave way to a contribution to integration, a reassessment of values which tended to unify cultures. Field-work, on the other hand, allowed an encounter between researchers and subjects, respectful of the self-perception of their own identities. Today, the cultural kaleidoscope has been amplified and the methodology diversified, hence the research has become enriched and open to conceptualizations which, are slowly adjusting the image of reality, so necessary to the understanding of multiculturalism. The researcher, a mere mediator in this process, must continue to exalt the relevance of diversity and intercultural connection.

Thus, Rodriguez de la Vega (2011) points out that university activity, inserted in community life, is closely related to citizenship and spaces for public action, at the same time she sustains that university education which acknowledges and implies varieties of learning and forms of apprehension of reality, contributes to the articulation of citizens and professionals in the construction of knowledge that may account for a world of diversity. The author points out that the option is a university which eludes immobility and recovers its place as the critical conscience of each historical time, while recovering historical memory, re/establishing ethical values that consider a plurality of views regarding the citizens' professionalization/action relationship; monitors the extent of integration; undertakes the social impression of the production and transmission of knowledge; articulates a conscious competence of diversity, and the need for team-work, thus articulating one another's access, with equal enunciation.

In a similar line of thought, El Ghali (2011) adds that the relationship between university and society must complement each other, though not based on university-productive sector concept, and he quotes Olivé by sustaining that the fundamental role of university is to produce knowledge in order to extend it to society and include the outcast.

Regarding the political dimension, Mojica Mendieta (2011) sustains that globalization implies an epistemological challenge to social sciences, that is to generate new analytical categories which may explain the space-time transformations of the social processes, and political conditioning in people's activities. Thus, it is important to re-elaborate new innovative forms of social research in order to understand and explain the structural violence within each culture, and among different cultures. Likewise, he explains that the knowledge and recognition of the political processes and conditioning of scientific practice may contribute to eradicate determinism, relativism, and pretended objectivity in the different axioms of political sciences.

Retamozo (2007) points out that the construction of epistemic subjectivity springs from an attitude which articulates will-power and conscience, non-dissociable from an ethical-political position, which considers that social knowledge must be function as to social projects that tend to fulfill political axioms (Dussel 2006). Therefore, the construction of this subjectivity contradicts a presumed neutrality of values and assumes knowledge as transformation praxis.

The impact on the different dimensions of qualitative researchers refers, in turn, to the possibilities and limitations of their task, in the scope of a permanent interpellation among the abovementioned dimensions. In this respect, Liamputtong (2010) emphasizes the interpretive and flexible approach of qualitative studies and makes allusion to a healing methodology which, paraphrasing Denzin et al. (2008), refers to a methodology of the heart [...], embracing the ethics of truth based on love, care, hope, and forgiveness; its principle being love, hugging, compassion, and seeking reciprocity. We believe that this is related to the reference given by Yáñez del Pozo (2010), who, quoting Estermann (1998), points out that the primal wish of the Andean human being (or rune) is not the acquisition of abstract knowledge of the world around him but "a mythical insertion, a cult representation, and a symbolic celebration of this reality". Hence, we consider that research emerges as a task of interpretation and explanation of the universes under consideration, in a process in which people emerge as agents of knowledge.

Regarding symbolism, it is understood by Giménez (2005), following Geertz, as the world of social representations, materialized in sensitive forms, which refers to a set of social processes of significance and communication, illustrated by a fellow historian, a 55 year old female, who undertakes the question of language:

> From History which is my field of expertise, studies the human beings' past through ruins, written documents, oral tradition, and other traces that human action leaves behind. Though there is a quantitative line of work, our techniques are, without a doubt, essentially qualitative. And it is from those traces left by human action that we make a selection, classify, reconstruct, interpret, and explain. When we study the past of "others", we must also add the action "translate" to that of interpreting. The mastering of the language is important, though the actual task of translation is very complex. Although the process of acquiring the code must be linked to a profound knowledge of that "other culture" to attempt to understand the connotations of their expressions, it is obvious that it will never be exact [...] those who have no notion about that code will evidently be at a disadvantage, for they will have to depend on another interpreter, and that will mean a new filter will be added [...]

In this sense, the symbolic aspect is perceived in this context as a constituent dimension of social life, as a whole; furthermore, the reality of the symbol does not end in its function as a significant, but also as a means of becoming immersed in the world, as well as a mechanism of power.

Temple et al. (2006) point out that the discussion on translation/interpretation evidences an increasing number of comments opposing the idea that whoever interprets or translates the text is irrelevant, so long as the translation in question is "objective". They quote Venuti (1998) who sustains that the predominant translation practices result in the rewriting of the text rather than in a transference of meaning, since the translators select the words and concepts in their attempt at reconstruction, and more than one choice may be considered correct in that process. In other words, translators and interpreters are part of the context in which the information is produced.

On the other hand, the contact with "the others" is fundamental, for their mutual understanding constitutes a central epistemological principle (Mojica Mendieta 2011) which derives in a dialogic relationship, in an unimposed contemporaneity which, in turn, implies a quest for intersubjective knowledge. A fellow 55 year old female historian expresses the following:

> Experience—field work—in the society under study, is also vital. Still, it is also true that though we may spend many years immersed in that "other" society, and even be lucky enough to get to know its members day by day, and its culture from practice, it will always be a fragmentary vision in space, limited in time.

In that respect, Christians, 1997 (quoted in Christians 2011), points out that, considering that all human cultures have something important to tell, social science research acknowledges individual values, without overlooking universal human dignity.

Focusing on a cultural context intimately related to the researchers' own origin often makes this fact evident, by the opposition of different knowledge. The same colleague sustains that:

> We are not exempt from these risks even if we are lucky to be a sort of cultural "bridge" because of sharing the "other" culture's family origins, or being acquainted with it through

> the culture we received by birth and up-bringing. It is a fact that systemic research and studies cannot be replaced by origin.

In this connection, Chaitin et al. (2009) agree with Sansonse (2003), who regards ethnic identity as a process affected by history and contemporary circumstances, as well as by local and global dynamics, and other matters such as hierarchy and power. They further add that Banks (1996) considers that it is more useful for researchers to regard ethnicity as something that exists in the "observer's head" as well as an analytical device or tool used by academics to explain the actions and feelings of the subjects under study.

A critical attitude towards self-formation—a permanent characteristic—together with research work in general and personal development in particular, seem to seek the insurance of an acceptable trajectory in terms of related knowledge and ethics. In this connection, a fellow 55 year old female historian points out:

> I've began to study the history of the Japanese people and their culture, over 30 years ago, informally at first and later on systematically, gradually learning from contact with Japanese colleagues (their points of view), also through Latin-American colleagues, other experiences and warnings to avoid falling into traps set by our own culture [...] our critical vision is also enhanced as we increase our knowledge, it sometimes leads us to overrate negative aspects in the worst of cases, or simply to highlight them, in order to break with stereotypes—only to end up creating new ones.

Pedulla (2012) reminds us that stereotypes may play a central role in molding attitudes and behaviors, thus often being related to prejudice and discrimination. On the other hand, Dovidio et al. (2010), give more precision to these interrelated terms. Regarding stereotypes, they believe that the latter are cognitive schema used by social percipients to process information about others, which not only reflect beliefs regarding the characteristic features of typical group members, but also contain information about the different qualities of those "others" who influence the emotional reactions towards the members of the group in question. They further make allusion to prejudice, indicating that the latter is conceptualized as an attitude which, like some others, possesses cognitive components (beliefs regarding a certain group), affective (dislike), and co native (a negative disposition towards the group under consideration). As to discrimination, they sustain that it implies more than social distinction among social objects, it also refers to inappropriate and potentially inappropriate treatment towards other subjects, on account of their being members of some community.

This critical attitude and permanent reflective state of alert is evidence of the amalgam of our work with the researchers' own private lives. Thus, a 57 year old fellow historian describes it, on the basis of his research study of Japan which has gone through several stages:

> Firstly, in my stage of academic formation, approaching the "other" represented approach challenges which left their marks. Doubtless, Saïd's work was essential and, though it was not directly related to Japan, it opened a space for reflection in order to attempt to make a careful approach of the study of the "Japanese". Probing into the history of Japan was another watershed, for the mere acquaintance with that country broke with the preconceived classification of the world's historical evolution (Western) which had, so far, determined my vision of the world (non-Western peoples also had history, as Georg Iggers, accurately

expresses in "La historiografía del siglo XX"). Finally, another essential element was the fact that Japan was my place of residence and I was directly related, not only to academic life and the Japanese's own focus on study but, to a greater degree, everyday "contact" with the "other", and waking up and going to sleep in a "space" that was molding and constructing the ways to approach.

Taking these theoretical and practical elements helped me challenge the chief assumption of a certain history conceived under a presumed "objectivity", understanding that there is no such thing as an "object of history". Yet another even more determinant element was a more personally intense and direct approach to the social history of the Japanese in Mexico. The connection to "social movements" which I had upheld since my early years as a student, were broadened by of the migrants of that nationality in my own country, particularly the stage of vigilance and confinement they had to undergo at the outbreak of World War II. [...] This put an end to a stage and gave way to another: the gist of the first stage was my living experience in Japan; while the second hinged upon the way in which migrants displayed the reproduction of two societies in their everyday lives. Thus, "culture" revealed itself in the complexity of the actual world of economy, politics and social sciences which I had conceived as "historical science" fields. The social and intellectual framework of my research, so far, was an INTERNAL and CONSTITUENT part of the study of the first 40 years of the twentieth century, joining two temporal spaces of my research and of my own life. The spaces, daily controversies in which I dwelt in the last decades, were not separate, much less alien to what I had been studying and researching: historiography and reality had taken my academic world by storm.

In the same line of thought, another fellow, 44 year old female historian, points out that, to the work done in this field she could add her marriage to a Japanese immigrant, together with her artistic side "my artistic vein was another contribution to the events during the Conferences on Japan, by singing Japanese Songs or lecturing on the Colonia Urquiza Community I was able to illustrate it".

That dynamic of interlacing with one's private life is reflected in long range influential challenges, in life itself, and in research work. Dickson-Swift et al. (2007) focused on the challenges experienced by qualitative researchers who deal with sensitive themes, but we believe that their impressions may apply, in general. They show the challenges faced by qualitative researchers, like intruding in people's lives, sometimes in critical moments, requiring them to talk in detail about their experiences, sometimes even during long periods of time; constructing rapport with the interviewed subject, which may even lead to information, not necessarily related to the research topic, but relevant since it has generated this rapport; generating a dynamic of reciprocity between the researcher and the subject of research, involving the necessary care that this requires; the researcher's vulnerability; developing bonds with the participants; keeping their distance; appreciating the privilege of taking part in this kind of study and the responsibility it implies. Different authors give a broader view on the themes mentioned herein; some of them are: Dickson-Swift et al. (2006), Liamputtong and Ezzy (2005), Ceglowski (2000), Daly (1992).

To sum up the views of the aforementioned colleagues, the 55 year old female historian, mentions that

The Nigerian writer Chimamanda Adichie, spoke, in a TV conference, of the peril of a single story, making reference to a negative vision that predominates in the Western World on the Sub-Saharian African peoples [that we extend to any disciplinary outlook of a qualitative approach]. In that sense, so long as we fail to produce a great number of studies from the broadest variety of perspectives, we shall never be able to approach each other in a full dimension. Finally, we may conclude that it is important to run the risk of making mistakes, while being conscious of our subjectivity and conditioning factors, although the knowledge of the language continues to be fundamental because if we persist in resorting only to the available translations as a means of getting to know others, we will merely be recycling information, thus contributing to the preservation of only one story/history.

3.5 Summing Up

The assessment that the subjects (and/or groups) make of their quality of life is related to their cultural background, situated in a specific point of time and space. Likewise, the practice of qualitative research and its results are socially constructed and also determined by space and time.

The researchers' task is developed in this context which refers to the consideration of plural conceptions of reality—which, in the Jaina theory of Multilateralism, is known as anekāntavāda and considers such conceptions as valid, even when they contradict each other (Tola and Dragonetti 2009)—that, in fact, refers to the way in which we approach and construct the other and therefore ourselves, in the background of social research projects that aim at transformation.

In other words, researchers express themselves within specific interpretive communities and give a personal configuration to the cultural elements of their research, thus offering their observation and interpretation which are socially situated between the world of the researcher and that of the subjects under study; therefore there cannot be a unique true interpretation. Corbin Dwyer and Buckle (2009) embrace the theme of "space between" and follow Kanuha (2000) who points out that it is important to consider more comprehensive forms of acquaintance and understanding of people, practices, and cultures, so similar yet so different from what we are.

That construction we make of ourselves, which takes place in our dialogue with others constitutes, according to Taylor et al. (1994), relationships in a space of self-assertment and self-discovery. Denzin and Lincoln (2011), point out that qualitative research not only involves a scientific project but also a moral, therapeutic, and allegorical one; and, in that respect, our own moral dimension is nurtured by the social connections which bring us closer to the different known conceptions of Good and creates a commitment that urges us to be active participants of the moral articulation of a community.

Lincoln and Denzin (2000 quoted in Christians 2011) consider that the challenge to those who write about culture is the act of becoming involved in the same moral space as the people subject to their research and, from that perspective, the research strategies are legitimated in terms of vitality in order to shed light on the best way of generating human welfare.

All in all, "the problems of the social sciences must be, ultimately, related to the visions of the world they are contained in" (Guba and Lincoln 1994, quoted in Christians 2011, p. 322).

Acknowledgement I am particularly thankful to Drs. Carmen Dragonetti and Fernando Tola for anticipating all discussions on culture, its diversities, and the position of researchers about it, making of contemporary dialogue with others their starting point for the interpretation of other cultural contexts. Their teachings excel academic level and allow us a return to life with higher knowledge, greater pleasure, and huge pride in been their student.

I am, further, very thankful for the generous contributions made by Cecilia Onaha, Sergio Hernández Galindo, Eugenia Arduino, Irene Cafiero, Miguel Marlaire and Vilma Carrizo de Hadat.

References

Banks, M. (1996). *Ethnicity: Anthropological constructions*. London: Routledge.

Bassand, M., & Hainard, F. (1985). *Dynamique socio-culturelle régionale*. Lausanne: Presses Polytechniques Romandes.

Berry, J. W., Trimble, J. E., & Olmedo, E. L. (1986). Assessment of acculturation. In W. J. Lonner & J. W. Berry (Eds.), Field methods in cross-cultural research. Newbury Park: Sage.

Bourdieu, P. (1980). *Le sens pratique*. Paris: Editions de Minuit.

Bourdieu, P. (1987). *Choses dites*. París: Les Editions de Minuit.

Ceglowski, D. (2000). Research as relationship. *Qualitative Inquiry, 6,* 88–103.

Chaitin, J, Linstroth, J. P., & Hiller. P. T. (2009). Ethnicity and Belonging: An Overview of a Study of Cuban, Haitian and Guatemalan Immigrants to Florida. Forum: Qualitative Social research, 10, 3, 12. http://www.qualitative-research.net/index.php/fqs/article/view/1363/2856. Accessed 10 Feb 2014.

Christians, C. G. (2011). La ética y la política en la investigación cualitativa. In N. K. Denzin & Y. S. Lincoln (Eds.), *Manual de investigación cualitativa. Volumen l. El campo de la investigación cualitativa* (pp. 283–331). Barcelona: Gedisa.

Christopher, J. C. (1999). Situating psychological well-being: Exploring the cultural roots of its theory and research. *Journal of Counselling and Development, 77,* 141–152.

Corbin Dwyer, S., & Buckle, J. L. (2009). The space between: On being and insider-outsider in qualitative research. *International Journal of Qualitative Methods, 8*(1), 54–63.

Daly, K. (1992). The fit between qualitative research and characteristics of families. In J. F. Gilgun, K. Day & G. Handel (Eds.), *Qualitative methods in family research*. Newbury Park: Sage.

Denzin, N. K., Lincoln, Y. S., & Smith, L. T. (2008). Introduction: Critical methodologies and indigenous inquiry. In N. K. Denzin, Y. S. Lincoln, & L. T. Smith (Eds.), *Handbook of critical and Indigenous methodologies* (pp. 1–20). Thousand Oaks: Sage.

Denzin, N. K., & Lincoln, Y. S. (2011). Introducción general. La investigación cualitativa como disciplina y como práctica. In N. K. Denzin & Y. S. Lincoln (Comps.), *Manual de investigación cualitativa. Volumen l. El campo de la investigación cualitativa* (pp. 43–101). Barcelona: Gedisa.

Dickson-Swift, V., James, E. L., Kippen, S., & Liamputtong, P, (2006). Blurring boundaries in qualitative research on sesitive topics. *Qualitative Health Research, 16,* 853–871.

Dickson-Swift, V., James, E. L., Kippen, S., & Liamputtong, P. (2007). Doing sensitive research: What challenges do qualitative researchers face? *Qualitative Research, 7*(3), 327–353.

Diener, E., Emmons, R. A., Larsen, R. J., & Griffin, S. (1985). The satisfaction with life scale. *Journal of Personality Assessment, 49*(1), 71–75.

Diener, E., & Diener, M. (1995). Cross-cultural correlates of life satisfaction and self-esteem. *Journal of Personality and Social Psychology, 68,* 653–663.

Diener, E., & Fujita, F. (1994). Social comparisosns and subjective well-being. In B. P. Buunk & F. X. Gibbons (Eds.), *Health, coping and well-being* (pp. 329–357). Mahwah: Lawrence Erlbaum.

Diener, E., & Suh, E. (1997). Measuring quality of life: Economic, social and subjective indicators. *Social Indicators Research, 40*(1–2), 189–216.

Diener, E., Gohm, C. L., Suh, E., & Oishi S. (2000). *Journal of Cross-Cultural Psychology, 31*(4), 419–436.
Dovidio, J. F., Hewstone, M., Glick, P., & Esses, V. M. (2010). Prejudice, stereotyping, and discrimination: Theoretical and empirical overview. In J. F. Dovidio, M. Hewstone, P. Glick & V. M. Esses (Eds.), *Handbook of prejudice, stereotyping, and discrimination* (pp. 3–28). London: Sage.
Dube, S.-coord- (1999). *Pasados Poscoloniales*. México. El Colegio de México.
Dussel, E. (2006). *20 tesis de política*. México: Siglo XXI-Crefal.
El Ghali, K. (2011). Los retos de la universidad marroquí en la sociedad del conocimiento. *Magriberia, 4,* 61–71.
Estermann, J. (1998). *Filosofía andina. Estudio intercultural de la sabiduría autóctona andina.* Quito: Ediciones Abya-Yala.
Finlay, L. (2005). 'Reflexive embodied empathy': A phenomenology of participant-researcher intersubjectivity. Paper for 2005 *Methods* issue #4 *The Humanistic Psychologist.* http://www.google.com.ar/url?sa=t&rct=j&q=&esrc=s&frm=1&source=web&cd=1&ved=0CC4QFjAA&url=http%3A%2F%2Fwww.lindafinlay.co.uk%2FReflexive_embodied_empathy_new.doc&ei=fILAUuCxI461kQf9ooD4Cg&usg=AFQjCNFtavDiu2ALApCvtxhuPYImczxqEg. Accessed 12 Feb 2014.
Finlay, L. (2009). Embracing researcher subjectivity in phenomenological research: A response to Ann Scott. *European Journal for Qualitative Research in Psychotherapy, 4,* 13–20.
Forougui, E. (1995). Cross-cultural quality of life among Persians. Master Thesis of Clinical Psychology. School of Psychology, Deakin University, Australia.
Frost, N., Nolas, S-M., Brooks-Gordon, B., Esin, C., Holt, A., Mehdizadeh, L., & Shinebourne P. (2010). Pluralism in qualitative research: The impact of different researchers and qualitative approaches on the analysis of qualitative data. *Qualitative Research, 10*(4), 1–20. http://eprints.mdx.ac.uk/5000/1/QRJ366802.pdf. Accessed 26 Jan 2014.
Giménez, G. (2000). Identidades en globalización. *Espiral, 7*(19), 27–48.
Giménez, G. (2004). Culturas e identidades. Revista Mexicana de Sociología. http://www.redalyc.org/articulo.oa?id=32109908. Accessed 23 Jan 2014.
Giménez, G. (2005). La concepción simbólica de la cultura. In G. Giménez (Ed.), *Teoría y análisis de la cultura* (pp. 67–88). México: CONACULTA e Instituto Coahuilense de Cultura.
Gokdemir, O., & Dumludag, D. (2011). Subjective well-being among ethnic minorities: the Dutch case. MPRA Paper No. 38691. http://mpra.ub.uni-muenchen.de/38691/.
Goodenough, W. H. (1975). Cultura, lenguaje y sociedad. In J. S. Khan (Ed.), *El concepto de cultura. Textos fundamentales* (pp. 157–249). Barcelona: Anagrama.
Grimson, A. (2012). *Los límites de la cultura.* Buenos Aires: Siglo Veintiuno Editores.
Grossber, L. (2003). Identidad y estudios culturales. In S. Hall & du P. Gay. *Cuestiones de identidad.* Buenos Aires: Amorrortu.
Guba, E., & Lincoln, Y. S. (1994). Competing paradigms in qulitative research. In N. K. Denzin & Y. S. Lincoln (Comps.), *Handbook of Qualitative Research* (pp. 105–117). Thousand Oaks (California): Sage.
Hofstede, G. (1984). The cultural relativity of the quality of life Concept. *The Academy of Management Review, 9*(3), 389–398.
Kanuha, V. K. (2000). "Being" native versus "going native": Conducting social work research as an insider. *Social Work, 45*(5), 439–447.
Kawana-Singer, M., Padilla, G. V., & Ashig-Giwa, K. (2010). Health-related quality of life and culture. *Seminars in Oncology Nursing, 26*(1), 59–67. http://www.seminarsoncologynursing.com/article/S0749-2081(09)00115-6/fulltext. Accessed 28 Dec 2013.
Liamputtong, P. (2010). Cross-cultural research and qualitative inquiry. *Turkish Online Journal of Qualitative Inquiry, 1*(1), 16–29.
Liamputtong, P., & Ezzy, D. (2005). *Qualitative research methods.* South Melbourne: Oxford University Press.
Lincoln, Y. S., & Denzin, N. K. (2000). The seventh moment: Out of the past. In N. K. Denzin & Y. S. Lincoln, *Handbook of Qualitative Research* (pp. 1047–1065). Thousand Oaks: Sage.

Lipiansky, E. M. (1992). *Identité et communication*. París: Presses Universitarires de France.
Mojica Mendieta, F. J. (2011). Investigación cualitativa, epistemología y poder simbólico. Trama. Revista de Tecnología, cultura y desarrollo, ll, 2, pp. 7–20. http://www.tec.ac.cr/sitios/Docencia/cienciassociales/revista_trama/pdf/revista.pdf. Accessed 20 Dec 2013.
Oishi, S., Diener, E. F., Lucas, R. E., & Suh, E. M. (1999). Cross-cultural variations in predictors of life satisfaction: Perspectives from needs and values. *Personality and Social Psychology Bulletin, 25*(8), 980–990.
Owusu-Ansah, F. E. (2004). Cultural orientation and subjective well-being. *Journal of Science and Technology, 24,* 76–83.
Pedulla, D. S. (2012). The positive consequences of negative stereotypes: Race, sexual orientation, and the job application process. Working Paper. Center for the Study of Social Organizaton, Department of Sociology, Princeton University. http://www.princeton.edu/csso/working-papers/WP7.pdf. Accessed 8 Jan 2014.
Restrepo, E. (2010). Identidad: apuntes teóricos y metodológicos. In G. Castellanos Llanos, D. I. Grueso & M. Rodriguez (Eds.), *Identidad, cultura y política. Perspectivas conceptuales, miradas empíricas* (pp. 61–70). México: Honorable Cámara de Diputados-Universidad del Valle-Miguel Ángel Porrúa.
Retamozo, M. (2007). *Cuaderno de Trabajo n 9. El método como postura. Apuntes sobre la conformaqción de la subjetividad epistémica y notas metodológicas sobre la construcción de un objeto de estudio*. México: Universidad Nacional Autónoma de México.
Rodriguez de la Vega, L. (2011). Diversidad cultural, "sociedad del información y el conocimiento" y universidad. *Magriberia, 4,* 95–104.
Russell, D., Peplau, L. A., & Cutrona, C. E. (1980). The Revised UCLA Loneliness Scale: Concurrent and discriminate validity evidence. *Journal of Personality and Social Psychology, 39,* 472–480.
Sansone, L. (2003). *Blackness without ethnicity: Constructing race in Brazil.* New York: Palgrave Macmillan.
Schumaker, J. F., Shea, J. D., Monfries, M. M., & Groth-Marnat, G. (1993). Loneliness and life satisfaction in Japan and Australia. *Journal of Psychology, 127,* 65–71.
Schütz, A. (1974). *El problema de la realidad social*. Buenos Aires: Amorrortu.
Scott, A. (2008). The effect of doing qualitative research on novice researchers. *European Journal for Qualitative Research in Psychotherapy, 3,* 10–18.
Sewell, W. H. Jr. (1999). The concept (s) of culture. In V. E. Bonnell & L. Hunt (Eds.), *Beyond the cultural turn* (pp. 35–61). Berkeley: University of California Press.
Shin, D. C., Rutkowski, C. P., & Min, P. (2003). *The quality of life in Korea. Comparative and dynamic perspectives*. USA: Kluwer Academic.
Skevington, S. M. (2002). Advancing cross-cultural research on quality of life: observations drawn from the WHOQOL development. *Quality of Life Research, 11*, 135–144.
Taylor, C., Appiah, K. A., Habermas, J., Rockefeller, S. C., Walzer, M., & Wolf, S. (1994). *Multiculturalism: Examining the politics of recognition*. Princeton: Princeton University Press.
Temple, B., Edwards, R., & Alexander C. (2006). Grasping at context: Cross language qualitative research as secondary qualitative data analysis. Forum: Qualitative Social Research, 7, 4, 10. http://www.qualitative-research.net/index.php/fqs/article/view/176/393. Accessed 6 Jan 2014.
Theuns, P., Baran, B., Van Vaerenbergh, R., Hellenbosch, H., & Tiliouine H. (2012). A cross-cultural experimental approach to the contribution of health, religion and personal relations to subjective satisfaction with life as a whole. *Psicológica, 33,* 591–608.
Thompson, J. B. (1998). *Ideología y cultura moderna*. México: Universidad Autónoma Metropolitana- Unidad Xochimilco.
Tola, F., & Dragonetti, C. (2009). El Milenio de Oro de la filosofía de la India. *Ilu. Revista de Ciencias de las Religiones, 14,* 199–214.
Tonon, G. (2013). *La integración de métodos de investigación en Ciencias Sociales: la triangulación y los métodos mixtos*. Documento de investigación número 135. Serie Documentos de investigación del Colegio Mexiquense. Toluca México. Mayo 2013.
Triandis, H. C. (1995). *Individualism and collectivism*. Boulder: Westview.

Triandis, H. C. (1996). The psychological measurement of cultural syndromes. *American Psychologist, 51*, 407–415.

Triandis, H. C. (2000). Cultural syndromes and subjective well-being. In E. Diener & E. M. Suh (Eds.) *Culture and subjective well-being.* Cambridge: MIT Press.

Venuti, L. (1998). The scandals of translation: Towards an ethics of difference. London: Routledge.

Verkuyten, M., & Kwa, I. (1994). Ethnic self-identification and psychological well-being among ethnic minority young people in the Netherlands. *International Journal of Adolescence and Young people, 5,* 19–34.

Yáñez del Pozo, J. (2010). El pensamiento andino y la construcción de país plurinacionales y sociedades interculturales. ALAI, América Latina en Movimiento.

Chapter 4
Integration of Qualitative and Quantitative Methods in Quality of Life Studies

Graciela Tonon

The decision to use a certain research methodology is no minor question on the contrary it implies a philosophical, theoretical, political, and operative decision.

The path towards method integration sprang from triangulation, as far as the validation process of the completed research is concerned, and converged in the use of mixed methods as a strategy to complement and expand the combination of the quantitative and qualitative methods.

In 1978 Denzin defines triangulation as the combination of methodologies for the study of the same phenomena or process. Some decades before, Creswell, Felters e Ivankova (2004) explained that in triangulation each method has the same importance and the work is organized in different sections, with a final discussion at the end, in which the researcher combine the results of the use of both methods.

As the idea of triangulation develops, it gives way to the idea of mixed-methods. Apart from Sieber (1973) different authors have proposed this new methodological strategy in which researchers can combine both methods at different stages of the project. Actually, mixed-methods are considered a kind of theory and practice analyses in the research field, from different points of view, with the aim of achieving depth and corroborating the results.

Achieving method integration in the field of research on quality of life requires that the researcher should articulate the data obtained through qualitative and quantitative means, and produce an integrated analysis of the said data.

G. Tonon (✉)
UNICOM, Faculty of Social Sciences, Universidad Nacional de Lomas de Zamora, Lomas de Zamora, Argentina
e-mail: gracielatonon@hotmail.com

CICS, Faculty of Social Sciences, Universidad de Palermo, Ciudad Autónoma de Buenos Aires, Argentina

G. Tonon (ed.), *Qualitative Studies in Quality of Life*,
Social Indicators Research Series 55, DOI 10.1007/978-3-319-13779-7_4

4.1 Perspective and Points of View in the Quality of Life Research

Doing research on quality of life implies a series of theoretical and methodological decisions that must be undertaken by the researcher on the point of developing his project. As to the methodological alternatives, it is optional whether to use the quantitative method or the qualitative method, or both.

The possibility to use both methods has been developed from the use of a process known as triangulation, as well as the use of the so-called mixed methods, both questions that will be developed in the following items. Nevertheless, before becoming immersed in this subject, it is interesting to reflect upon two concepts which play a major role in the process leading to methodological decision-making: the concepts of perspective and of points of view (Tonon 2013).

According to Lechner (2002)

> … perspective allows us to take a step back and raise our eyes beyond immediacy, assuming a point of view from which to look, since there is no longer a neutral view, hence all perspectives are situated (concerned) and imply a project, i.e. an intention towards the future. For, creating a certain perspective, is the same as creating a narration that situates the present in relation to the past and the future. (Lechner 2002, p. 124).[1]

Bourdieu (2008, p. 17), on the other hand, calls our attention to the fact that "there is no such thing as a research object without a point of view, even when the object in question, has been produced with the intention of revoking the point of view, an equivalent to "partiality".

In this line of thought, the consideration of the perspective chosen by the researchers and the considerations of their points of view, both sustain and mark the limits of their type of work.

Regarding the methods, the debate has traditionally been centered in the relevance of choosing the quantitative method or the qualitative method and, in this sense, we are aware that each of these options implies a number of specifications, characteristics, advantages and disadvantages.

In this case, we shall put forth the possibility of using both methodologies, not with a view on juxtaposition, but regarding it as an interchange leading to a possible integration.Thus, the choice of this perspective elicits the initial need to characterize and mark the difference between triangulation and the use of mixed methods.

4.2 Triangulation

In 1959, Campbell and Fiske, introduced the idea of triangulation based on the use of various methods to validate a process, with the ultimate object of demonstrating that the result obtained is not a mere product of the method used.

Metaphorically speaking, triangulation emerged from navigation and military strategy, in which cases it refers to the operation through which the situation of an

[1] Translation of the author of the original, in Spanish language.

object is defined by the crisscross pattern of lines drawn from different points, these latter being multiple points of reference which allow the localization of the exact position of the object. (Smith 1975, p. 273).

In 1978, Denzin defined triangulation as the combination of methodologies for the study of the same phenomenon, identifying four kinds: triangulation of data, triangulation of researchers, triangulation of theories, and triangulation of methodologies.Likewise, according to the author, triangulation has given way to three possible results: convergence, inconsistency, and contradiction.

Some years later, Kelbe (2001) would take up this idea by expressing that, if the quantitative and qualitative…methods are combined to answer a specific research question, three things may happen. They may:

- Converge: i.e., that the results of both methods will lead to the same conclusion.
- Complement: since, though the quantitative and qualitative results may relate to different objects or phenomena, they may be used to supplement each other.
- Contradict: a situation that takes place when the quantitative and qualitative results are divergent.

In 1979, Jick acknowledged the advantages of triangulation by expressing that it allows researchers to be more confident of the results, stimulate the development of creative forms of gathering data, facilitate the synthesis and/or integration of theories, and contemplate possible contradictions.

In 1991, Morse enunciated two types of methodological triangulation: simultaneous triangulation and sequential triangulation. Simultaneous triangulation implies the use of quantitative and qualitative methods, with a limited interaction between both methods during the stage of data gathering, and complementing each other's results at the moment of their interpretation. Sequential triangulation is characterized by the use of the application of the results of one of the methods for the planning of the application of the other; since they are both necessary to the development of the research process.

Finally, in 1995, in his joint work with Field, Morse defined triangulation as the simultaneous or sequential use of two or more methods in order to examine the same phenomenon.

When triangulation is used in research, it is characterized by the fact that it gives equal importance to both methods, and is organized in separate sections: on the one hand, the gathering of data and qualitative analysis, and quantitative analysis on the other; this is followed by a final discussion of the results obtained by both. (Creswell et al. 2004, p. 11)

Considering that the concept of triangulation has acquired different meanings, Morgan (1998) has recommended the use of the concept of convergence or confirmation, in concurrence with Campbell who, in 1959, had emphasized the fact that triangulation referred to the convergence or confirmation of results in different methods.

Finally, Kelbe (2001, p. 5), identified two meanings of the word triangulation:a validation process, or a process that generates a new framework for the researched phenomenon.

4.3 Mixed Methods

The origin of the so-called mixed methods is simultaneous with the development of the idea of triangulation. In 1973, Sieber had already pointed out the reasons for the combination of quantitative and qualitative methods, without using the term triangular; only explaining how this combination might be effective to the different stages of research, i.e., the moment of making the design, when collecting data or when proceeding to analyze them.

Later on, in 1989, Greene, Caracelli and Graham identified five purposes in the studies made through mixed methods. They consider that the latter facilitate:

- triangulation (in terms of convergence),
- complementation, allowing a classification of results,
- development of the use of the results of the application of one method as a contribution to the information provided by the other,
- initiation, which reaffirms the initial question of the research by describing paradoxes and contradictions, and
- expansion, which allows probing into the research development.

Collins, Onwuegbuzin and Sutton (2006) identified four rational expositions to sustain the use of mixed methods:

- enrichment of the participants
- fidelity of the instruments
- integrated treatment, which allows to determine fidelity in the operation
- enhancement of significance, since they increase and allow interpretation and use of the results.

Mixed methods are plural and complement each other, and they allow the researcher an eclectic approach. (Johnson and Onwuegbuzin 2004). The importance of their usage lies in the initial question of the research, and the mixture of methods may take place at the stage of data collection, at the stage of analysis, or both.

Johnson and Turner (2003) constructed what is known as "the fundamental principle of mixed methods" which requires the researchers to collect a great amount of data through different strategies, thus strengthening the research study, which implies that the resulting product will be superior to the one derived from the application of individual methods, i.e., by using only the quantitative or the qualitative method.

Concerning the strong points and weaknesses of mixed methods, Johnson and Onwuegbuzin (2004) have identified some strong points:

- the use of words and images may complement figures, just as figures may give precision to words and images,
- researchers may broaden and complete research questions,
- the strong points of one of the methods may compensate the other's shortcomings,
- access to stronger evidence in the conclusion and more thorough results,
- Eliciting of more complex knowledge, both in the fields of theory and practice, as a result of the use of mixed methods.

As regards weaknesses, the authors mention that:

- It requires team research work because it is difficult for a single researcher to use this approach,
- It is necessary that all the researchers should be acquainted with and master both methodologies,
- The use of this type of approach requires more time and is more expensive.

Morgan (1998, p. 364) pointed out two difficulties in the use of mixed methods, the first one is the fact that combining qualitative with quantitative generates a technical problem and a methodological challenge; and the second one implies taking into account the conflicts between the paradigms related to the origin of knowledge and the manner in which knowledge is produced.

These last decades have shown the advantage of using a combination of quantitative and qualitative methods and, in this sense, the opinions of the interviewed subjects across demographic variables, have facilitated the understanding of the situations in which these persons live. (Santos et al. 2007 in Tonon 2012).

Mixed methods are a form of research which implies much more than a mere collection of quantitative and qualitative data, it indicates that the data may be integrated, related, and/or mixed at some stage in the process. (Creswell et al. 2004, p. 7). The mix may occur both at the stage of data collection, at the stage of analysis, or both.

Nowadays, mixed research methods are considered an approach to knowledge, both in theory as well as in practice, from multiple points of view, perspectives, positions and outlooks (both qualitative and quantitative), with the purpose of probing more deeply into understanding and in the corroboration of the results, once they have been acknowledged as the third approach or paradigm of social research. (Johnson et al. 2007, p. 123).

4.4 Studies on Quality of Life Though Mixed Methods in the Applied Research in Quality of Life

During the period between 2006 (when the Journal appeared) and June 2013, *Applied Research in Quality of Life* has published four articles dedicated to the study of quality of life through mixed methods.

The first one, entitled *Kinship foster care from the perspective of quality of life: research on the satisfaction of the stakeholders*, Carmen Montserrat and Ferrán Casas, was published in September, 2006 and presents the results of a research with three main stakeholders: kinship caregivers, children who are placed in extended families and practitioners of the EAIAs (Childhood and Adolescence Interdisciplinary Care Teams). During the research the authors collected quantitative and qualitative data. For quantitative data collection they used a questionnaire for each stakeholder. The questionnaire included items about the personal characteristics of the respondents and items about their satisfaction according to the specific objectives.

All these items were measured through a five point Likert scale. For qualitative data collection they included: field observations throughout a year during the meetings of six existing caregivers support groups in the city of Barcelona (a total of 109 meetings were observed with the participation of 57 caregivers) and six caregivers focus group results with the participation of 40 caregivers.

The second article is entitled *Development of the measure of adaptation for pelvic symptoms (MAPS): the importance of incorporating the female patient's voice* by Patricia Wren, Nancy Janz, Linda Brubaker, Diane Borello-France, Catherine Bradley, Kathryn Burgio, Geoffrey Cundiff, Anne Weber, Jhon Wei, and it was published in September, 2006. The research aimed at extending women's health literature and expanding the registry of available measures to assess pelvic floor disorders. It was developed by following a specific sequence of steps utilizing quantitative and qualitative methods. First, a pilot study was carried out to explore the feasibility and utility of the first version of MAPS (measure of adaptation for pelvic symptoms) a questionnaire directed to 42 women with pelvic floor disorders who had already undergone surgery. Then, separate focus groups were conducted over a two week period with volunteer female clinic patients presented at Loyola University Medical Center outside Chicago.One of the conclusions of the authors was that the combination of quantitative pilot data and the descriptions of adaptations that women provided in the focus group enhanced the development and refinement of this new measure. (Wren et al. 2006, p. 249).

The third article, *A Mixed Methods approach to vulnerability and quality of life assessment of waste- picking in urban Nigeria* was written by Thaddeus Chidi Nzeadibe, Raymond Anyadike, Roseline Njoku-Tony. This paper identifies predominant social indicators relevant to the Aba scavengers, waste pickers' perceptions of quality of life expectations, and potential outcomes of meeting the quality of life expectations of waste pickers in the area. The authors approached the use of mixed methods by implementing different qualitative techniques such as focus group, oral statements, observation and interviews of key informants, and the later application of a questionnaire to 401 waste pickers. There were 2 sessions of focus groups, each composed of 6 subjects; 15 oral statements were taken; as well as 10 interviews of key informants (local authorities, residents, university professors, and ONG representatives). The article shows the need to apply quantitative and qualitative research methods in assessment of quality of life in the informal waste recycling system.

The fourth article written by Fahad Manee, Mohammed Nadar, Musaed Al-Naser, Khadijah Al-Ramezi, is *Quality of Life among Kuwaiti women living with chronic neuromuscular conditions.* The authors developed a mixed method design to describe the participants' perspectives of their functional impairments, level of activities and participation, and life satisfaction. They worked with a sample of 50 women with chronic neuromuscular conditions that live in the community, using the Barthel Index (Mahoney and Barthel 1965), the Role Check List Arabic (Yazdani et al. 2008) and the Arabic Version (Halabi 2006) of the Ferrans and Powers Quality of Life Index (Ferrans and Powers 1985). They completed the study with a phenomenological approach developing a semi-structured interview with five women selected from the sample of 50. The use of both methods allowed a better understanding and analysis of the research problem.

4.5 Final Reflection on the Integration of Methods in Quality of Life Research

Reflecting on the possibility of integrating methods in the quality of life research field first implies remembering that the quantitative and qualitative methods play specific roles in the research process and, in this respect we coincide with Strauss and Corbin (2002) when they point out that "each form of research must receive due recognition and must be valued for its specific contribution". (p. 36).

The path towards method integration began with triangulation in the validation of the accomplished research, and led to the use of mixed methods as a strategy to complement and expand the combination of the quantitative and qualitative methods. In this context we may state that integration, in terms of methodology, refers to the moment in the research process when the researcher articulates the collected data obtained through quantitative or qualitative means, and produces an integrated analysis of them. (Creswell et al. 2004, p. 10).

The complex social reality we live and work in should be approached and studied, not only through triangulation methods, but also by achieving their complementation and integration.

The decisions taken by every one of the researchers, according to their stock of acquired knowledge, technical training and philosophical-ideological outlook on the research subjects and the research itself, will (or will not) allow them to advance in the process towards methodological integration in the quality of life research field.

References

Bourdieu, P. (1990). *Sociología y cultura*. México: Editorial Grijalbo.

Bourdieu, P. (2008). Homo Academicus. Buenos Aires. Siglo XXI Editores Bryman, A. Integrating quantitative and qualitative research: How is it done? Qualitative Research 2006 SAGE Publications. London, 6(1), 97–113.

Campbell, D. T., & Fiske, D. W. (1959). Convergent and discriminant validation by the multitrait-multimethod matrix. *Psychological Bulletin, 56,* 81–105.

Creswell, J., Felters, M., & Ivankova, N. (2004). Designing a mix-methods study in primary care. *Annals of Family Medicine, 2*(1), 7–12.

Denzin, N. K. (1978). *The research act: A theoretical introduction to sociological methods*. New York: Praeger.

Greene, J. C., Caracelli, V. J., & Graham, W. F. (1989). Toward a conceptual framework for mixed-method evaluation designs. *Educational Evaluation and Policy Analysis, 11,* 255–274.

Jick, T. D. (1979). Mixing qualitative and quantitative methods: Triangulation in action. *Administrative Science Quarterly, 24,* 602–611.

Johnson, R. B., & Turner, L. (2003). Data collection strategies in mixed methods research. In A. Tashakkori & C. Teddlie (Eds.), *Handbook of mixed methods in social and behavioral research* (pp. 297–319). Thousand Oaks: Sage.
Johnson, R. B., & Onwuegbuzie, A. (2004). Mixed methods research: A research paradigm whose time has come author(s): R. source: Educational Researcher, Vol. 33, No. 7 (Oct., 2004), pp. 14–26 Published by: American Educational Research Association.
Johnson, R. B., Onwuegbuzie A., & Turner, L. (2007). Toward a definition of mixed methods research. *Journal of Mixed Methods Research, 1*, 112
Kelbe, U. (2001). Sociological explanations between micro and macro and the integration of qualitative and quantitative methods. *Forum Qualitative Social Research, 2*(1), 1–23
Lechner, N. (2002). *Las sombras del mañana. La dimensión subjetiva de la política*. Santiago de Chile: Lom Ediciones.
Montserrat, C., & Casas, F. (2006). Kinship foster care from the perspective of quality of life: research on the satisfaction of the stakeholders. *Applied Research in Quality of Life, 1*, 227-237.
Morgan, D. (1998). Practical strategies for combining qualitative and quantitative methods: applications to health research. *Qualitative Health Research, 8*, 362–376.
Morse, J. (1991). Approaches to qualitative-quantitative methodological triangulation. *Nursing Research, 40*, 120–123.
Morse, J., & Field, P. (1995). *Qualitative research methods health professionals*. Thousand Oaks: Sage.
Nzeadibe, T., Anyadike, R., & Njoku-Tony, R. (2012) A mixed Methods approach to vulnerability and quality of life assessment of waste picking in urban Nigeria. *Applied Research in Quality of Life, 7*, 351–370.
Santos, L., Martins, J., & Brito, P. (2007). Measuring subjective quality of life: a survey to Porto residents. *Applied Research in Quality of Life, 2*(1), 51–64
Sieber, S. D. (1973). The integration of fieldwork and survey methods. *American Journal of Sociology, 73*, 1335–1359.
Smith, H. (1975). *Strategies of social research. The methodological imagination*. Englewood Cliffs: Prentice Hall.
Strauss, A., & Corbin, J. (2002). *Bases de la investigación cualitativa. Técnicas y procedimientos para desarrollar la teoría fundamentada*. Colombia: Universidad de Antioquia.
Tonon, G. (2012). *Young people's quality of life and construction of citizenship. Series SpringerBriefs in Well-being and quality of life research*. Dordrecht: Springer.
Tonon, G. (2013) *La integración de métodos de investigación en Ciencias Sociales: la triangulación y los métodos mixtos. Documento de investigación* número 135. Serie Documentos de investigación del Colegio Mexiquense. Toluca- México. Mayo 2013
Wren, P., Janz, N., Brubaker, L., Borello-France, D., Bradley, C., Burgio, K., Cundiff, G., Weber, A., & Jhon Wei. (2006). Development of the measure of adaptation for pelvic symptoms: The importance of incorporating the female patient's voice. *Applied Research in Quality of Life, 1*, 239–251.

Part II
Cases: Qualitative studies in quality of life in Geography, Health, Communities, Youth, Childhood and Yoga in Labor Life

Chapter 5
Qualitative Methodologies in Geography, Contributions to the Study of Quality of Life

Claudia Mikkelsen and Josefina Di Nucci

Quality of Life lessens intimate space to a minimum
(Woman 66 years of age, San Eduardo de Chapadmalal, Partido de General Pueyrredon, 2008)

5.1 Introduction

Methodological reflection accompanied the evolution of geographic thinking from its roots, although since the second half of the twentieth century, it significantly deepened. Such Geography, conceived basically as a science of space, was presented as a discipline which epistemological and ontological basis was supported on logical positivism, and therefore provided predictive explanations through the creation of laws and quantitative theories.

It is relevant to point out that over the past decades, with the development of Humanistic Geographies (based on more subjective Philosophies) and Human Geographies of critical style, it was necessary to review the already developed qualitative methodological field, both because of the discipline itself and because of other disciplines related, especially Anthropology and Sociology.

Additionally, visions of geographical space as lived, felt, perceived and socially constructed space, have led geography to think about the need to know other individual and social aspects in its studies, for which it started opening up to qualitative and interpretative approaches.

C. Mikkelsen (✉)
Study Group on Population and Territory, Geography Department, Universidad Nacional de Mar del Plata, Buenos Aires, Argentina

Geographic Research Center, Geography, History and Social Sciences Institute, Universidad Nacional del Centro de la Provincia de Buenos Aires, Buenos Aires, Argentina
e-mail: claudiamikkelsen@gmail.com

J. Di Nucci
Geographic Research Center. Geography, History and Social Sciences Institute, Universidad Nacional del Centro de la Provincia de Buenos Aires. CONICET, Buenos Aires, Argentina
e-mail: josedinucci@yahoo.com

G. Tonon (ed.), *Qualitative Studies in Quality of Life*,
Social Indicators Research Series 55, DOI 10.1007/978-3-319-13779-7_5

From this viewpoint, the way to grasp the meanings and uses of space in Geography departs from a set of qualitative techniques that trace three possible paths: the observation of territory utilization or the spatiality of the acts; the use of documents, contents and images that account for this; and the study and analysis of the discourse of people that occupy and build the space.

The improvement observed in the set of theoretical and methodological contributions converged to give precision and complexity to the geographical investigations, which is an observable condition, for example, in the study of quality of life.

Although the concern of humanity about their quality of life is old, its scientific treatment is new; it was in the 1960's that it began to be included in various disciplines and in various fields: politics, economics, geography, planning, architecture, environmental studies, psychology, medicine, education, among others.

As Gómez and Sabeh (2007) point, it was not until the late 1970's that the concept achieved its own identity and is defined "as an integrative concept that involves all areas of life (multidimensional character) and refers to both objective conditions and subjective components" (p. 1)[1]. It is a multidisciplinary and multidimensional concept comprising the satisfaction of material and non-material needs, desires and ambitions of individuals, and which is culturally and territorially defined.

In this work we are interested in reflecting on the methodological background disciplines considered in the studies of quality of life, which were specially developed from the elaboration of objective indices. Nevertheless, we want to consider that by applying certain qualitative techniques (focus groups, analysis of documents and objects, and interviews, among others) it will be possible to perceive and search other aspects of quality of life, thus contributing to understand the well-being of the population and the complexity of its knowledge.

We seek to contribute to the generation of knowledge, reflecting on a theoretical-methodological approach, able to combine lifestyles, value systems, living conditions of individuals, and on the use and appropriation of space, both in an objective mode as well as in a symbolic evaluative manner.

The chapter is organized into four sections: along the first section it describes the theoretical background and qualitative existing contributions in Geography; in the second section it resumes the notion of quality of life, reflecting on its definition; the third part presents, in general terms, the methodological approaches applied to the study of quality of life; finally, in the fourth section, our proposal for a qualitative approach to the geographical study of quality of life is outlined, ending with a series of integrating reviews.

[1] Translation of the authors of the original, in Spanish language.

5.2 The Background and Qualitative Contributions to the Geographical Thought

The evolution of theoretical thinking in Geography was accompanied by changes in the methodological aspects. In Geography the positivist view dominated authoritatively for most of the twentieth century, however:

> from the dawn of Modern Geography, at the beginning of the nineteenth century, another current can be detected that, without denying the importance of reason, aims to build a different Geography, based on the "sensitive" reason, that is a reason that does not depreciate or forget the symbolic, emotional and human dimensions of life in its spatial dimension (Hiernaux 2008, p. 29)[2].

In the history of thought we find stimulating background to the use of what we today call qualitative methodologies or techniques, yet it was not until recent decades, with the development of the Humanistic Geographies of idealistic, phenomenological and existential styles, and Human Geographies of critical trends, that it became necessary to review the qualitative methodological field achieved by other disciplines, especially Anthropology and Sociology.

Among the historical antecedents we must highlight the use of methods of observation and the realization of field work from travelers and historians such as Herodotus and Marco Polo, which have been recognized as the geographers of those times.

In Greek Geography we find a literary heritage, under the trend of "qualitativist geography, the science of the places and the conception of the Earth, in which mythical, philosophical and metaphorical speech occupies a fundamental place" (Lévy 2006, p. 460)[3]. It is the geography of Strabo against that of Tolomeo, becoming the first in a literary center and the second in a scientific one.

On the other hand, and as a reference which exceeds Geography as a discipline, the classic study of Le Play (1855) must be mentioned, which profits from what today is called 'participant observation', known as "the study of the community technique", which comprises an exhaustive inventory of the conditions of daily life of working families in different cultural contexts.

It can be recognized in some classical authors like Ratzael, Schlüter, and Brhunes that in their geographical studies related to human nature and landscape there is the presence of culture as an explanatory factor. As Claval (1999) explains: "the way in which geographers apprehend culture at the beginning of the century is not different from the one adopted by ethnographers and anthropologists: ones and others were primarily interested in tools, artifacts, the fields, the habitat" (p. 51)[4]. With the contributions of Boas and Malinowski, on field work, participant observation and familiarity with other languages, ethnologists incorporate the way they say things, the interpretations made by individuals of history and reality.

---

[2] Translation of the authors of the original, in Spanish language.

[3] Translation of the authors of the original in Spanish language.

[4] Translation of the authors of the original, in Spanish language.

But as Claval (1999) states:

> Geographers are unaware of this evolution. Their field work keeps different: in the regions of the world where humanity is fragmentized and languages are numerous, their concern for comparison forbids them to limit to the analysis of a community: they do not always make the effort to master at least one indigenous language (p 51)[5].

It should be noted that Geography (as other disciplines related) in the positivist context of change from the nineteenth century to the twentieth, was concerned to find a place within the natural sciences, and therefore, to formulate general laws for natural as well as human phenomena.

During the 1920 and 1930 decades in the twentieth century, the "Chicago school" was developed in the United States, with substantial input for the further promotion of a Geography that we can call Pragmatic or Quantitative, notably urban geography, given the progress of ecological type models. However, this school also employed, in its research, participant observation, in-depth interviews, the development of life histories and the use of personal documents as a source of qualitative information.

However, it will only be with the Classical, Human and Regional French Geography from the beginning of the twentieth century that this discipline perceives the need to apply some methodologies which today we call qualitative. That Geography, following the basic guidelines of the functionalism of Durkheim, planned to study the influences of the environment on man within a defined geographical framework: the region, proposed to interpret these relationships based on distinctive life groupings, i.e. the way that "man has the environment humanized for their own objectives" (Vidal de la Blache 1931, p. 202, quoted by Gregory 1984, p. 143)[6]. Nevertheless, de la Blache avoided any internal tests over those genres of life, i.e. studying the interior links, only to develop empiricist typologies and not structural explanations (Gregory 1984). You can see in this Geography Bergson's philosophical methods, with their emphasis on the role of intuition to learn the particular truth of individual beings, in particular region and landscapes. Thus this geography was more inclined to "understand their own cognitive practice as an 'art' dedicated to descriptively 'evoke' the 'life'of the regions" (Gómez Mendoza et al. 1988, p. 68)[7].

Vidal de la Blache himself had referred to a "geography made from the feet", "as argument of the centrality of the direct work of the geographer with places, and the personal and experiential geographer contact with space through his field work" (Hiernaux 2008, p. 38)[8].

His concern for the detailed observation of the region and the genres of life, encouraged a methodology in which field work is a fundamental share. It also used more or less qualitative surveys, a wide range of documentary techniques, to expose

[5] Translation of the authors of the original in Spanish language.

[6] Translation of the authors of the original in Spanish language.

[7] Translation of the authors of the original in Spanish language.

[8] Translation of the authors of the original in Spanish language.

well-informed regional analysis and literary works to provide data that denote social facts of a region or descriptions of a landscape (Carreras 1998).

During the same years, but in the German School of Geography, we must mention Hettner, who proposed Geography as a chorological discipline of the Earth's surface, according to a regionalist concept of idealistic neo-kantian basis that tried to differentiate themselves from the positivist basis in vogue at that time.

Between Ist and IInd World Wars, another kind of Geography is originated, which attempted to differentiate itself even more radically from the scientific rationalist perspective and that intended to be a geography separated from science. This "artistic geography", as it announced itself, (linked to the German Bance and the Italian Gribaudi) claimed an artistic geography nature, because they conceived it as an aesthetic discipline, associated to emotional satisfaction, to subject's sensitivity (Ortega Valcarcel 2000). That Geography pretended to be art, literary endeavor, result of aesthetic and intuitive, individual and group perceptions and experiences of the landscape. It was also, known as the "geography of the landscape", since the personality of the region and of the landscape should be found through creative description.

Such geography laid the groundwork for development since about the 1920s, it was the Historical Geography, a distinctive product of British geography and the Cultural Geography born in a North American context.

Following two prominent British Geographers, East and Darby, a Classic Historical Geography was developed until the 1960s. East studied the European historical landscape and Darby turned his attention to Britain. Roughly, you could say they were looking for analysis over time of spatial-geographical type variations in landscape (García Ramón 1985). This geography had and still has an interesting methodological challenge since it took ancient documentary sources for his research, which was a customary qualitative technique among historians and archaeologists of the period, and this "geographic history" (as East named it) should use it. García Ramón (1985) puts forward that these geographers faced "primarily a problem of interpretation as it has to be able to infer the spatial dimension of its documentary sources without the possibility of checking on the ground" (p. 14)[9].

Cultural Geography was born in 1920 at Berkeley School's with Sauer and became a very accepted proposal in all North American geography. It proposed studies of a globalizing and integrative character, for which they drew nearer a human geography in which cultural aspects were the last phase of those studies. Cultural Geography seeks "understanding of the differentiation of the Earth according to the different cultures and the establishment of a critical system covering the phenomenology of landscape as a method of apprehending all the meaning and richness of these diversities" (García Ramón 1985, p. 16) [10]. It sought to find the "historicist character, which seeks to discover the genesis of landscapes, as a result of a process

[9] Translation of the authors of the original in Spanish language.

[10] Translation of the authors of the original in Spanish language.

of adaptation of social groups to their environment, in accordance with their cultural, ethnic, or social characteristics" (Sauer 2010)[11].

Sauer and his disciples put emphasis in field work and the relationship with other disciplines, particularly with Economy, Anthropology and History.

These classical geographers used different literary accounts as essential sources for their landscape descriptions but, apart from this, their own works had high quality and literary richness, accompanied by images of great beauty and precision (Carreras 1998).

It should be noted that Sauer at the end of his career introduced some very interesting questions in the context of logic quantitative domination in Geography. He says:

> beyond all that can be transmitted through instruction and can be mastered using the techniques, it is the domain of individual perception and interpretation, the art of geography. Really good regional geography is finely figurative art, and creative art is not constrained by the guideline or method (…). While field work is performed, more than a letter is written that gives life and illustrates the study, but there is no trace of it in the final report (Sauer 1985, pp. 52–53)[12].

Middle twentieth century found Geography again involved in the search for "objectivity" through the accurate use of quantitative techniques and methodologies, which have been widely developed in different areas of geographical interest until now. It was precisely this geographical neo-positivism which led many geographers to look for other alternatives; on the one hand, a broad humanistic perspective, and on the other hand, the neo-Marxist historical materialistic radical approach (Unwin 1995).

Studies on the development of critical-radical-Marxist Geography are abundant, and even more the different authors of that tendency who have written works central to the development of that theoretical proposal.

In a simple and general way we can declare that this perspective focused, from the beginning, at the end of the 1960s, on studying reality from the interrelationship between social processes (in the broad sense of the term that includes what is economic, political, cultural, etc.) and the processes of space, being the analysis and discussion of the social processes previous to that of the space. The thematic studies established in Economical, Urban, Historical, and Cultural Geography, among others, were central to this perspective.

Critical Geography made fundamental contributions to Geography as a social discipline in terms of: the vision of the space as a social product; the linking of Geography with Philosophy and other disciplines related to a global Social Theory; the incorporation of new focuses of attention more committed to reality; and the progress in conceptual theoretical formulations, among others. However, neither the discussions nor the methodological contributions, particularly qualitative, have been central, as developed from this vision of Geography.

---

[11] Translation of the authors of the original in Spanish language.

[12] Translation of the authors of the original in Spanish language.

It is Humanistic Geographies, in their theoretical, philosophical and thematic explorations, which have advocated a methodologically renewed development for our discipline, either by examining their own qualitative disciplinary bases, or by resorting to advances in other related disciplines with longest tradition on the subject.

Humanistic Geography, based on philosophical approaches of Humanism, denounces the primacy of reason and science, as equivalent concepts, and the existence of a scientific and rational pattern as a validity standard of knowledge (Unwin 1995). The term Humanistic Geography was definitively introduced in 1978 with the publication of the book Humanistic Geography of Ley and Samuels, considered the forerunner classical work of this geography. The exclusive entitlement of rational or scientific knowledge is there criticized; the individual and his personal experience being vindicated instead.

Several papers have studied the theoretical, conceptual and thematic contributions to this perspective (García Ramón 1985; Unwin 1995; García Ballesteros 1998; Gregory 1984; among others).

Phenomenology is considered a fundamental instrument in Humanistic Geography, vindicating the everyday experience of the subjects as a essential feature to the understanding of the place of human beings in the world.

Ultimately, it is to overcome the dichotomy between objectivity and subjectivity. If we add some features of Existentialism to this, which embrace being and existing, a Geography not only focused on the individual and the fragmentary will be obtained. All this is framed in a strongly idealistic conceptual context. Thus Guelke (1985) states that:

> the nucleus of the idealistic position requires a method of interpretation, quite different from the one that is suited to the non-rational human and non-human phenomena (…). The idealistic sustains that the rational action is explained when thoughts behind it are understood (p. 195–196)[13].

Tuan (1985) poses that Humanism in Geography should reflect "on the geographical phenomena with the purpose of achieving better understanding of the man and his condition" (p. 143)[14], because of which he differentiates from the traditional geographical view by stating that:

> scientific approaches to the study of man tend to minimize the role of awareness and human knowledge. Humanistic Geography, on the contrary, is committed specifically to understand how activities and geographic phenomena reveal the quality of human awareness (Tuan 1985, p 146)[15].

This Geography postulates the need to seek the understanding of phenomena to be studied, therefore far from minimizing the role of consciousness and human knowledge, it tries to understand specifically how activities and geographic phenomena reveal the quality of human consciousness (García Ballesteros 1998).

---

[13] Translation of the authors of the original in Portughese language.

[14] Translation of the authors of the original in Portughese language.

[15] Translation of the authors of the original in Portughese language.

Links between individuals and the material environment become central, once expressed in the definition of site. The place is unique and complex, being a special set, characterized by being rooted in the past and develop towards the future (Tuan 1985). The place takes on a value that results from the perception of its own residents and the meaning they attribute to it; in addition, it represents the embodiment of the experiences and aspirations of the people. The place as a physical entity, such as a point or an area, as a simple objective, acquires a subjective dimension, becomes an individual image taking into account aspects such as its emotional, aesthetic and symbolic charge. A fundamental work that reflects this model, where subjective experience is central in the everyday space is Tuan's (1974) "Topofhilia". It refers to a set of affective and emotional relationships that man, through his five senses, keeps with a place.

This geography reflects on spaces linked to the existence of each individual, to his specific experiences, his personal relationship with the environment, to the perception he has of it, according to cultural and personal circumstances.

They argue that there is no unique world of objective character, but different worlds in relation to pluralities of attitudes, feelings, and intentions of individuals. So it is central the notion of an undergone world, that can be defined as the amalgam of facts and values encompassed by the everyday personal experience. In the words of one of the leading exponents of the phenomenology in Humanistic Geography:

> for phenomenology, the world is the context within which principles are revealed (…). It is anchored in the past and addressed to the future; it is a shared horizon, although each individual can build it in a unique personal manner. Once conscious of the world as lived through personal experience, an individual should recognize the shared horizons of the world of other people and of society as a whole (Buttimer 1985, p. 172)[16].

This proposal is supported by a vision of geographical space as subjective space, i.e. the scope of lived experiences, of subjective experience. The space is considered a mental reality subject to the particular perception of each individual, product of experience and individual conscience. Although the concept of space as social product includes the society as producer of that space, from the subjective point of view of the discipline it is argued that it is not including the individual who designed it; "the subject that made the space distorted in the geographical analysis by the preeminence of the space produced. When the subject is included, it is usually as an attribute of space" (Lindón 2008, p. 6)[17]. In other words, this concept spreads the idea of geographical space to non-material dimensions that have always been the classic components, and includes the notion of space as experience (Tuan 2007).

Thus, Lindón (2008) argues:

> finding a midpoint that neither puts aside the materiality of space for the sake of a theory exclusively subjective or idealistic, nor forgets everything immaterial with which subjects give sense to space (to space forms), considering that building it socially precisely implies doing it physically and also giving it sense (p. 7)[18].

---

[16] Translation of the authors of the original in Portughese language.

[17] Translation of the authors of the original in Spanish language.

[18] Translation of the authors of the original in Spanish language.

This involved new approaches and spheres of interest especially devoted to the conception of place as a space for individual and collective experience, lived space linked to the individual and subjective experiences, i.e. a particular relationship with the environment and with the pursuit of symbolic dimensions of space. Although concepts of place and landscape were the most influenced by Humanistic Geography, we must also mention the work of Frémont (1976), who studied the region as lived space.

A Humanistic Geography,

> open to the study of the arrangement of meanings, exploring them in relation to places and to practices people set up in each place (…) therefore the key trilogy to decode in geographic qualitative research is "spatial practices, spatial forms and significance of places" (Lindón 2008, p. 12–13)[19].

Thus Geography goes into the meanings of places, and then the discipline challenge is to be able to "read" the meanings materialized in practices.

These new visions involved changes in the discipline as a whole, and we want to especially emphasize that, in actual Cultural Geography, it is possible to find extensive conceptual and thematic discussions with interesting approaches to a methodological renewal in Geography. Cultural Geography takes into account "the committed and interdisciplinary character of the production of knowledge, the interaction of culture with economic and political domains, and the critical connection between space and culture" (Clua and Zusman 2002, p. 105)[20]. In this sense Claval (2011) points out that, more than being a sub-area within Geography, it is a type of approach, since facing different themes or classical problems of Geography, for example rural, economic and political Geography, among others, it brings about new perspectives and cultural aspects for their studies.

It is worth emphasizing the type of qualitative inquiry widely used in Geography, influenced by the proposal of Geertz (1973), based on descriptions in depth that he calls thick description; the ethnologist gives the word to observed persons and cares for their speeches and reactions in various circumstances (Claval 1999).

The speech and language of the subjects become important taken from their own narratives, images, creative features, directing to the way in which people speak about the world or speak the world (Claval 1999).

In these humanistic and cultural proposals of Geography, "the novel sometimes becomes a document: novelists subtle intuition helps us feel the place through the eyes of their characters and across their emotions" (Claval 1999, p. 52)[21, 22].

There is a renewed Cultural Geography, Zusman and Haesbaert (2011) distinguish between: the cultural Geography of the French tradition, from contributions of the Vidal de la Blache School, and the recovery of reflections on Existentialism based on Eric Dardel, who have diversified their subjects and objects of interest

---

[19] Translation of the authors of the original in Spanish language.

[20] Translation of the authors of the original in Spanish language.

[21] To read about the connection between Geography and Literature, we propose to refer to the article by Bertrand (2006).

[22] Translation of the authors of the original in Spanish language.

towards representations, myths, landscapes, passions and people's likes, discourses of different cultures and an interest in literary sources, among others (Claval 1999). Secondly, the new Cultural Geographies displayed in the Anglo-Saxon world (Duncan 1990; Cosgrove 2002) where Marxist and phenomenological positions live with different post-structuralist perspectives that try to understand the symbolic interpretation that groups and social classes give to the environment, the aesthetic or ideological justifications they propose and the impact of representations about collective life (Claval 1999); furthermore they have recently incorporated the relationship between the body, the emotions and the environment to the analysis (Lorimer 2007). Thirdly, Zusman and Haesbaert (2011) highlight the contributions of Latin American works on Cultural Geography (Barbosa 1999; Carney 2007; Corrêa 2011; Rosendahl 2011) who:

> Wished to move away from the Eurocentric views and understand the peculiarities of the subcontinent from their own history and the syncretism of their popular cultures. Second, we remark the interest in building a critical perspective of global processes and thinking culture as an element of social transformation (p. 10)[23].

These new objectives, arguments, views, can only be apprehended with qualitative methodologies which comprise getting to understand meanings, values, goals and intentions of the subjects, and their inquiry in relation to the places and practices that people display in each location, becoming central to two issues: geographic language and communication.

As indicated by Lindón (2008), it is necessary that Geography be "closer to hermeneutics, within the connotation of the interpretation of the other, or more precisely, of the interpretation of interpretations of the other" (p. 9)[24], causing another type of approach to the subject of study, to "otherness". Thus the perspective of "experiential" field developed by the geographer Rowles (1978) is a proposal of this type[25].

Experiential field work, clearly humanist biased, carries with it the essence of qualitative approaches in the Social Sciences. It is the importance of getting closer to the other, to allow for empathy, even though the creation of these bonds can prolong the time needed for field work (Lindón 2008, p. 10)[26].

The set of theoretical and methodological contributions so far raised converge to give precision and complexity to geographical investigations, which is an observable condition, for example, in the study of quality of life.

---

[23] Translation of the authors of the original in Spanish language.

[24] Translation of the authors of the original in Spanish language.

[25] To go deeper into field work in Geography we suggest reading Katz (1994); Pedone (2000) and Zusman (2011).

[26] Translation of the authors of the original in Spanish language.

5.3 Defining Quality of life From a Geographical Perspective

Studies on quality of life are neither new nor recent in Geography as they are in other related disciplines which worried about the methodologies related to the well-being of man. Although Geography has had much to say about these studies, we must state that quality of life is a multidisciplinary and multidimensional category (without existing agreement with respect to the number and definition of the dimensions and domains), therefore it is transversal in its contribution to the construction of this knowledge.

In the beginning of the diversity of definitions is the conceptual positioning of the researcher, the heterogeneity of contexts in which the concept is used, the measures to be used, the purpose of the evaluation and the subject who performs the assessment (Albert and Logsdon 2000, cited by Fernandez Mayoralas et al. 2005, p. 122)[27].

Well, as we have pointed out in the previous section, the Chicago School has been a central source of inspiration for Social Sciences and there we can find fundamental quantitative and qualitative methodological background for Geography. Likewise, it was in that school that the academic interest in quality of life around the movement of social indicators started. These studies emerged as a critique of consumption, to the society of opulence, to the need of prioritizing quality over quantity and superfluous consumption in the societies of the developed countries "where despite high levels of comfort, symptoms of social breakdown, loss of the sense of life, intensification of suicide, violence, drug addiction, etc, were increasing" (Palomino and López 2000, p. 33)[28].

Since the 1940s several researchers from different social disciplines have undertaken the work of developing research tools that could effectively assess the ability of Nations to meet the basic needs of their population (Estes, 1989). Thus "all evaluation of human well-being approaches tried to combined different indicators of social welfare into composite indicators, which could be used for international comparative analysis" (Estes 1989, p. 131)[29].

In that decade such investigations addressed the strictly quantitative and economic study of the development of the countries, using objective indicators such as the gross domestic product (GDP), "however, this was not successful at the time of measuring social aspects, since it was linked to monetary values and did not allow assessment of behavior of the determining social variables on the welfare of populations" (Estes 1989, quoted by Camargo Mora 1999, p. 251)[30]. Tonon (2008) indicates that it was the English Economist Pigou who first used the term "quality

[27] Translation of the authors of the original in Spanish language.

[28] Translation of the authors of the original in Spanish language.

[29] Translation of the authors of the original in Spanish language.

[30] Translation of the authors of the original in Spanish language.

of life" referring to the possibility of quantifying social services or social costs of Governments' decisions to calculate the net social product.

In the 1950s, and following the economistic view of these studies on the development of Nations, the concept "standard of living" was incorporated, a notion coming from Economy, referred to aspects of monetary nature which support the idea of consumption of goods and services, purchasing power becoming a mechanism allowing the achievement of personal development. The standard of living allows for distinction of a set of individuals deprived of those who have a series of material possessions and capabilities to acquire them, differentiating, in this sense, social classes. Critics and limitations to this conception have been pointed out. Espinosa (2000) argues that what is known as luxury and abundance does not necessarily mean having the optimum in reference to quality of life, and that these aspects will only provide social status.

It was from the 1960s since another perspective in the studies of quality of life began to be included, both in different disciplines and in various fields, such as politics, economics, geography, planning, architecture, environmental studies, psychology, medicine, education, among others. The central objective was to do research that went beyond the importance and centrality that had been previously given to the economic growth and development, and to include topics related to the well-being of societies.

In this way, the term quality of life corresponds to the idea, conception and implementation of the Welfare State, developed from the second post-war period, mainly in the core countries. It should be noted that the notion of welfare, according to Camargo Mora (1999), presents two different views throughout the twentieth century. At first, it is identified from a mainly quantitative perspective associated with the level that individuals acquire from the economic and social points of view, measured on the basis of education, nutrition, employment accessibility, health, among others. Until the 1970s this utilitarian approach whereby what is central is to maximize the well-being of the population prevailed, being known as welfare. In this sense, welfare is similar to the idea of living conditions and standard of living, while its arrival is associated with the implementation of economic and social policies which make sustainable consumption of goods and services most relevant as the engine of the economy.

At a second instance, welfare reaches a more humanistic meaning (in the sense of well-being), beginning with Sen (Sen 1996; Sen and Nussbaum 2001) postulates about human development and quality of life. Welfare is interpreted in a broader sense, associated with capacities, opportunities and advantages of individuals. This approach, known as the capabilities one, dares overcome the perspective of basic needs, proposing as essential the discussion about the person and his abilities, and not about the goods he should attain. Sen (Sen 1996; Sen and Nussbaum 2001) argues that a set of capabilities should not be assessed in accordance with actual achievements (welfare achievements), but according to the set of real opportunities (freedom to achieve well-being). In this way, the discussion focuses not only in knowing what a person achieves but also what the options were, among which that person had to choose. To include in the studies of quality of life the perspective of capabilities and skills of the subjects implies a change of approach or perspective given that:

> It is not the same to assess the achievements made by individuals as a reflection of the access that they have to the use or consumption of any good or service, than as through the capacities that they have to apply or use those goods or services specifically, in order to meet their needs (Camargo Mora 1999, p. 254)[31].

Having said that, to trace the central background in Geography, as regards the studies of quality of life, we must go back to the 1970s, in the context of the critical-radical Geography, which began to worry about the relevant social issues of the time. As pointed out in previous attempts by Smith (1980)

> to widen the field of interest of the human geographer, we must include suggestions for possible uses of the index of the standard of living in regional delimitation (Lewis 1968) and the efforts of Gould (1969) to associate the spatial preference with a "social welfare indicator" (p. 26)[32].

Themes of poverty, crime, black ghettos, health care and issues began to be developed, which related Geography with what Knox and Smith called Geography of Well-being. The work of Smith (1980) must be highlighted, entitled 'Human Geography a Welfare Approach', being him the same Smith who first talked about Radical Geography, and proclaimed it as "geography corresponding with the end of the continuous growth experienced by the real standard of living in the postwar period, and with a time in which the issues about the distribution of wealth became urgent" (Smith 1980, p. 27)[33].

Smith (1980) proposes a new way of structuring Human Geography around welfare, considering that this subject is integrative and brings together the contributions of the geographical currents of the previous 20 years (quantitative geography and radical geography, especially), to constitute a social science for the benefit of the age.

For Smith (1980), Human Geography should be defined as "the study of "who gets what, where and how"" (p. 30)[34], and this is the meaning of the question of social welfare in a spatial context. It is significant to remark that the author uses the term social welfare including "all things through which human satisfaction (positive or negative) is obtained, and also their distribution within society" (Smith 1980, p. 32)[35].

It is particularly interesting the distinction that this author makes when he uses the terms quality of life or social welfare, the first being "to describe the state of the population ranging from a set of territories" and the second to refer "not only to what but also who gets this what and where he gets it" (Smith 1980, p. 32)[36]. Then,

[31] Translation of the authors of the original in Spanish language.

[32] Translation of the authors of the original in Spanish language.

[33] Translation of the authors of the original in Spanish language.

[34] Translation of the authors of the original in Spanish language.

[35] Translation of the authors of the original in Spanish language.

[36] Translation of the authors of the original in Spanish language.

he holds that the quantity and quality of goods consumed and supported disadvantages are the result of the system of production and distribution. García Ramón (1985) summarizes this proposal of Human Geography, asserting that:

> the productive system must take decisions about the type of goods produced, its quantity as well as the techniques used to produce them, and the location of the production process. Each of these dimensions of the production system generates goods but also troubles, because of its effects over both the differential availability of goods and the geographically distinguished external effects (p. 144)[37].

It is this way, considering that the production not only engenders division of work and differences in levels of development, i.e. geographical inequality implications, but also that it is a process that contributes to the increase or decrease of human well-being in each of its phases.

Evidently, Geography of well-being is a theoretical discipline essential to current studies on quality of life. Caution must be taken that, from a more objective point of view, closer to Quantitative Geography or its latest variety, the Automated Geography (Buzai and Baxendale 2006), the study of quality of life can be condensed in the construction of macro-variables which bring together diverse indicators. Through mapping of elaborated groupings, it is possible to detect areas or regions formed by spatial units in which data have a fairly homogeneous inner distribution.

In this respect, the contributions of Velázquez (2001) in Argentina should be mentioned, having defined quality of life as "a measure of achievement with respect to an established optimal level, taking into account socio-economic and environmental dimensions that are dependent on the scale of values prevailing in society, and which vary according to the expectations of historical progress" (p. 15)[38]. The concept quality of life would make it possible to accomplish convergence between quantitative analysis and geographical interpretation of the social processes (Boroni et al. 2005).

Questions made by Bailly (1998) to studies based on objective indicators become interesting from a more humanistic attitude of Geography. They can be summarized in three points: (a) is it possible to use the same dimensions and variables in different socio-spatial contexts?; (b) statistical series in general fail to respond to the data requirements to explain problems in micro-geographical ratios; finally, (c) of all the indicators with data availability, which one should we choose?. In this way this author claims that:

> not every indicator can be objective, since it must reveal the internal subjective framework on which all behaviors stand. The environment reveals to whoever studies it through observation or interpretation. Both methods are very important, allowing you to seize the emphatic relationship environment-subject and, therefore, the way in which the environment is perceived and lived (Bailly 1998, p. 49)[39].

[37] Translation of the authors of the original in Spanish language.

[38] Translation of the authors of the original in Spanish language.

[39] Translation of the authors of the original in Spanish language.

In relation to this outlook, and trying to give greater prominence to the subjective components of quality of life, Liberali and Massa (1986) argued that it includes not only material or economic needs, but it also comprises what makes men happy (agreeing with Nuvolati 2002, 2006). There appears affection and leisure as subjective components of quality of life.

To conclude this section, we synthesize some central ideas about the concept of quality of life.

Abaleron (1999) considered that:

> quality of life in a territory is the degree of excellence that a given society, precisely located in a particular time and a specific geographical space, offers in the supply of goods and services, in order to satisfy certain range of human needs for all its members, and the corresponding level of individual and group satisfaction or dissatisfaction, according to the perception held on that offer, accessibility and use, by the population involved (p. 8)[40].

Therefore it is not a universal category, but it is cultural and territorially defined.

UNESCO defines quality of life as:

> the satisfaction of needs which represent the requirements that must be fulfilled to make a person physically and psychosocially healthy. The components of quality of life and the degree of well-being of people are determined by the perception of the relationship between the desired satisfiers (which meet human needs) and those actually obtained. Implicit is the adaptation between the characteristics of the reality that surrounds them and the expectations, capabilities and needs of individuals, such as they and their social group perceive them (Pérez Maldonado 2002, p. 22)[41].

It is interesting to reflect here on the definition of quality of life of the Dictionary of Human Geography of Johnston et al. (1987):

> Quality of life: psychological and individual aspects of social welfare. It reflects a frame of mind that depends on the socio-economic position and the individual characteristics. Therefore the conception of what a high life quality is will be based on the unchallenged conformity with the existing state of things. In a more general sense, quality of life can be evaluated with respect to environmental factors such as pollution, energy and nutrition. In this way, it can be used as a general term to compare the prevailing situation in different Nations (p. 65)[42].

Therefore, quality of life concerns both satisfaction of material needs as well as subjective and symbolic desires of the people. This sort of satisfaction is not preferring one over the other, meeting them separately or in steps, as they are strongly linked and associated (Palomino and López 2000), the spatial dimension being fundamental to be taken into account. The options present in the territory are not the same for all subjects; the geographical space offers potential of uneven value, by which there are disputes and competitions (Santos 2000). Feu (2005) warns that the space is unequally provided with infrastructure, and that it conditions the individual or group access to essential services.

---

[40] Translation of the authors of the original in Spanish language.

[41] Translation of the authors of the original in Spanish language.

[42] Translation of the authors of the original in Spanish language.

It should be noted, matching what Alguacil Gómez (2001) points out, that quality of life is at the same time synthesis and expansion between the individual and the collective subject, between personal and objective character, between small scale or great scale social analysis, circumstances that make it possible to overcome the traditional breakdown between scientific technical and scientific humanistic culture.

5.4 How do We Study Quality of Life? Objectivist Traditions and Subjectivist Potentials

Studies on quality of life, based on the proposal of the Geography of Welfare, have traditionally built indexes held on secondary data coming from various statistical sources, official and unofficial, i.e. from the generation of quantitative indicators. Objective quality of life refers to how individual life is evaluated by the outside world, influenced by the culture in which population resides, and it is usually based on social indicators. As Diner and Suh (1997) express, the trademark of social indicators is that they are based on quantitative criteria, statistics and not on subjective perceptions of individuals, according to their social environment.

Objective questions are transformed into a search of a series of goods and services provided by the constructed environment to meet the so-called basic needs (housing, education, health and work). In this sense, objective quality of life discloses a person's ability to adapt to the values of a culture, but tells us little about the life of that person. In this regard, if we try that the quality of life consider the appreciation and understanding of individuals and societies, it is here where a necessary subjective nature of the concept appears, which implies both interpersonal and inter social strata relationships. As Abaleron expresses (1999), the qualitative posture, non-measurable, subjective…

> emphasizes the internal environment of people, their vision of the world, their beliefs, their values, aspirations and desires, culminating in exclusively perceptive aspects of preference or disapproval, happiness or unhappiness, satisfaction or dissatisfaction, pain or pleasure to different dimensions of life, in general, and of those goods and services located in the geographical area in particula (pp. 4–5)[43].

According to Gallopin (2006), "qualitative indicators may be preferable to quantitative indicators in at least three situations: when there is no availability of quantitative information; when the attribute of interest is inherently non measureable (such as it happens with many variables of cultural or political nature); and when cost considerations become determinant" (p. 16)[44].

In this way, it is possible to work with micro geographic scales of primary data gathering, which allow a direct approach to the subjects and their evaluations with respect to quality of life. Subjective well-being means to contemplate subjective

[43] Translation of the authors of the original in Spanish language.

[44] Translation of the authors of the original in Spanish language.

experience of life that persons have, thus to understand the quality of the experiences of individuals. It is convenient to examine directly how a person feels about his life in the context where it is developed (Diner and Suh 1997).

In this sense, the subjective quality of life is what is good in life for each individual. The quality of existential life means that one's life is good on a deeper level. It assumes that the individual has a more intense nature that deserves to be respected.

In recent years, the number of investigations which include subjectivity in the study of quality of life, focusing on the assessment of life satisfaction made by the same subjects has increased. When referring to life satisfaction this is valued globally (satisfaction with our lives as a whole) or for particular domains, i.e. family, education, work, health, friendship, income, among others, "these conditions, in particular those enabling human behavior as soon as they meet requirements, are called satisfiers (…)" (Abaleron 1999, p. 7)[45]. The possibility and availability of satisfiers will allow to cover the requirements of individuals and communities, thus "the balance between the desired satisfiers and those actually obtained will indicate the degree of satisfaction (or dissatisfaction) of each component of necessity involved in the quality of life concept" (Leva 2005, p. 34)[46]. As Schalock & Verdugo Alonso claim "satisfaction has been used to examine the subjective nature of the quality of life, usually asking people their degree of satisfaction with various aspects of their lives" (2006, p. 34)[47].

As Vega Rapun and Lamote de Grignon Pérez (2008) hold, that the

> objective and subjective indicators of wellbeing are partly interrelated, insofar as the objective indicators refer to the coverage of basic needs, it is expected that the objective and subjective indicators have a close connection. However, as countries develop and income is intended to cover fewer basic needs, less clear the relationship between both. It is precisely for this reason that subjective indicators of well-being have gained importance in recent years (p. 13)[48].

Subjective measurements have become a complement of objective indicators where assessment surveys of different domains characteristic of quality of life of subjects try to find the perceptions that individuals have with respect to their lives, and to their lives in places of residence (Matijasevic et al. 2010). The subjective approach is specifically designed to collect primary data at a disaggregated level into microranges (districts, cities, towns) or at the level of the same subjects, using social surveys, where attention is focused on the behavior of the population and in the evaluations they make with respect to their quality of life (Marans and Stimson 2011). It is possible to "go directly to the opinion of individuals to know what they think about the most important aspects of their lives, such as their health, their education, their jobs and their homes, and how they perceive the main aspects of public policies and the social and economic environment where they live" (Lora 2008, p. 5)[49].

---

[45] Translation of the authors of the original in Spanish language.

[46] Translation of the authors of the original in Spanish language.

[47] Translation of the authors of the original in Spanish language.

[48] Translation of the authors of the original in Spanish language.

[49] Translation of the authors of the original in Spanish language.

From this view, Cerda and Vera (2008) pose that any social indicator is the result of a question made to social reality, and that each question initiates from a certain implicit or explicit tendency, or a hypothesis, or a problem. When planning a project of social indicators, researchers make theirs and explicit, the proposal by Smith (1980), which can be considered as the paradigm of social welfare: "who gets what, where and how". As we have already explained, each one of the words: "who", "what", "where" and "how" raises its own set of dimensions.

> Empirical studies carried out seem to indicate that the seven major factors affecting the subjective well-being are (Layar 2005a): family relationships, finances, work, community and friends, health, personal freedom, personal value (the first five shown in order of significance) (Ansa Eceiza 2008, p. 22)[50].

In this sense, what was customary in the creation of information related to the subjective assessments of individuals and of communities or places with respect to their quality of life, was to apply more or less closed questionnaires, from which people are consulted about how they evaluate various aspects of their lives, those questions presented as domains or dimensions of quality of life. Roughly, those questions are linked to levels of satisfaction and are held with closed or fan-like answers, being the Likert scale shown as one of the more exploited options (McCrea et al. 2011a, b; Marans and Kweon 2011; Lucero et al. 2008a; Sirgy et al. 2006), placing 7 points in the measurement of satisfaction, which range from completely satisfied to fully unsatisfied.

As established by Lora (2008), one of the pioneering works in terms of the measurement of the quality of life considering the subjectivity of the persons was the "comparative welfare study" for Scandinavia, directed by Allardt. In this work, the relieved criteria were: income, housing, political support, social relations, being unique, doing interesting things, health, education, and satisfaction with life.

These indicators allow distinguishing between "having", "loving" and "being", considered as the three basic dimensions of well-being based on humanistic psychology then in fashion (Lora 2008).

"A scale of measurement of the quality of life recognized in the world of psychology is the proposal by Cummins (1997), that considers quality of life as an aggregate of objective and subjective components" (Lora 2008, p. 10)[51]. Each component includes seven aspects:

- Material well-being; measured by income, quality of dwellings and possessions.
- Health: measured by the number of disabilities and medications.
- Productivity: measured by the work, education and leisure activities.
- Privacy: contacts with close friends, availability of support.
- Security: perceived at home, sleep quality, safety concerns.
- Place in the community: social activities, responsibilities, being requested for advice.
- Emotional well-being: opportunity to have/ do things desired, enjoying life.

---

[50] Translation of the authors of the original in Spanish language.

[51] Translation of the authors of the original in Spanish language.

It is also likely to involve the Index of Satisfaction with Life, created by White of the University of Leicester, a social psychologist who measures satisfaction with life in a subjective way, or the Happy Planet Index, conducted by the New Economics Foundation, which includes 178 Nations, designed to measure development according to life expectancy, the subjective perception of happiness and the ecological footprint.

As Lora (2008) designates an:

> underlined effort of measuring progress of societies is that promoted by Estes, University of Pennsylvania, by means of the Weighted Index of Social Progress (WISP), covering 163 countries. The WISP includes 40 objective indicators that comprise 10 sub-indices on the following components of quality of life: education, health, status of women in society, defense efforts, economy, demography, environment, social chaos, cultural diversity and efforts in social welfare programs (p. 10)[52].

You could build a long and rich list of valuable contributions in terms of the measurement that combines objective and subjective aspects, at various scales (neighborhoods, cities, metropolitan areas and countries), however it must be indicated that, in most of these works, there is a quantitative analysis of the information achieved, i.e. the exercised operationalization is statistical in nature, for example, establishing percentage, offsets and counts of how many subjects of the prospected samples say they are more or less satisfied with their lives, given that broadly, in an overall analysis of data created through the surveys, they are addressed from statistical packages.

Therefore, while there is today some agreement with regard to dealing with the study of quality of life from the objective and the subjective sides, where the objective refers to social welfare, the material environment, the constructed environment; and the subjective or psychosocial refers to satisfaction with life, analyzed on the basis of the valuations of their lives that the same subjects perform (Tonon 2005), we consider necessary to reflect on the qualitative analysis of data obtained directly from the everyday experiences of subjects and their actions in a lived space.

Complementarity between objectivity and subjectivity becomes increasingly a possibility, in this way, quantifiable measurable outcomes that are obtained through objective criteria can be used to judge the conditions of a society and allow obtaining a first approximation to reduction or case study. This could then be enhanced through a qualitative approach to the study of quality of life. As noted in Diner and Suh (1997), the parallel use of objective and subjective indicators is important from methodology, since both provide alternative views of quality of life, breaking thus the opposition of purely quantitative or qualitative approaches, since each of them captures a different aspect of the welfare of society. As established by Díaz (1985):

> Obviously the opinion of the people is essential to be able to evaluate the level of needs satisfaction. For this purpose, the best way to identify and prioritize needs consists of using various methods and different categories of needs (p. 59)[53].

[52] Translation of the authors of the original in Spanish language.

[53] Translation of the authors of the original in Spanish language.

On this path of analysis, Chacon (1998) establishes that the most important problem at present is the need for further studies on a theoretical and methodological approach able to combine lifestyles, value systems and living conditions of individuals in an objective and perceptive way, where self-assessment, or self-definition, processes of welfare are respected.

We uphold with Lindón (2008) that the way to capture meanings and spatial practices in Geography is from a set of techniques that spot us three possible paths: the observation of practices and its spatiality; the use of content and images that account for such practices; and the study and analysis of discourses of the subjects who carry out these practices.

5.5 Quality of Life and Everyday Space: A Qualitative Proposal

We start from the concept of quality of life as:

> perceptions, aspirations, needs, satisfaction and social representations that members of any social grouping experience in relation to their environment, and the social dynamics into which they are submerged, including the services that are offered to them and the social interventions to which they are eligible and which come from social policies (Ferran Casas 1996, quoted by Tonon 2010 p. 26)[54].

It is a concept that involves the undergone experiences of the subjects in everyday space, their possibility of access to goods, services and the use of the territory. It involves multiple dimensions considered fundamental in the experiences of the subjects in their lived, felt, and perceived space. Accordingly, it should be pursued to jointly consider the material environment, i.e. the created environment, the territory and the psychosocial environment; thus bringing together, the study of living conditions (objective aspect) and the valuations, images, and perceptions of satisfaction with life that subjects have (subjective aspect) (Tonon 2010). In Geography, this conception of quality of life leads us to think in socially constructed space in which the material and non-material or symbolic dimensions are articulated from the perspective of spatial experiences of the subjects (Lindón 2008).

Therefore, to consider quality of life as a sensitizing notion, a social construct (Verdugo et al. 2006) takes us to reflect on the possibility of including the valuations of subjects from new questions and techniques. We are not underestimating the major achievements from the construction of objective social indicators, but it is the challenge of managing a different proximity with the object of study.

The qualitative leap means starting from a first approximation, provided by the objective indicators, in order to study later, in a different mode, other dimensions that contribute to the quality of living of the subject, i.e. to survey and analyze what statistics don't show us.

---

[54] Translation of the authors of the original in Spanish language.

The proposal is to add to the dimensions that are traditionally studied on the quality of life, other dimensions that we understand put together fundamental elements for their study, and those altogether are: family, education, health, work, recreation, safety, territoriality or everyday space.

The purpose is to obtain other types of information, to empathize with subjects, enhancing the possibility of increasing the scale of analysis, and to apply different techniques of a qualitative nature, such as, among others, the gathering of documents, the straight observation, focus groups, in-depth interviews and life stories.

The basic unit of all subject reference is the family,

> the family context is a privileged space for social development, being an area where multiple interrelations occur, where spaces, time, outings, entertainment, experiences are shared, where everyone learns through confrontation with others, where everybody can learn to live together and be with others (Romera Iriuela 2003, p. 53)[55].

We understand that to achieve a good life or a worthy life is a commitment of the subjects, and of the subjects with and in their families, independently of the family model, i.e. nuclear, without children, single parent families, assembled, among others.

The family dimension, which as designated by Madariaga and D'Arterio (2008), little of it is included in the works on quality of life, is of utmost importance in achieving a better quality of life, given its importance as a cell which mingles the individuals who constitute it, containing, supporting, advising and developing them in a first instance. Words like "*being together*", "*having a well-established family*", "*meeting at the table*" (Mikkelsen 2010), appear as important signals and as justification enough to be incorporated as a dimension of the quality of life, understanding that it refers to more subjective, spiritual or emotional conditions. Within the family dimension, in objective type studies, the following indicators have been employed: single, nuclear, extended, female parental homes, which can be obtained from national censuses (Madariaga and D'Arterio 2008; Velázquez and Mikkelsen 2010).

We look at education as a dimension of the quality of life in the sense of present and future possibility of legal rights, of freedom, of accomplishment, for individuals and families, since it allows the subjects "to be an element of and participate in life in society" (Lucero et al. 2008b, p. 98). There is a relationship, although not decisive, between education and the possibility of carrying out a good life since, when you think of this pair, the level accomplished may not be the source of satisfaction, but what is really achieved through the level of instruction, promoting awareness in subjects to interpret education as improvement of their quality of life, and thus also enhancing the education of future generations. Such as Velázquez expresses (2004, p. 179), the low educational level "…tends to provide a vicious cycle feedback that reduces the possibilities of development and social promotion of massive sectors of society". For the elaboration of objective indices of quality of life, it is customary to use variables belonging to the educational pyramid, these being: alphabetization rate of population over 6 years old; percentage of population over 25 years old having

[55] Translation of the authors of the original in Spanish language.

completed a university level degree; educational level of the head of the family (Madariaga and D' Arterio 2008; Velázquez et al. 2013; Velázquez 2008; Lucero et al. 2005, among others).

In terms of the quality of life related to health, two situations are evident, on the one hand to enjoy good health and, secondly, in case of illness, to have the possibility of being properly attended. Testimonials attained in various field works claim that "*health is everything*" "*health is to have social security,*" "*at least, to have health*", "*an installed water pump running is health*" (Mikkelsen 2010). According to Fernández Mayoralas Fernández et al. (2005, p. 126) health is defined as "the value assigned to the duration of life, modified by social opportunities, perceptions, functional status and disability, caused by diseases, accidents, treatments or policies (Patrick and Erickson 1993)"[56]. We believe that it is important to consider not only the conditions of disease or the presence and possibility of access to centers and/or health services, but that is also of interest to reflect all around prevention, and this is strongly related to food, hygiene, the habitability of dwellings and even education. With respect to the Health dimension, indicators utilized, among others, are: percentage of population with social health security coverage; percentage of homes with access to drinking water outside the house; percentage of houses with access to water for cooking from automatic pumping water; child mortality rate (Velázquez et al. 2013; Velázquez 2008 and 2004; among others).

In terms of work, in general the subject finds it positive to achieve a salary-based employment or to perform a salary-based activity, since it enables the acquisition of goods and services, constitutes a forethought both for the present and for the future, adding other benefits linked directly with the satisfaction of needs associated with health and education, especially. According to Lucero (2008), "the dominant cultural model in the Argentine society requires to recognize the role attributed to the employment of the active members of the community as a necessary means for access to goods and services and as a key value of emancipation and realization" (p. 253).

Moreover, employment should beunderstood as a social construct, yet it is referred to a historical context, to a specific culture, to experience and to a way of life of the subjects, as well as a system of symbolic relations which develop in its surroundings (Alonso 1999).

In previous works (Mikkelsen 2010), words such as "*having a job, which provides you with the basics*", "*working is essential,*" "*having money*", appear, phrases that are reiterated without distinction of social groups, regarding work as a value that dignifies in addition to enabling personal maintenance.

In the Work dimension, it is possible to refer to the following indicators, which result from the Homes Permanent Enquiry (HPE) and/or the national censuses: Non-demanding Unemployment Rate; Employment Rate; percentage of population incorporated to the retirement system; households heads only workers; home heads in the retirement system; home heads classified as qualified professional or technical

[56] Translation of the authors of the original in Spanish language.

workers (Mikkelsen et al. 2013; Lucero 2008; Velázquez and Mikkelsen 2010; Ares and Mikkelsen 2007, among others).

Time devoted to leisure and recreation, as designated by Yanes and Liberali (1986) "a compulsion of renewal of one's self, which promotes values, closer relationships, increases performance in the workday, contributes to education and primarily to physical and mental health" (p. 159).

Security, understood as feelings of danger experienced by subjects in their homes, neighborhoods, cities, therefore thinking of places they escape from, in the times they elude (spaces of the day and night routine, (Lindón 2010), and in practices they apply not to be part of a criminal act. Feeling latent threats, mistrusting places they walk and trying to avoid them, organizing special methodologies to enter and exit their homes, using security systems or finding alternative locations: all this leads to the terms "topophilia" or "topophobia". The first "can be defined broadly to include all human emotional links with his material environment" (Tuan 2007, p. 130)[57]. 'Topophilical' ties can be developed by the aesthetic appreciation, by tactile feelings (as when you enjoy the pure air) or by personal and national history built in direct relation with the territory. In the opposite direction, 'topophobical' relations refer to negative relationships between the subject and the space.

In terms of daily life or personal space, it is directly linked to the place in which individuals or families reside, to services present there, combined with the identity and the sense of belonging, that give social significance to the territory. To inquire the territory (Haesbaert 2004) from the perspective of its inhabitants is the right way to observe and interpret their lived spaces, their temporary space trajectories and their spatial practices. Daily life can be defined by the plot constituted by diverse social practices located in the territory at a specific time, and through which it would be possible to find new meanings of the place, by means of geographical studies of the experienced world that consider the role of objects, actions, techniques and time (Santos 2000). The site expresses the relationship among individuals and the material environment, therefore, the study of that link is a basic starting point.

From these dimensions we intend to review the implication that subjects have on their quality of life, now turning to determine "how" they are valued individually and collectively, i.e. how we approach empirically the construction of evidence, information, trying to question subjects according to their values and needs.

In such sense, a way to be closer to what subjects lived on a daily basis is to capture their views and observe them in a given context and time, focusing especially on the significance of the selected dimensions. Guber says (2001) "the only means to accede to those meanings that subjects negotiate and exchange, is the experience, the possibility of experiencing firsthand those senses as it happens in socialization" (p. 60)[58].

A first exercise is to use the technique of analysis of written documents, in this case maps, photographs, satellite, flat images, illustrations, information from the press, objects which analysis will facilitate the construction of a mental perspective

[57] Translation of the authors of the original in Spanish language.

[58] Translation of the authors of the original in Spanish language.

and a relational position referring to persons and places involved in the study, just for mentioning some examples: location maps of public spaces for recreation, location maps for educational institutions and providers of health services, both public and private, maps of the routes of public transport, among others.

Then, if we take each dimension in an individual way, we understand that *direct observation*, one of the more formerly employed techniques in Geography, will allow not only the visual collection of information, but also the evidence seized by the other senses, i.e. all that is potentially relevant apart from the direct vision, which may add pictures and videos. Hence it is possible to create information concerning leisure as a dimension, from observing persons in public places intended for recreation and their enjoyment of leisure time, paying special attention to the constituent elements of the place, to the handling of the space, to the activities carried out, to the way subjects communicate, to distances that they keep while doing so, to the representation of the roles that correspond to each one of them, to the differences in their behavior and their activities, among others. As González expresses (2005) the geographical observation is neither a simple task, nor a passive or completely objective one, it is a comprehensive systematic operation, and it is an action to include reality in its real dimension, i.e. to scale 1:1. In this sense, you come in touch with the everyday life of the subjects, their actions and practices materialized in the everyday space, you watch them, you see them, you observe them within a geographic matter, being aware in such practice of the overlapping of interpretations, since the subjectivity of the researchers strongly comes into play in the interpretation of the interpretation of the subjects studied. "The main tools are: the experience, the sensory organs, and the affections which, far from ruining, approach the object of study" (Guber 2001, p. 60)[59].

The survey, in order to obtain meaningful information, requires at least a minimum degree of participation; that is, to play whichever role and therefore to influence the behavior of informers, and reciprocally the researcher's. Without thinking in participant observation, it intends "talking" with subjects, who enjoy of recreation spaces on different days of the week and at different times. This allows restructuring the reasons for choosing these places, time of year, forms of amusement, the methods and modes of arrival to the place, as well as the frequency, asking them about the elements that must be present in a place of recreation, if they consider leisure time significant to hold a good life, and other issues that the same subjects identify as interesting in this joint research. To watch them taking pictures and also to photograph them, consists of an exercise of contemplation which involves several visits, on different days and times, taking records in the field, asking and occasionally interacting with the subjects present in the area, attempting also to observe the movements and dynamics of a zone designed for the leisure of the population.

Local newspapers have a fundamental role, especially in the **Security** dimension, since based on the analysis of their contents, we can recognize, rebuild and observe security/insecurity cuttings. Reading a text, in this case written press, has been the most extensive and universalized form of survey. Ruiz Olabuenaga (1996) establishes that "content analysis is nothing but a technique to read and interpret the

[59] Translation of the authors of the original in Spanish language.

contents of all kind of documents, specially written documents" (p. 192)[60], in this sense, a text or an object cannot be interviewed but it can be interpreted.

The possibility of having the perception and assessment of the inhabitants in these places allows underlining the importance given to language, a component showing what people do and what they think about the places. According to Di Meo (cited by Lindón 2007), the permanent building of the territory is engendered in everyday practices, which are not strange to the interaction between objective structures (built by society) and cognitive structures (individual, but influenced by the social constituents).

In this context the *individual and group interviews* will be the best option to collect verbal information from subjects with regard to the health, work, education, and security dimensions. Interviews are the most utilized instrument in empirical social research, defined as a purposeful conversation between two partners, which is comprehensive, since during the meeting held by interviewed and interviewer, the dialogue about the purpose that brings them together, must be exhausted: talking with goals, the interviewer knows the objective of his interview and his research problem deeply.

In this case we propose to employ individual in-depth interviews aimed at representative qualified informants for each dimension to deal with: hospitals managers, health centers, clinics, and first aid small quarters, school headmasters representing various levels of instruction, social workers, dining rooms, and inspectors, just to mention some of them. The snowball technique could be used for the elaboration of this qualitative sample, i.e. the selection of qualified informants, which allows choosing subjects who have special characteristics and who, because of their knowledge of the subject to be addressed, may point to other subjects for interviews, who could provide valuable information to the problem in research.

Later the health, work, education and security dimensions will also be treated in *discussion groups* formed by subjects with different roles in the analyzed society, since one of the key elements that have an important impact on the type of material obtained by this technique is the design of the groups (Colectivo IOE 2010). The proposal is to form a heterogeneous group of discussion, establishing as the meeting space, an emotionally representative site for the local society: a school, a social club or a neighborhood association. The dynamics of the group will be observed, for which the purpose of the meeting and the issue of research are made explicit, opening the possibility of the debate addressed by a series of structured lines, while researchers perform the role of guides of the story, writers, inviting everyone to reflect on the issue that brings them together, their well-being. As established by Scribano (2008):

> the central idea that motivates its use is to catch the view that a group of individuals in interaction elaborate on certain issues that constitute their social reality… [since]… the discussion group is a scaled representation of the forms of production, circulation and reproduction of social discourse (p. 116)[61].

[60] Translation of the authors of the original in Spanish language.

[61] Translation of the authors of the original in Spanish language.

The family dimension can be worked through the use of *stories of life* applied to women between 50 and 60 years of age being part of a family which, even though it is relevant to reconstruct the story of their lives around the family dimension, will be guided so that it is possible to renovate the meaning of the past and the present with regard to the concept of quality of life, taking care to observe continuities and changes in their social and individual well-being. The story of life

> implies a combination between what their individuality and their place are in a network of interpersonal and social relations. Therefore, a story of life is presented as the coming and going through different levels: the individual's own and those in which his life was inserted (Scribano 2008, p. 99)[62].

In this way, as García Ferrando et al. (2005) express that,

> when surrounded by social reality, the researcher can select a single perspective or overlap several. And, although he will never solve the paradox that the closer to social reality, the farther it will be—because his own approach is part of social reality-; if the researcher puts together several perspectives, he can at least have access to a greater number of dimensions of that everlasting complex social reality (p.11)[63].

Then the information obtained must be properly systematized by building codes and labels that simplify the understanding of the problem considered, interpreting it and trying to find its meanings. Thus, the surveyed information receives a double treatment for its interpretation: on the one hand, it is decoded in order to establish broad categories; secondly, it focuses on the analysis of the evidence, now transformed into first-hand documents, central inputs in the achievement of a compromise between research theory and practice.

When employing a methodology of a qualitative nature, data are analyzed as stories, vignettes and short stories which ideal is the so-called "dense description", i.e. the interpretation of the interpretations of subjects taking part in a social action. Thus the analysis and interpretation of qualitative information is accomplished at the intersection of field work and processing, i.e. survey of data and its analysis are exchanged since the beginning of the qualitative research, in a process from the field to the text to the reader. As a result, the ultimate goal is the apprehension of meanings, a claim that was present throughout the entire investigation.

To analyze discourses on the quality of daily life is the central work back to our office; we have created information that comes from the spatial practices of subjects, using various techniques, since Lindón says (2010)

> the subjects not only construct their places when they build houses, buildings, cut down forests, open roads, cultivate land. Places are also built when talking about them and doing it in a certain way, emphasizing some features, ignoring anothers, associating with certain phenomena to others"…"Places are also built by the senses and meanings attributed to them (p. 32)[64].

[62] Translation of the authors of the original in Spanish language.

[63] Translation of the authors of the original in Spanish language.

[64] Translation of the authors of the original in Spanish language.

So in the words of Velázquez (2008), the

> concept of life quality that, from a certain point of view, we can assimilate to "everyday life", will become, from each of the notions of population and its reference groups, a subjective quality of life. Each assessment will largely focus on the individual experiences, environment, culture, etc, of each group. This sort of self-diagnosis can partly take 'objective' elements as: provision of services, infrastructure, landscape, etc. But, however, it will always be present in perceptions—sometimes with greater power—factors such as: memories, associations, emotional ties, ideologies and beliefs, among others (p. 20).

Quality of life is then conceived as a sensitizing, sensitive, emotional, sentimental notion that provides reference and guide on what is "important" in the daily life of individuals and society, i.e. that it can reflect the space socially lived.

5.6 Conclusions

Resuming the objective that guides this study, we want to emphasize that in recent decades, the inclusion of renewed forms of addressing the object of study is evident in the geographic community, penetrating into the interpretation of the meaning of the places as they are materialized in the spatial practices of the subjects. One of these realizations comes concurrently with the study of the quality of life of the population. In this sense, the possibility of methodological complementarity allows a multiple approach to the concept of quality of life, promoting an appreciation of micro-geographical type studies in combination with those of macro-geographical nature. In this way, the conjunction of both modes of study, objective and subjective, can help provide clarity to the explanation of how and why people live every day in certain places.

Thus, the employment of objective indicators, statistical techniques and macro-geographical scales can be unpredictable at the micro-social level, where lived experience, the relationship subject-place, and spatial practices provide new answers to the social-territorial problematic in research.

As we have seen, quality of life is a concept consisting of multiple and varied dimensions that are interrelated in a complex way, according to the prevailing historical context in each of the places, but above all it is a highly sensitizing concept, as it refers to the life of the subject, to our own lives, to analyze it and analyze us, to study it and study us, and that is why sometimes it can be difficult to focus our lens, and in this sense, to consider objective measures as much as subjective appreciations animate us in the path of the understanding of the well-being of the population as a dynamic and controversial construct.

We understand the concern for the quality of life of the population as a practical sensitive issue currently always present in political debates; in the discussion forums; in the aspiration to solve education, health, work, environment, among others, for specific age groups (young people, children, older adults, women), therefore the fact of being present works as "evidence", as a track, a sign, which in the different academic disciplines attracts your attention, appears as an issue needed to be addressed, and it becomes the object of study which must be accompanied by methodology.

In this way Geography has much to provide and offer, beginning by turning back to the central categories, bearing in mind a problem that is at right angles with scientific knowledge, reviewing the methods for knowing, apprehending this subject from "how", from methodology, from a methodological convergence, so to contribute with ideas, understanding, knowledge that, in the field of decision-making, allow contributing to "live a life of virtue", since we as human beings aspire to welfare, to happiness, to a meaningful life full of significance with ourselves, with our communities, with our daily lives.

References

Abaleron, C. A. (1999). Calidad de vida como categoría epistemológica. Area, Architecture, Design & Urban Planning Magazine, No. 6, August, National University of Buenos Aires.

Alguacil Gómez, J. (2001). Calidad de Vida y modelo de ciudad. Ciudades para un futuro más sostenible, CF+S bulletin, Number 15, March 2001. http://www.habitat.aq.upm.es/boletín/n15/ajalg.html. Accessed 4 Aug 2006.

Alonso, L. E. (1999). *Trabajo y ciudadanía. Estudios sobre la crisis de la sociedad salarial.* Madrid: Trotta.

Ansa Eceiza, M. M. (2008). Economía y felicidad: Acerca de la relación entre bienestar material y bienestar subjetivo, 11th Critical Economy Conference, Bilbao. http://pendientedemigracion.ucm.es/info/ec/ecocri/cas/Ansa_Eceiza.pdf. Accessed 23 Aug 2013.

Ares, S., & Mikkelsen, C. (2007). Segregación espacial de la población en Localidades Menores del Partido de General Pueyrredon. Argentina. 2001. 11th Geographic Information Systems Iberoamerican Conference, Department of Social Sciences, National University of Luján. 29th to 31st May, 2007. Buenos Aires.

Bailly, A. (1998). Los indicadores sociales: medidas objetivas de las ciencias duras en las evaluaciones subjetivas de las ciencias blandas. In C. García Ballesteros (Ed.), *Métodos y técnicas cualitativas en Geografía Social*. Barcelona: Oikos-Tau.

Barbosa, J. (1999). Geografia e cinema: em busca de aproximações e do inesperado. Alessandri Carlos, Ana Fanni. (Comp.)

Boroni, G.; Gómez Lende, S., & Velázquez, G. (2005). Geografía, calidad de vida y entropía. Aportes de la Teoría de la Información para la construcción de un índice de calidad de vida a escala departamental (1991–2001). In G. Velázquez & S. Gómez Lende (Eds.), *Desigualdad y calidad de vida en la Argentina (1991–2001). Aportes empíricos y metodológicos.* Tandil: UNCPBA.

Buttimer, A. (1985). Apreendendo o dinamismo do mundo vivido. In A. Christofoletti (Ed.), *Perspectivas da Geografia*. 2nd ed. Rio Claro: UNESP. [Originally, 1976].

Buzai, G., & Baxendale, C. (2006). *Análisis socioespacial con Sistemas de Información Geográfica*. Buenos Aires: Lugar Editors.

Camargo Mora, M. G. (1999). Calidad de Vida y Capacidades Humanas. Venezuelan Geographic Magazine. 40(2) 1999. http://www.saber.ula.ve/db/ssaber/Edocs/pubelectronicas/revistageografica/vol40num2/articulo40–2-4.pdf. Accessed 28 April 2007.

Carney, G. (2007). Música e lugar. In L. Corrêa & Z. Rosendahl (Eds.), *Literatura, música e espaço*. Rio de Janeiro: EdUERJ.

Carreras, C. (1998). El uso de los textos literarios en Geografía. In A. García Ballesteros (Ed.), *Métodos y técnicas cualitativas en Geografía Social*. Barcelona: Oikos Tau.

Cerda, T., & Vera, X. (2008). Indicadores Sociales y Marcos Conceptuales para la Medición Social. Documento de Trabajo. Instituto Nacional de Estadísticas (INE). Chile. http://www.ine.cl/canales/sala_prensa/revistaseconomicas/documentostrabajo/30_06_09/documento_de_trabajo_indicadores_sociales.pdf. Accessed 28 Aug 2013.

Chacon, R. M. (1998). La dimensión cualitativa en la definición de indicadores de calidad de vida urbana. 4th Latin American Urban Life Quality Seminar, UNCPBA, Tandil.

Claval, P. (1999). *La geografía cultural*. Buenos Aires: EUDEBA.

Claval, P. (2011). ¿Geografía Cultural o abordaje cultural en Geografía? In P. Zusman, R. Haesbaert, H. Castro, & S. Adamo (Eds.), *Geografías culturales, Aproximaciones, intersecciones y desafíos*. Buenos Aires: UBA. (Edition of the Department of Philosophy and Language).

Clua, A., & Zusman, P. (2002). Más que palabras: otros mundos. Por una geografía cultural crítica. A.G.E. N 34 bulletin.

Colectivo IOE. (2010). ¿Para qué sirve el grupo de discusión? Una revisión crítica del uso de técnicas grupales en los estudios sobre migraciones. Empiria: N° 19 Methodologies in Social Sciences Magazine. National University of Distance Education. http://www.colectivoioe.org/uploads/d70e92469ea5d534c31d5b25acaf48ae0c593b25.pdf. Accessed 26 Oct 2013.

Corrêa, R. L. (2011). Las formas simbólicas espaciales y la política. In P. Zusman, R. Haesbaert, H. Castro, & S. Adamo (Eds.), *Geografías culturales, Aproximaciones, intersecciones y desafíos*. Buenos Aires: UBA. (Edition of the Department of Philosophy and Language).

Cosgrove, D. (2002). Observando la naturaleza: el paisaje y el sentido europeo de la vista. A.G.E. N 34 bulletin.

Díaz, K. (1985). Los estudios geográficos sobre la calidad de vida en Venezuela. Revista Geográfica, 102.http://www.jstor.org/discover/10.2307/40992499?uid=2129&uid=2&uid=70&uid=4&sid=21102810054987. Accessed 23 Sept 2013.

Diener, E. y Suh, E. (1997). Measuring quality of life: economic, social, and subjective indicators. Social Indicators Research 40. http://link.springer.com/article/10.1023%2FA%3A1006859511756#page-1. Accessed 26 Sep 2013.

Duncan, J. (1990). *The city as text: The politics of landscape interpretation in the Kandyan Kingdom*. Cambridge: Cambridge University Press.

Espinosa, O. M. (2000). Enfoques, Teorías y Nuevos Rumbos del Concepto Calidad de Vida. www.naya.org.ar/congreso2000/ponencias/Oscar-Mauricio-espinosa.htm. Accessed 22 March 2006.

Estes, R. (1989). Hacia un índice de calidad de vida: enfoques empíricos para la evaluación del bienestar humano a nivel internacional. (Kliksberg, B comp). Pobreza un tema impostergable, FCE-PNUD, Caracas.

Fernández Mayoralas Fernández, G., & Rojo Pérez, F. (2005). Calidad de vida y salud: planteamientos conceptuales y métodos de investigación. Territoris 5, Universitat de les Illes Balears. http://www.raco.cat/index.php/Territoris/article/viewFile/117017/147939Consulted. Accessed 24 Oct 2013.

Feu, R. (2005). A noção de qualidade de vida: uma revisão. 10th Latin American Geographers Meeting, Geography Department, Faculty of Philosophy, Language and Human Sciences, University of São Paulo.

Frémont, A. (1976). *La région, espace vécu*. París: PUF.

Gallopin, G. (2006). Los indicadores de desarrollo sostenible. Aspectos conceptuales y metodológicos, Santiago de Chile, Fodepal. http://www.cusur.udg.mx/fodepal/Articulos%20referentes%20de%20Des%20Susr/otros%20art.%20de%20Des%20Sut/gallopin.pdf. Accessed 22 Oct 2013.

García Ballesteros, A. (1998). Métodos y técnicas cualitativas de investigación en geografía social. In A. García Ballesteros (Ed.), *Métodos y técnicas cualitativas en Geografía Social*. Barcelona: Oikos Tau.

García Ramón, M. D. (1985). *Teoría y método en la Geografía Humana Anglosajona*. Barcelona: Ariel Geographic.

García Ferrando, M., Ibáñez, J., & Alvira, F. (Eds.). (2005). *El análisis de la realidad social. Métodos y técnicas de investigación* (3rd ed.). Madrid: Alianza Editors.

Geertz, C. (1973). *The interpretation of cultures* (Institute for Advanced Study). Princeton: Basic.
Gómez Mendoza, J., Muñoz Jiménez, J., & Ortega Cantero, N. (1988). *El pensamiento Geográfico. Estudio interpretativo y antología de textos* (De Humbolt a las tendencias radicales). Madrid: Alianza Editors.
Gómez Vela, M. y Sabeh, E. Calidad de vida. Evolución del concepto y su influencia en la investigación y la práctica http://campus.usal.es/~inico/investigacion/invesinico/calidad.htm. Accessed 10 Oct 2013.
González, E. (2005). La observación directa base para el estudio del espacio local. Geoenseñanzas, Vol. 10, University of Los Andes, Venezuela, 2005.
Gregory, D. (1984). *Ideología, ciencia y Geografía Humana*. Barcelona: Oikos-tau.
Guber, R. (2001). *Observación participante. La etnografía. Método, campo y reflexividad*. Buenos Aires: Norma.
Guelke, L. (1985). Uma alternativa idealista na Geografía Humana. In A. Christofoletti (Ed.), *Perspectivas da Geografía* (2nd ed.). Rio Claro: UNESP. [Original, 1974].
Haesbaert, R. (2004). *O mito da desterritorialzaçao. Do "Fim dos Territorios" á Multiterritorialidade*. Rio de Janeiro: Bertrand.
Hiernaux, D. (2008). Geografía Objetivas versus Geografía Sensibles: Trayectorias divergentes de la geografía humana en el siglo XX. *ANPEGE Magazine (Associaçao Nacional de Pós Graduaçao em Geografía), 4*. www.anpege.org.br/revista/ojs-2.2.2/index.php/anpege08/article/viewArticle/8. Accessed 10 May 2009.
Johnston, R., Gregory, D., & Smith, D. (1987). *Diccionario de Geografía Humana*. Madrid: Alianza Diccionaries.
Katz, Cindi. (1994). Playing the field: Questions of fieldwork in Geography. *Professional Geographer*, *46*(1), 67–72.
Leva, G. (2005). Indicadores de Calidad de Vida Urbana. Teoría y Metodología. Metropolis Habitat. niversidad Nacional de Quilmes.
Lévy, B. (2006). Geografía y Literatura. In D. Hiernaux & A. Lindón (Eds.), *Tratado de Geografía Humana Autonomous Metropolitan University*. México: ANTRHOPOS.
Ley, D., & Samuels, M. (1978). *Humanistc Geography*. Londres: Croom Helm.
Liberali, A. M., & Massa, C., (1986). Los indicadores de calidad e vida en la Argentina. In L. Yanes & A. Liberali (Eds.), *Aportes para el estudio del espacio socio-económico* (*I*). Buenos Aires: El Coloquio.
Lindón, A. (2007). Los imaginarios urbanos y el constructivismo geográfico: los hologramas espaciales. Eure, Vol. 33, núm. 99. http://www.scielo.cl/pdf/eure/v33n99/art04.pdf. Accessed 18 Aug 2013.
Lindón, A. (2008). De las geografías constructivistas a las narrativas de vida espaciales como metodologías geográficas cualitativas. *ANPEGE Magazine, 4*. www.anpege.org.br/revista/ojs-2.2.2/index.php/anpege08/article/viewArticle/8. Accessed 14 May 2009.
Lindón, A. (2010). Los giros teóricos: textos y contextos. In A. Lindón & D. Hiernaux (Eds.), *Los giros de La Geografía Humana*. Barcelona: ANTHROPOS.
Lora, E. (2008). Calidad de vida más allá de los hecho. BID. Fondo de cultura económica. http://www.fundacionpobreza.cl/biblioteca-archivos/calidad_de_vida.pdf. Accessed 15 Sept 2009.
Lorimer, H. (2007). Cultural geography: Worldly shapes, differently arranged. *Progress in Human Geography, 31*(1), 89–100.
Lucero, P. (2008). Geografía del Trabajo y Calidad de Vida: contrastes socio-territoriales en Mar del Plata. In P. Lucero (Ed.), *Territorio y Calidad de Vida: una mirada desde la geografía local*. Mar del Plata: EUDEM.
Lucero, P., Riviere, I., Mikkelsen, C., & Sabuda, F. (2005). Brechas socioterritoriales vinculadas con la Calidad de Vida en Mar del Plata. In G. Velázquez & S. Gómez Lende (Eds.), *Desigualdad y Calidad de Vida en la Argentina* (1991–2001). (Aportes empíricos y metodológicos. CIG). Tandil: UNCPBA.
Lucero, P., Mikkelsen, C., Sabuda, F., Ares, S., Ondartz, A., & Aveni, S. (2008a). Calidad de Vida y espacio: una mirada geográfica desde el territorio local. In P. Lucero (Ed.), *Territorio y Calidad*

de Vida, una mirada desde la Geografía Local. Mar del Plata y Partido de General Pueyrredon, GESPyT. Mar del Plata: EUDEM.

Lucero, P., Riviere, I., Ares, S., Aveni, S., Celemín, J. P., Mikkelsen, C., Ondartz, A., & Sabuda, F. (2008b). Perspectiva geográfica de la satisfacción vital: salud, seguridad y vivienda en la ciudad de Mar del Plata. In G. Tonon (Ed.), *Desigualdades Sociales y Oportunidades Ciudadanas*. Buenos AiresL: Espacio Editorial.

Madariaga, H., & D'Arterio, J. (2008). Propuesta de medición de la calidad de vida en las localidades rurales y su implementación en la provincia de Tucumán. In G. Velázquez & N. Formiga (Eds.), *Calidad de Vida, diferenciación socio-espacial y condiciones sociodemográficas. Aportes para su estudio en la Argentina*. Bahía Blanca: UNS Editors.

Marans, R., & Kweon, B. (2011). The Quality of Life in Metro Detroit at the Beginning of the Millennium. In R. Marans & R. Stimson (Ed.), *Investigating quality of urban life*. Londres: Springer.

Marans, R., & Stimson, R. (2011). An overview of quality of urban life. In R. Marans & R. Stimson (Ed.), *Investigating quality of urban life*. Londres: Springer.

Matijasevic, M. T., Ramírez, M., & Villada, C. (2010). Bienestar subjetivo: una revisión crítica de sus resultados, alcances y limitaciones. Revista RegionEs, Vol. 5, N. 1. CRECER.INER. Universidad de Antioquía. http://issuu.com/guerrerortiz/docs/bienestar_subjetivo_regiones_volumen_5_n_1__caroli. Accessed 22 Aug 2013.

McCrea, R., Stimson, R., & Marans, R. (2011a). The Evolution of Integrative Approaches to the Analysis of Quality of Urban Life. In R. Marans & R. Stimson (Ed.), *Investigating quality of urban life*. Londres: Springer.

McCrea, R., Marans, R., Stimson, R., & Western, J. (2011b). Subjective Measurement of Quality of Life Using Primary Data Collection and the Analysis of Survey Data. In R. Marans & R. Stimson (Ed.), *Investigating quality of urban life*. Londres: Springer.

Mikkelsen, C. (2010). Movilidad territorial y Calidad de Vida en los espacios rurales del Partido de General Pueyrredon. Tesis doctoral. Departamento de Geografía y Turismo. Universidad Nacional del Sur. Bahía Blanca.

Mikkelsen, C., Ares, S., Sabuda, F., & Lucero, P. (2013). Calidad de Vida Urbana en la Argentina de la postconvertibilidad. Procesos sociales y territoriales en el período 2003–2012. XII Jornadas Argentinas de Estudios de Población. Bahía Blanca, 18th, 19th and 20th, September, 2013.

Nuvolati, G. (2002). Qualità della vita e indicatori social. Modulo di didattica per ildottorato di ricerca in Scienza, Tecnologia e Società, presso l'Università della Calabria, Cosenza. Italia. http://www.sociologia.unical.it/convdottorati/nuvolati.pdf. Accessed 3 Dec 2006.

Nuvolati, G. (2006). La qualità della vita delle cità. Metodi e risultati delle ricerche comparative". Milano. Dipartimento di Sociologia e ricerca sociale. UniversitÃ degli studi di Milano Bicocca. Online http://www.sociologia.unimib.it/wcm/file/materiali/3584.pdf. Accessed, november 2006.

Ortega Valcarcel, J. (2000). *Los horizontes de la Geografía. Teoría de la Geografía*. Barcelona: Ariel Editors.

Palomino, B., y López, G. (2000). La calidad de vida: expresión del desarrollo. En: Calidad de vida, salud y ambiente. México: UNAM, INI.

Pedone, C. (2000). El trabajo de campo y los métodos cualitativos. Necesidad de nuevas reflexiones desde las geografías latinoamericanas. Scripta Nova. Geography and Social Sciences Electronic Magazine N. 57. Universidad de Barcelona.

Pérez Maldonado, A. (2002). La calidad de vida en los asentamientos rurales de Iberoamérica. *Revista Geográfica Venezolana, 43*(1). http://www.saber.ula.ve/bitstream/123456789/24502/1/articulo43-1-1.pdf. Accessed 11 Sept 2012.

Romera Iruela, M. J. (2003). Calidad de vida en el contexto familiar: dimensiones e implicaciones políticas. Psychosocial Intervention, Colegio Oficial de Psicólogos de Madrid, España. http://www.redalyc.org/pdf/1798/179818041002.pdf. Accessed 14 Sept 2013.

Rosendahl, Z. (2011). Religión, bienes simbólicos, mercado y red. In P. Zusman, R. Haesbaert, H. Castro, & S. Adamo (Eds.), *Geografías culturales, Aproximaciones, intersecciones y desafíos*. Buenos Aires: (Department of Philosophy and Language Editors), UBA.

Rowles, G. (1978). Reflections on experiential fieldwork. In D. Ley & M. Samuels (Eds.), *Humanistic geography: Prospects and problems*, London: Croom-Helm.

Ruiz Olabuenaga, J. (1996). *Metodología de la investigación cualitativa*, (Serie Ciencias Sociales) Vol. 15. Bilbao: Universidad de Deutso.

Santos, M. (2000). *La naturaleza del Espacio. Técnica y Tiempo. Razón y Emoción*. Barcelona: Ariel Editors.

Sauer, C. (1985). La educación de un geógrafo. In M.D. García Ramón (Ed.), *Teoría y método en la Geografía Humana Anglosajona*, p. 38–53. Barcelona: Ariel Geografía. [Originally published in Annalss of A.A.G., 46, p. 287–299, 1956].

Sauer, C. (2010). Hacia una geografía histórica. Geografía en Español. Traducciones. Colombia, N 4. http://www.geografienespanol.net/Sauer_GeE_4.pdf, [Original in Annals of the Association of American Geographers, 31, p. 1–24, 1941]. Accessed, Sept 2013.

Schalock, R. & Verdugo Alonso, M. (2006). Revisión actualizada del concepto de calidad de vida. http://jalvaro.files.wordpress.com/2009/02/concepto_cv-revision_2006_schalock_r.pdf. Accessed 13 Aug 2013.

Scribano, A. (2008). *El proceso de investigación social cualitativo*. Buenos Aires: Prometeo.

Sen, A. (1996). Capacidad y bienestar. (Nussbaum, M. y Sen, A. Comp.) La calidad de vida. Fondo de Cultura Económica. México D. F.

Sen, A. & Nussbaum, M. (2001). Calidad de Vida. Reseña a cargo de Montesino Jerez, J.L., published in Polis, Bolivar University Academic Magazine Vol. 1 N. 2. 2001. http://www.revistapolis.cl/2/monte.pdf. Accessed 15 April 2011.

Sirgy, M. J., Michalos, A. C., Ferriss, A. L., Easterlin, R. A., Patrick, D., & Pavot, W. (2006). The Qualityity-of-Life (QOL) Research Movement: Past, Present, and Future. *Social Indicators Research, 76*(3), 343–466.

Smith, D. (1980) *Geografía Humana*. Barcelona: Oikos-Tau.

Tonon, G., (2005). Apreciaciones teóricas del estudio de la calidad de vida en Argentina. El trabajo que desarrolla el Internacional Wellbeing. Hologramática Magazine, Dpartment of Social Sciences, UNLZ, Year II, Number 2 V 1.

Tonon, G. (2008). Los estudios sobre Calidad de Vida en la Aldea Global, en América Latina y en Argentina. Revisión conceptual, avances y desafíos. In P. Lucero (Ed.), *Territorio y Calidad de Vida, una mirada desde la Geografía Local. Mar del Plata y Partido de General Pueyrredon, GESPyT*. Mar del Plata: EUDEM.

Tonon, G. (2010). La utilización de indicadores de calidad de vida para la decisión de políticas públicas. Revista *Polis,* Centro de Investigación Sociedad y Políticas Públicas (CISPO). http://polis.revues.org/820. Accessed 8 June 2013.

Tuan, Y- F. (1985). Geografía Humanística. In A. Christofoletti (Ed.), *Perspectivas da Geografía* (2nd ed). Rio Claro: UNESP. [Original, 1976].

Tuan, Y-F. (2007) *Topophilia. Un estudio de las percepciones, actitudes y valores sobre el entorno*. España: Melusina. [Original, 1974].

Unwin, T. (1995) *El Lugar de la Geografía*. Madrid: Cátedra.

Vega Rapun, M. & Lamote de Grignon Pérez, J. (2008), Los indicadores de bienestar desde una perspectiva de género en España. http://www.ub.edu/tig/GWBNet/docs/Social%20Indicators/ReportSocialIndicators%20SP%201esp.doc.pdf. Accessed 14 Aug 2013.

Velázquez, G. (2001) Geografía, Calidad de Vida y Fragmentación en la Argentina de los noventa. Análisis regional y departamental utilizando SIG's, CIG-FCH-UNCPBA, Tandil.

Velázquez, G. (2004). Calidad de vida en la Argentina. Elementos de diferenciación socio-espacial. In Otero, H. Dir. (Ed.), *El mosaico argentino. Modelos y representaciones del espacio y de la población, siglos XIX–XX*. Buenos Aires: Siglo Veintiuno de Argentina Editors.

Velázquez, G. (2008). *Geografía y Bienestar. Situación local, regional y global de la Argentina luego del Censo 2001*. Buenos Aires: EUDEBA.

Velázquez, G., & Mikkelsen, C. (2010). Comparación entre índices de calidad de vida. La población rural del Partido de General Pueyrredon, 2001–2007. Norte Grande Geographical Magazine, Pontificia Universidad Católica de Chile, N. 45.

Velázquez, G. A., Linares, S., Mikkelsen, C., & Celemín, J.P. (2013). Calidad de vida en la República Argentina (2001 y 2010). Una primera aproximación a escala provincial. Actas IV Congreso Nacional de Geografía de Universidades Públicas, Mendoza, 23rd to 26th October.
Verdugo, R., Schalock, K., Keith, R., & Tancliff, R. (2006). La calidad de vida y su medida: principios y directrices importantes. *Intellectual Disabilities Spanish Magazine, 37*(2), 218.
Zusman, P., & Haesbaert, R. (2011). Introducción. In P. Zusman, R. Haesbaert, H. Castro, & S. Adamo (Eds.), *Geografías culturales, Aproximaciones, intersecciones y desafíos*. Buenos Aires: (Department of Philosophy and Language Editors). UBA.

Chapter 6
Qualitative Studies in Health-Related Quality of Life: The Case of Young People Living With HIV/AIDS

Milton Décima

6.1 Health-Related Quality of Life

Traditionally, health has been approached from a medical point of view and its discussion has been mainly limited to the detection and treatment of disease, pain relief and healing. As medical science has been developing, that approach has proved to be inadequate and it has been necessary to extend the concept of health to the entire life of the subject, not restricted only to the biological manifestations.

The term Quality of Life is difficult to define since it is a global and multidisciplinary term which must be considered from a cultural point of view, the historical moment and the society in which it operates (Ardila 2003).

In 1945 the World Health Organization (WHO) defined the term health as a *state of complete physical, mental and social well-being and not only the absence of disease*. This concept was pioneering at that moment but at the same time only an expression of desire but a reality and that eventually went away from that meaning and taking other dimensions the concept of health.

However, years later, the Quality of life Group at WHO took up that idea and defined health as the individual's perception of their position in life in the context of culture and value system that the subject lives in relation to their targets, expectations, patterns and concerns (WHO QoL Group 1995).

After nearly 20 years, there is still a lack of consensus on the exact meaning and evaluation of QoL. Consequently, many authors developed the concept, especially in terms of personal satisfaction in different areas, ranging from physical and financial aspects to politicians and others, relating to the physical, social and emotional well-being.

So, Ardila (2003) himself proposes a more inclusive and modern definition of quality of life as a general state of satisfaction derived from the realization of the

M. Décima (✉)
Lord's Miracle Hospital, Salta, Argentina
e-mail: miltondec@hotmail.com

G. Tonon (ed.), *Qualitative Studies in Quality of Life*,
Social Indicators Research Series 55, DOI 10.1007/978-3-319-13779-7_6

individual potential. It is a subjective feeling of psychological and social well-being that includes physical and subjective aspects of emotional expression intimacy security perceived personal productivity and objective health. Thus it could be argued that quality of life includes both objective and subjective aspects as the study refers to the physical environment (social well-being) and the psychosocial environment (psychological well-being) based on experience and global vision of life or life satisfaction.

The latter concept has been analyzed from different perspectives and two main approaches that can be recognized on this regard. First, it comprises the affective or emotional approach, from which the quality of life is understood as a balance between positive and negative affect (Bradburn 1969). Second, the cognitive approach focuses on how individuals evaluate their own life in general or some aspects of it such as family, health, work and leisure (Diener 1984).

The cognitive component of well-being would be life satisfaction, globally or for specific areas and the affective component refers to the presence of positive feelings, called happiness by some authors (Arita 2005) In a different direction, some authors define happiness as a greater concept, including welfare and satisfaction (Cuadra and Florenzano 2003).

Some authors suggest that quality of life includes well-being as the subjective component of the concept (Liberalesso 2002; García-Viniegras and González 2000) which would consist of cognitive and affective aspects (Diener 1994; Diener et al. 1999).

In short, it can be said that the QoL refers to the global evaluation each subject does of his own life in general. To some extent, this satisfaction is the result of a combination between the perception of the subject itself and its environment at a micro and macro level so some variables like self-esteem and some personal characteristics are the basis of life satisfaction (Diener et al. 1999).

Regarding the importance of the components of quality of life, health is one of the leading and influencing directly and indirectly in that way. Directly, since the daily activities of the human being depend on the health status and indirectly because it affects other aspects present in the quality of life of people such as social relationships, leisure, autonomy and others (Moreno Jiménez and Kern 2005).

Currently, the area that arouses more interest and that more research is being devoted to is health. Thus, it is important to distinguish between quality of life and HRQOL.

The concept of HRQOL was included in the Index Medicus in 1966 and although some authors identify it as part of the quality of life, others report interchangeable meanings. Despite these discrepancies, the concepts must be differentiated in practice.

Patrick and Erickson (1988) specified it as a value given to life expectation and its modification by impairment, functional status, perception and social opportunities influenced by disease, injury, treatment or policies.

Shumaker and Naughtozn (1995) define it as the subjective evaluation of the influence of the current health status, health care and health promotion activities, the ability to achieve and maintain a level of general functioning allowing valued life goals and that this is reflected in their general well-being.

Other authors such as Fernández et al. (2001) state that HRQOL should comprise at least the perception that the person has of the impact that caused the disease or its treatment on his sense of well-being and ability to act (functionalism) These basic dimensions should be analyzed in the physical, emotional and social aspects.

Finally, Schwartzman (2003), from a subjective point of view, states that HRQOL is the evaluation done by an individual, according to his own criteria of physical, emotional and social state at a certain moment and reflects the level of satisfaction with a personal situation at a physiological, emotional and social level.

As it can be seen in the definitions of the above authors, they first share the idea of HRQOL as a perception, experience or subjective evaluation. Second, it is influenced by health status and, finally, that perception affects the functionality or performance of relevant activities or goals in life of a subject.

Based on the above considerations, it is important to emphasize the differences between HRQOL and quality of life. First, HRQOL is expressed based on the impact of the disease, evaluating the possibility of the presence of satisfaction of the person in a subjective way, while the quality of life emphasizes the analysis of psychosocial aspects and subjective well-being including both objective and subjective aspects (Vinaccia et al. 2007).

Throughout the statements that have been made, although there is no conceptual model of HRQOL unanimously accepted by the scientific community and there is no consensus on a quality of life meaning as well, the HRQOL could be defined as a subjective, multidimensional concept that the individual perceives about their level of physical, emotional and social well-being to understand the influence of the health condition in their life closely related to the context and the time determined where the subject is found.

There are some dimensions of HRQOL studied and related to each other in varying degrees that measure different aspects of life and autonomy of the subject. Some of the most relevant are:

Physical Functioning This dimension limited aspects of health and fitness and the impact of clinical symptoms on health or specific treatment, the personal care, performance of physical activities and autonomy. It also examines the discomfort which produces symptoms in daily life:

Psychological Factors This dimension reflects the impact of cognitive functioning and emotional state. The first refers to the ability to evoke memories at a short and long-term and the ability to think clearly. It also collects the energy and vitality or perceived competence to deal with problems arising from the illness or treatment. The emotional state includes analysis of depression, anxiety, and what concerns to the patient.

Social Aspects It analyses the impact of health status on the usual performance of social relationships, social isolation due to physical disability and altered performance of social roles in work and family life, as well as the activities and interactions of the patient with friends, family, co-workers or others.

Other particular areas of HRQOL explored by some researchers are pain, sexual function, satisfaction with life, the impact on labor productivity and activities of daily living. The number of visits to the physician for illnesses or medical problems and the need to use drugs has also been frequently used as indicators of HRQOL.

Notice that HRQOL dimensions should not be confused with other measures reported by the patient and used in Health Outcomes Research, such as satisfaction with medical treatment and medication, the preference for treatment, adherence and treatment compliance or expectations regarding treatment, although some of these concepts share dimensions with HRQOL.

From the above mentioned it can be deduced that the HRQOL directly involves the definition of health. However, among the definitions of health, HRQOL and quality of life, a variety of related terms can be found in the literature. These concepts are health, functional status and personal well-being. While those were used as synonyms and sometimes they are still used this way, their definitions are indeed different and have different meanings.

The *health status* is a definition derived directly from the concept of health, it was defined by Bergner (1989) according to five dimensions corresponding to: (I) genetic or hereditary characteristics (basic structure that supports the others); (II) biochemical, anatomical and physiological of a patient (associated with disease, the deterioration, disability and handicap or disadvantage); (III) functional status (activities of daily living); (IV) mental status (perception of health and mood); (V) potential of individual health (longevity and prognosis of the diseases and disabilities). The term was defined in a more direct and consolidated way by others authors who consider health as a component of the quality of life.

Meanwhile, the *functional status* refers to the evaluation of abilities and disabilities and got impulse enough to establish criteria for inclusion in clinical trials. Their evaluation instruments are described as brief, specific (for each disease) and subjective (performed by the physician)

Finally, the state of *personal well-being* refers to the general perception of the patient on their health or disease without discriminating the different aspects that determine it.

According to the arguments that have been made in all such conceptions it is important to distinguish these definitions and when to apply them in research although there will always be disagreements.

6.1.1 Psychosocial Aspects

Above mentioned dimensions of HRQOL, there are several variables that can affect the perception that a subject on its HRQOL has been assessed. Some of them are sex (among other things, by the different pain tolerance), the age (by the deterioration of the body and the loss of mobility and autonomy), marital status (for his relationship with aspects of social and sentimental support), education (by differences in the scales of social valuation and its relationship with the socio-economic level), the socio-economic level (by the health access capacity) rural or urban habitat (by the environmental influence of the stress, noise and pollution) and the cognitive disorders (for the decline to assess reality).

In the HRQOL of people living with HIV/AIDS (PLWA) are some factors socio-demographic and psychosocial that can distress it. The first include advanced age, female sex, unemployment and low income, which would affect it negative way. Nevertheless, are the psychological problems which occur more frequently in PLWA such as anxiety, depression, and behavioural disorders.

At the time of diagnosis the subjects not only experience a feeling of uncertainty relating to the hope and expectation of life in general, if not also uncertainty as to the quality and length of life, the effects of treatment and the reaction of the society of the condition. The vital events, such as the diagnosis of HIV, are relevant and crucial facts in the life of the person, affecting the evolutionary process and the valuation which the person engages in the event. These events are related to its capacity to meet it, depending on the personality, level of self-esteem and social support.

Fierro (1997, cited by Arjona and Guerrero 2004), defines the *coping* as a skill of the subject in the acquisition of some control or mastery of a given stressful situation. It also includes efforts cognitive and behaviour to mastering, tolerating or reducing internal and external demands. Consequently, it is a personal and psychological characteristic of each individual variable. Thus, Lazarus (1988, cited by Font 1990), postulated coping as intrapsychics (cognitive and affective) action-oriented efforts, in order to manage demands internal and environmental that they test or exceed the personal resources. That it to say, coping is a skill that takes on the subject of some control or domain of a given situation stressful through cognitive efforts and behaviour.

Effective coping in the PLWHA consists of generating greater adaptive in situations of stress responses as it is the diagnosis of HIV/AIDS; i.e., to the extent that there is an effective coping with stressful situations and a greater repertoire behavioural oriented to meet the demands of the middle, slowing the evolution of HIV/AIDS infection. At the same time, coping, according to the theory *coping effectiveness training*, it centres on the one hand, in strategies of the person to change the negative aspects perceived a situation and, on the other hand, in the management of the emotional responses to a stressful situation (Chesney 2003).

Similarly, there is a lack of social support from family, friends, or co-workers in the diagnosis of sickness impact, also in HRQOL. According to Brannon and Feist (2001), *social support* refers to the feeling of acceptance, affection or appraisal by others people. It is a practice of care that occurs in the exchange of relations among people and is characterized by expressions of affection, support of different behaviours, symbolic or material assistance to another person. In fact, social support is expressed as an interpersonal transaction that includes three aspects: the expression of affection from one person to another *(emotional support)*, the adoption of behaviour, thoughts, or points of view of the other person (*confidential support*) and the provision of material assistance (*instrumental support*).

With regard to the functions of social support are recognized that there are four types: the emotional providing the individual feelings of esteem, affection, trust and security; the assessment, which represents the sensations experienced by the individual which can count on someone, and feel accompanied socially; the informational, also known as advice or cognitive guidance, which helps to define and address the problematic events using advice from the network and finally the instruments constitute tangible aid and material in the solution to a problem.

Likewise, the stigma and discrimination affects in transcendental form HRQOL in PLWHA. Rejection, abandonment and alteration of functionality family are associated.

Stigma is a condition, attribute, trait or behaviour that makes the individual to be included in a social category whose members is generated a negative response and are seen as culturally unacceptable or lower. Indeed, it is an attribute that "discredits deeply", society applies it and they bear it or they have stigmatized people and groups. It can be linked to specific actions, such as adultery, sexual preferences, psychoactive substance abuse or delinquent behaviour; with innate, as the sex or colour of skin, or features almost innate, such as religion or nationality and in certain infectious diseases such as HIV/AIDS, tuberculosis and leprosy. Now the stigma also is a means of social control, which defines social norms and punishes those who deviate from these. The reasoning of the stigma is the fear of the stigmatized to threaten society.

The basis of that fear is often ignorance as in the case of HIV is stigmatized where about the way of life of vulnerable groups or the realities of the sexual behaviour of people.

Additionally, stigma has been linked in the history of mankind with diseases that cause intense emotional reactions by his relationship with physical deterioration, death and sexuality as in the case of HIV, where these three components are associated with a single virus.

Although the concept is pejorative, the stigma can have positive consequences and manages to create a sense of community among the stigmatized, motivating them to rest and change to improve their lives.

Another aspect psychosocial undoubtedly affecting the HRQOL in PLWHA is *discrimination*. It can be spoken that the original "discriminate" meaning was to observe the differences. However, with the passage of time, the word has acquired the meaning of taking active or passive attitudes that adversely affect persons belonging to, or believed that they belong to a particular group, in particular to a stigmatized group.

In other words, discrimination may be the end result of a process of stigmatization which refers to unfair and different treatment that is given to a person on the basis of their membership, or alleged membership, a group in particular. It can be legislative (sanctioned by laws or policies) or community, action or lack of action in less formal contexts, such as workplaces or social settings, such as markets, sports, commercial centres or bars, among others. It consists of three components: discriminatory attitudes (also known as prejudices), discriminatory behaviour and discrimination. The first two apply to persons who are within the social norm; on the other hand, the latter refers to the relationship between those who are within the social norm and the stigmatized. So, when it talks about HIV discrimination, it is referring to different deal, usually harmful, who a person receives (Foreman et al. 2003).

Unmistakeably, stigma and discrimination are intimately related and generated an incremental and interactive circle among the subjects. Thus, stigma facilitates or promotes discriminatory attitudes and these attitudes are often reflected in the behaviour giving rise to acts of discrimination and these in turn accentuate or favour the stigma.

Finally, it is important to mention that social representations that have the HIV-infection, is a determining factor in all the above-mentioned aspects of HRQOL in these subjects.

The social representation is referring to a set of concepts, perceptions and meanings that shares a particular human group in relation to its members and to the surrounding environment, i.e. buildings that structure the information that a cognitive process organized by categories and classifications, providing a communications code sharing and involving everyday knowledge that exist in the minds of the people. They are socially produced and shared expertise that form from the experiences, information, knowledge and models of thought received and transmitted through tradition, education and social communication.

From these it is understand and interprets reality, is thought, organizes and apprehends everyday life; it unifies and integrates the individual and the collective, symbolic and social, thought and action. Serves as guide on social responses generated by this disease as a phenomenon the social representation permit recognition of modes and processes of Constitution of social thought, approaching people world view and understanding of social behaviour.

By all perspectives above mentioned HIV/AIDS can be seen not only as a condition from the biological, but also as a purely psychosocial phenomenon which is characterized by different behaviours, attitudes, beliefs and feelings influenced largely by the environment socio-historical-political in that develops.

6.1.2 Physical Aspects

As a final point, in assessing the physical dimension of the HRQOL in PLWHA, include aspects related to the perception of the physical condition that causes the infection itself in the subject and effects of new therapies antiretroviral (HAART) that produce changes in body morphology.

With regard to the first aspect, it can express that HIV causes in some stages of the disease, if it is not diagnosed in time or not carried out specific treatment, referred to as wasting syndrome. It is usually one of the first symptoms of AIDS, and may also occur during the period of latency or asymptomatic phase with diffuse clinical signs.

Wasting syndrome is a process associated with symptomatic infection by HIV and is characterized by intense fatigue and mental depression deep caused by depletion of the neurotransmitters sympathomimetic. It is defined as the involuntary loss of more than 10% of body weight, along with more than 30 days of diarrhoea, weakness and fever. A portion of the weight lost during wear is fat but most importantly the loss of muscle mass. This is also called "lean body mass" or "mass of cells in the body."

On the other hand, although the treatments have caused a noticeable improvement in survival in patients affected by this condition, is known to cause toxicity in the long-term in a variable time between 12 and 24 months. This has allowed to observing changes in the appearance of the subjects developed an abnormal distribution of body fat, sometimes associated with syndrome of resistance to insulin, possible development of diabetes, and increases in the levels of cholesterol and triglycerides. This is called lipodystrophy syndrome and it has been studied in multiple investigations since the beginning of the HAART, in the 1990s (Lertora and Foster 2008).

Two components of the syndrome are described: the lipohipertrofia and the lipoatrophy. In the first, the distribution of fat has various ways to manifest itself in subjects: increase in deposits of fat in the abdomen, especially around the organ meats such as liver, kidneys and intestines, producing a very globular abdomen; breast growth by fat in men (in women without enlargement of the mammary gland); fat deposit in the cervical spine, which can be very important and it is called "Buffalo Hump" and finally, increased fat of the parotid glands.

In the lipoatrophy component fat loss occurs in areas of the body where it is normal to have it or where the fat has a protective role, specifically causes a loss of subcutaneous fat in the face, buttocks, arms and legs, simulating in these recent increases in the size of the veins of the members. Both problems are closely related and have to see activity of HIV itself on cell mitochondria and the distortion produced by the metabolism of adipose cells, with both the effect of antiretroviral drugs.

Although the direct mechanisms that trigger both are not well known, the various studies carried out so far is not conclusive.

The data accumulated after more than one decade of experience indicate that approximately half of the people who are under HAART could suffer at some time and in varying degrees of severity, both lipodystrophy as lipoatrophy. It has been observed that, in some patients, replacing those antiretroviral with greatest potential for mitochondrial toxicity, progression of lipoatrophy can be minimized and, in some cases, observed even a small recovery.

In summary, both wasting and the lipodystrophy syndrome can cause changes in the appearance of the subject. The first relates to the loss of weight, fever, chronic diarrhoea and loss of muscle mass; and the second to the loss of fat in different areas of the body, according to the predominant component.

For all the above, it is clear that HRQOL in people living with HIV/AIDS affect various dimensions, especially the factors psychosocial (social representations, coping, social support, stigma and discrimination) and alterations in the physical aspects caused by the own condition or specific treatment.

6.2 The Human Immunodeficiency Virus (HIV)

Since the discovery of the HIV that causes the Acquired Immunodeficiency Syndrome (AIDS) at the beginning of the 1980s, worldwide, the pandemic is not only a serious public health problem, but also a complex social, political, economic and cultural problem. HIV is a virus that affects the system of the body, called the immune system's defenses. The function of this system is to protect human infectious and tumoral diseases in general. All viruses are microorganisms that can only multiply to get into the cells, using the mechanisms of the same cell to reproduce and infect it.

Each virus has the ability to invade certain types of cells. Unlike other viruses, HIV has the particularity of invading the defences of the organism cells (so-called lymphocytes T CD4) destroying them progressively. For this reason, HIV can lead to AIDS, an infectious disease that means acquired (it is not hereditary, but caused by a virus) immunodeficiency (which attacks the immune system) syndrome (a set of symptoms). It is considered that HIV infection reaches the stage called AIDS when defences are weakened and cannot protect the body properly. Because of this so-called "opportunistic" diseases and tumours like Kaposi's Sarcoma could take place. The transmission route is mainly caused by unprotected heterosexual intercourse.

There are approximately 33.3 million PLWHA in the world. There are more than 7000 new infections per day according to data from the Joint United Nations Programme on HIV/AIDS (UNAIDS 2009). Of these, 97 % are in developing countries and about 1000 are younger than 15 years and 6000 are adults over the age of 15 years, in whom 51 % are women and 41 % are young people between 15 and 24 years of age. Nevertheless, the epidemiological situation in the world is very heterogeneous, as there are large differences between the various regions, especially in developed and underdeveloped countries. Thus, *prevalence* (Refers to the number of existing cases of HIV/AIDS over a period of time and place, which is usually expressed in percentage form) rates in people among 15–49 years old in Eastern Europe and central Asia range from 0.7 to 0.9 %, and that of Western Europe is at 0.1 %. However, there are regions that have higher rates, like sub-Saharan Africa, with a prevalence of between 4.7 and 5.2 %, followed by the Caribbean, Eastern Europe and Central Asia (UNAIDS 2009).

In Latin America the epidemic is moderate and low level of HIV transmission and it is stable since 2003 with an overall prevalence of 0.5 %. Brazil, Mexico, Argentina and Colombia are Latin American countries with the largest populations and, as a consequence, with the largest number of PLWHA.

In Argentina, as well as globally, unprotected sexual intercourse continues to be the main route of transmission. The prevalence in the general population is less than 1 % (0.4–0.5 %), but in so-called vulnerable group is greater, such as 12 % among men who have sex with other men, 7 % among injecting drug users, 6 % in sex workers/s and 34 % among transgender people. In that country, in 2009, the figures rise to 130,000 people and 20 % of which are under 24 years old. In turn, it was observed that 89 % of women and 86 % of the males became infected during unprotected sexual intercourse. In the case of males, 48 % contracted HIV sexually with a woman and 38 % with another male (National Programme of Fight against Human Retrovirus, AIDS and STDs 2011).

In summary, the epidemiological evidence of the situation in Argentina indicates that HIV affects increasingly the heterosexual population, women, urban and even rural areas and young people with the common denominator of the low socioeconomic level, although with different levels of vulnerability to HIV infection.

Ayres et al. (2006, p 380) in the context of HIV/AIDS, defined vulnerability according to:

> the different degrees and natures of the susceptibility of individuals and communities to become infected, sick or dying from HIV/AIDS, which depend on your situation against the integrated set of cultural, social, political and economic aspects that located them in relation to the problem and the resources to deal with.

In this way, this author suggests that it can be identified in two dimensions: an individual dimension and a collective dimension, which in turn, is divided into two: the social and the programmatic.

The individual dimension is defined by three assumptions: to) all people are vulnerable to HIV and its consequences; (b) in infected people, the potential for vulnerability is in inverse function to social support and assistance in health which has; and (c) the cognitive, behavioural and social affect individual vulnerability of everyone.

The social dimension is determined by the economic, political, cultural, moral and institutional situations that define greater or lesser protection of society against the epidemic. This dimension includes: social norms, relations of gender and generational, concerning cultural beliefs and religious regulations, stigma and discrimination, social well-being, employment, income, social support; access to health care, education, culture, leisure, sport and media in this context also refers to freedom of thought, of expression, political participation, citizenship rights, accountability of public and private sector, and, finally, access to the public system.

The programmatic dimension is determined by the strengths or weaknesses of the programs at systems and health services for the prevention, control and care to HIV/AIDS regardless if they come from the field of Government, non-governmental, or private; or if you belong to the territorial level (national, regional, or municipal).It should be noted that these actions are closely related to the social dimension and determine the individual dimension.

On the basis of the above considerations, it can currently recognize that HIV/AIDS is a controllable disease thanks to HAART that emerged in the 1990s, which attenuate the natural evolution of the infection. This makes that the prevalence rates remain relatively stable in places where there is access to treatment have a greater survival, although there are more new cases of disease.

In this way, with a powerful therapy, there has been a marked decline in hospitalization rates, morbi-mortality (Term used in public health that encompasses the concepts of morbidity and mortality). Morbidity describes the amount of individuals who are considered to be sick in a place and time certain, while mortality refers to the number of people who die in a place and in a certain period in relation to the total population

Turning to infection by HIV/AIDS, a serious, fatal acute illness to a chronic disease, i.e., long and slow, controllable progression long-term disease. As such a condition, it produces a progressive loss of functional capacity and autonomy of the individual, with a gradual deterioration of physical, psychological and social nature that determines a decrease in the feeling of well-being.

Taking into account then the TARGA has extended the life of these subjects, an important aspect that arises is the consideration of quality of life and especially the HRQOL in this population, since HIV/AIDS is a complex constellation of disease, stigma and discrimination that affect the family, work and social life of those affected.

6.3 Methodological Tradition in HIV Research

In recent years, different HRQOL in HIV research have been performed and published, especially with quantitative methods, but very few studies using qualitative approaches. Among the first, are registered strong and consistent associations between levels of social support, psychological disorders, clinical indicators and socio-demographic variables in levels of HRQOL.

In regard to studies using qualitative methods in HRQOL in people living with HIV are less and some of them found similar results, despite using different methodologies. Most evaluated dimensions mainly focus on the psychosocial aspects of HIV/AIDS infection.

In this ways, Jones et al. (2004) used the grounded theory based on the daily life of 20 people living with HIV, Hepatitis C Chronic (HC) and who are coinfected with HIV and HC, residing in the Metropolitan Area of the city of Buenos Aires. They used the interview in depth where evaluated six categories: knowledge of diagnosis, first reactions when they are diagnosed, predictability of infection, impact of the diagnosis in the life and immediate steps after the diagnosis.

When performing the analysis, draw attention that none of the subject take knowledge of his infection in an analysis of routine or have suspicions of your probable infection. The first reactions of the diagnosis, was different for both infections, HIV was the idea of death and in the HC a misunderstanding of what causes the disease. In the analysis of predictability, patients with HIV related more drug addiction as a way of transmission, the heterosexual sexual relations without protection. HC had no clear transmission ratio. The diagnosis of both pathologies caused an imbalance in their lives difficult to overcome, but to some it meant a continuity of life style, and to others it did not.

For his part, Cardona-Arias (2010), also based on the same theory, conducted an investigation with the aim of understanding the SR on people living with HIV in Medellin, Colombia, during 2009, through semi-structured interviews, field and both participant observation as a non-participating journals. Interviews were conducted at each of the patients three corresponding with open, axial and selective coding. The RS were addressed from the procedural approach, which focuses on the symbolic production of language, from hermeneutics. The RS of the HRQOL is understood based on biological, like the importance of HAART and the provision of health services, psychological, such as the acceptance of the diagnosis and the relevance of information on health, and determinants social, such as the stigma and social support.

In addition, described some strategies used by participants to improve their HRQOL. In total 19 people aged between 29 and 67 years old, average 48, 52% of men, 58% unmarried, 73% unemployed and 57% with primary studies were interviewed. A number of participants considered the therapy as a determinant of HRQOL in the AIDS phase, but not in the asymptomatic subjects. Changes to the project of life linked to the need to redefine priorities in the life of the subject and ways of taking the new reality of infected is referred in the psychological domain.

In the initial moments, diagnosis generated feelings of hopelessness and disappointment by what the priorities of the life project focused on ideas about death and the fear of the future. Socially, the RS interview revolved around the support of family and friends, and not to the stigma. For many infected one of the best strategies to protect their HRQOL is hide the diagnosis, support in love and perform activities that occupy the free time.

On the other hand, Cantú Guzman et al. (2012) search profile psychosocial variables such as emotions, social support and coping as well as the RS who have HIV in Monterrey, Mexico in 2003. They conducted semi-structured interviews with open-ended questions in eight subjects receiving medical treatment. He was a content analysis and their respective frequencies to determine which excelled. The emotional impact at the time of diagnosis was negative, characterized by sadness and fear, as well as thoughts related to the death. It could detect various actions by the subjects, as for example with anyone let alone the situation, talking only with some relatives because with other family members you suggesting rejection, this associated with social support.

In this study, the current individuals coping was oriented more towards positive behaviours and instrumental type, based on the search for professional care and adherence to treatments. Also among the factors that have helped the subjects beyond the instrumental aspects, is maintaining hope, which denotes the importance of psychological interventions covering the social environment of individuals.

Finally, Pecheny et al. (2012) in a quantitative-qualitative descriptive study of characterization of women recently diagnosed with HIV in Argentina, during May–July 2009, evaluated women's vulnerability to infection, the contexts in which know their diagnosis, the route of transmission of HIV, when and how access to the testing and initial news impact.

Surveys and additional interviews semi-structured women and also men, couples of the same, residents in the city of Buenos Aires, were districts in urbanized areas and main cities of the country. Following interview guides, explored the secret handling, the experiences of stigma and discrimination, the impact of the diagnosis and disease, recovering the words of men and women themselves. The sample was intentional, not probabilistic and was comprised of a total of 465 women surveyed over 15 years old with a diagnosis of HIV in January 2009 or later. The age range of those interviewed ranged from 17 to 70 years and the average age was 34 years old.

They were interviewed 31 women between 20 and 62 years old; most live in urbanized areas (city of Buenos Aires and suburbs), and the rest resides in other cities of the several provinces as Buenos Aires, Córdoba, Salta and Tucumán.

All patients were heterosexual, with different marital situations: single women, married or stable union, separated with boyfriend, and widows. The employment situation of these women was in general precarious: only half works and, just a few had a job in white. Less than half received any subsidy or social plan; the Universal allocation per child is majority.

Twelve males were also interviewed. Only one of those interviewed (in quality of partner of a woman newly diagnosed with) not living with HIV. The ages ranged between 18 and 50 years old, and live in different towns of the country. All were already partner with women today living with HIV at the time of diagnosis of the same. It is stable and lasting relationships (between 3 and 9 years of relationship, at the time of the interview).

In the most of cases, wives couples have received the diagnosis at the time of childbirth or during pregnancy. This leads to that, sooner rather than later, males also performed the testing and receive a positive diagnosis as well. In two other cases, the women have done the testing for other reasons.

Only in one case was the man who first received the diagnosis, at the time of plunging by different symptoms. Two men claimed to know their serological status in advance. In both cases, they had not communicated it to their partners. Some concerned have transmitted them the virus to their partners, while in other cases they claim other reasons (such as a transfusion), believe that they have been partners of women who have transmitted to them or directly do not know or do not want to talk about the issue. At the time of questioning how to believe they have contracted the virus, the responses also vary: in addition to those who are considered to have contracted the virus with its stable couples, some believe that they did this in the context of casual relationships, with women or men.

In accordance with the found data and the analysis of this research show that vulnerability to HIV is a complex phenomenon and that it involves individual, social and programmatic dimensions. The practices of each of the people, their social relations along in life and in the present, and the impact by action or omission of the State, all this is reflected in stories over time and focuses on vulnerable to infection by HIV, as well as other conditions and damage to health and social as other diseases use of substances psychoactive, social, sexual violence and gender.

With reference to studies using qualitative methods above mentioned, can be noted that they are mostly exploratory or descriptive studies, where evaluated primarily subjective aspects such as dimensions psychosocial and some socio-demographic. Biological or physical indicators of the disease were not valued.

How you can highlight, obviously there are a greater number of quantitative studies in the literature that dealt with HRQOL in subjects with HIV/AIDS, to qualitative research. Possibly this is due to different reasons, for example to the methodological difficulty of qualitative designs, the experience of the researcher in this field of research, the time of completion of the field work and sometimes costs that involve the qualitative studies, among other factors.

In addition, sometimes working with hospitalized people or with people in deteriorated health conditions requires the brevity of the study and low complexity of the application of research in subjects with HIV/AIDS.

6.4 A Qualitative Study in Young People With HIV

6.4.1 Methodological Design

A descriptive study using qualitative method was conducted. The objective of this work was to analyse the characteristics of the HRQOL of young people with HIV/AIDS identifying the psycho-social aspects. Qualitative research in HRQOL of young people with HIV/AIDS describes the qualities of a phenomenon, in this case the condition by HIV, with the intent to obtain an understanding and interpreting deep meanings and definitions of the situation as they face these subjects, rather than the mere production of a precise quantitative measurement of characteristics or behaviour. Qualitative research is presented as a flexible, interactive design, predominantly subjective and inductive.

In one way or another, attempted to find answers about what young people think and feel about HIV, treating the researcher go towards subjects or living among them, with emphasis on everyday social practices.

The study population was consisted of young people between 15 and 24 years-old, who attended the external office of Sexual Transmission Infections (STI) during June–October 2013 at Lord's Miracle Hospital of Salta city, Argentina. This hospice has a level of complexity III, i.e. only accomplishes non-surgical and clinical treatment. It depends on the Ministry of Public Health of the Salta province. The institution assists, carries out treatment, retrieves and rehabilitates acute and chronic diseases with particular emphasis on infectious and contagious, such as tuberculosis and HIV/AIDS diseases and other emerging and re-emerging diseases from the province.

Intentional non-probability sampling was performed, i.e., young participants randomly were selected based on the ability to provide important and substantial information of their HIV status. The final sample was consisted of ten subjects of both sexes. The most important consideration in qualitative sampling is the wealth or the value of the data. The validity and significance of the knowledge generated by qualitative inquiry have more to do with the wealth of information of the selected cases and the ability of observation and analysis of the researcher to the size of the sample. It is important to remember that the logic of the intentional sampling is different from the logic of sampling probability (Patton 1990), because that will be based on the purpose rather than the statistical probability of selection.

Young people between 15 and 24 years-old diagnosed with HIV/AIDS through Western Blott laboratory technique, in the last 5 years who are receiving or not treatment HAART were included. Pregnant woman, exposed perinatal (i.e., subjects infected by HIV since birth through pregnancy transmission mother to child), subjects with disabling physical conditions, and severe psychiatric pathologies associated or not with the HIV status, inmate people and individuals with refusal to participate in the study were excluded.

6.4.2 *The Field Work*

Semi-structured interviews during the field work for the study of HRQOL in young people with HIV/AIDS were used as data collection technique.

Taylor and Bodgan (2000) define the interview as a situation of direct interaction where a person (interviewer) explores the views or experiences of others (interviewed) from the perspective of the latter. It is considered as an interpersonal communication in order to "verbal" answers which is characterized by the flexibility to adapt to the different personalities of each subject. In addition, it works with the words of the interviewee and their ways of feeling, not being a technique that leads simply to collect data about a person, but that he tries to speak to this subject, to understand it from the inside.

Tonon (2009) says that the interview as a meeting between two people, where personal feelings, beliefs, desires, problems, experiences and behaviour reveal. In the semi-structured interview, also known as interview based on a script, the investigative work can be organised as thematic axes of reflection or based guiding questions. An interactive, circular, and incremental process is generated in this way.

In the present investigation of HRQOL in young people with HIV/AIDS have been investigated with the aim of assessing the ideas, beliefs, opinions or perceptions, the following topics with the subsequent guiding questions:

Coping with the illness:

- How have you carried your illness from the diagnostic?
- What have you done to be able to coping with?
- Have you taken any particular behaviour?
- Do you avoid, accept or forget that do you suffer from the disease?

Social support from family, friends or co-workers:

- Apart from professional staff, have you discussed your sickness with someone else?
- Whom with?
- Have you got support from a family member, friend or co-worker? Whereof way?

Life Satisfaction:

- Nowadays, how do you feel emotionally in relation to your disease?

- Do you feel that the illness has changed anything in your life?
- In a negative or positive way?

In the first instance was asked young people about identification data in order to know social-demographic profile of the sample, such as age, gender, marital status, level of instruction, occupation, date of diagnosis of HIV/AIDS and use of treatment HAART. Subsequently, subjects authorized the completion of the interview giving informed consent in writing (according to the regulations of ethics in health research) and voluntary participation. It was explain the potential risks and benefits of the research, guarantees of confidentiality, purpose of the study, how were chosen to participate and the procedure of collection of data was used.

The semi-structured interviews lasted 30 min and were conducted in external office of the Lord's Miracle Hospital of Salta city where usually carry out diagnostic and counselling on HIV/AIDS and sexually transmitted infections. We used a digital recorder and the interviews were audio-recorded, changing the names of the informants to ensure their anonymity. During the interviews each young man was encouraged to freely describe the experience of living with HIV/AIDS, and depending on the circumstances some questions were carry out. We used a field notebook as he interviewed the subjects to take additional notes describing non-verbal communication as emotions or attitudes that were shaped not structured during the interview.

Research design was approved for implementation by the Committee of Ethics, the Teaching and Research and the General management of the institution.

6.4.3 *Data Analysis*

Once those interviews were transcribed completely without deleting them in electronic format, it was proceeded to make the qualitative analysis of the data.

By talking about qualitative analysis, it means, not to the quantification of data, but not mathematical interpretation process, carried out with the purpose of discovering concepts and relationships of the data and then organize them into a theoretical explanatory scheme.

According to Tonon (2012) the process of data analysis requires both theoretical knowledge, and certain attitudes and skills. In this study we used the strategy of analysis within the framework of social phenomenology called thematic analysis to identify the essence of the phenomenon of study and transform the subjective experience of young people living with HIV/AIDS in their world or everyday life.

Braun and Clarke (2006) propose the use of thematic analysis as a method to identify, analyse and report issues and structures, and can thus reveal both the experiences, such as meanings and realities of the subjects, as well as to examine the ways in which events, realities, meanings and experiences are the effects of the speech of a society. Firstly, to carry out thematic analysis, was a reading detailed and repeated the information transcribed looking for structures and meanings. At the same time, also underwent a repeated reading of the notes made in field notebooks.

Then, the initial theoretical coding were performed using words or textual phrases of the participants, which were grouped according to similar meanings related to the established themes. Subsequently, were conducted the search for topics using pictures by setting definite hierarchies of topics and subtopics worked.

Ten young people with HIV/AIDS, eight of them men and two women, with an average age of 21 years old participated in this study. Seven of the subjects were reported as unemployed, while the other three mentioned engage as administrative in a company's phones, voluntary promoter in a society for the protection of animals and sex worker respectively.

Eight of the participants obtained a level of complete primary and secondary education. The remaining two participants had an incomplete tertiary level. Two young people were studying, one nurse and another social worker. All young men said to be singles, and seven of them referred to have homosexual practices. The two women were heterosexual and single mothers. They had one or two children, correspondingly. The average date of diagnosis was two years, while the rest was 4 months old. Only a single subject was specific in treatment with HAART, while the rest had not begun treatment yet.

First, when analysed the psychological aspects of HRQOL in young people, it was observed that in all subjects at the time of the diagnosis HIV provoked an emotional impact with negative feelings such as fear, sadness, and denial of the disease. In this way, the subject usually suffers from a state of crisis that manifests itself in a social, physical and psychological imbalance i.e. goes through what is called a Vital Event. One of the young people said in this regard:

> … I'm not going to lie, when they say to you that you have HIV you get upset, there everybody was upset, there you said positive, but in my case, Yes, I was obviously disturbed. I couldn't believe it… Typica reaction, crying all day, because you never know, there is no cure, only treatment; they take it badly, if the treatment lasts 10 years and then, you still die… (male, 24 years old)
>
> And mostly I try not to remember, I try to think that it didn't happen, I don't remember, no nothing. The first days with my husband crying every day… because to us? It was a thing which we couldn't, understand that it had happened to us… And, well, the first few days I was crying all the time, the first months… and after that I didn't cry any more… (female, 19 years old)

Other young people expressed, along with previous feelings, ideas of trying to damage his life or suicide:

> …and when they found out (parents)… they felt bad, very bad… At first I wanted to kill myself. They had to take stop me… (female, 24 years old).
>
> The truth, at the beginning I was scared, I started to cry… what would I do if I had HIV. I thought of this madness, of killing myself, I don't know… (male, 24 years old)

It is important to emphasize that there is a grieving process, which in the case of HIV, certain stages shows very well in every disease. This grief represents an imbalance of the health state and well-being that perceives the subject and usually requires a period of time to get the person back to this state of balance.

According to Kubler-Ross (1969, cited in Kuczewskiahe 2004), there are five stages of grief popularly known by the acronym DABDA, including denial, anger, bargaining, depression, and adaptation of the disease.

In relation to the current coping of the suffering in young people, i.e., the ability to have people in acquiring some control in a stressful situation, included both efforts to adapt both cognitive as behaviour among the first, it was observed that subjects most well accepted disease, after having experienced some stages of mourning. They took it as part of everyday life and continued their normal life performing routine without any interference. Some young peoples expressed:

> … I decided that it was alright…I have the disease, and that I'd go on as I am now but with more stack obviously, trying to brace myself, try not to be depressed "bajonearme". Really it's useless, so… (male, 17 years old).
> If obviously accept it and try to be calm… positive and everything'll be ok, if I'm calm out there….at first, I was "bajoneada", but now I've been thinking about everything; it's alright. I'm more concerned about it and so…(female, 24 years old)
> … I accept it, I had to accept it… because I have to live with the problem, it's in me… but obviously, as I say… not… in the meaning of life… I feel like a little… I'd say… disappointed… (male, 23 years old)

However, other subjects were difficult for them admit the sickness and they are with depressive pictures, while others deny it still… At the stage of depression the people realizes her illness and suffers loss of different aspects of life and demonstrate a depressive reaction accompanied by fear, loneliness and loss of ability to fight and will to live. Only three subjects felt these emotions:

> It's hard to accept. It was very hard. Out there the other day when I got the news I couldn't bear it. The truth is that I was lost. I didn't know… Out there… I try not to remember that and going on with my normal life. No, I don't want to think about it. And the truth is I'm feeling bad, depressed, but I try not to lie down because I'm a very depressive person… the truth is that I don't know if I'm accepting it or not, if I should change for good, I know I have to but… Or is it that you like me are just spending time… (male, 24 years old)
> The truth is that I'm feeling bad (distressing look with tears in his eyes)… I can't accept it yet… (male, 24 years old)

Some young people tried to not fall into depression and staying emotionally well either with its vital as small children, or in some cases links to the parents. A young man said:

> .. I don't let myself go for my children's sake,… I have my two little children and they are the only thing that I have and I have to be strong for them, because I know if I get to cry or anything like that, it's worse for me and my defences are low (female, 19 years old)

On the other hand, very few young people use work or study as a coping resource, since most were unemployed and not studying. Other young people used strategies of reasoned action, since they meant that they were suffering the consequences of certain behaviours and unsafe sexual practices which had been carried out, a young man said in this regard:

> … I, psychologically, accept it, I'm fine. Knowing the consequences I don't care myself… What I have to do is to resign myself to the fact… (male, 24 years old).

At the same time, certain positive and negative behaviours were generated to meet them. Among the first subjects demonstrated a greater commitment to continue studying or find employment and greater capacity for reflection in family relations to avoid conflicts:

> … Before, I didn't know anything, I used to answer my mom back and now it's like that… I'm like that… I try to live a better life. I try to live well. Avoid fighting, avoid… For example I used to argue about with my mom about little things and now I try to not get angry… (female, 24 years old)

However, the most important positive aspect that young people expressed is that from the HIV diagnosis generated positive attitudes of self-care with behavioural changes in sexual practices. In addition, they also expressed wanting to care for other people to prevent secondary transmission of disease. These individual resources generated promote what is called resilience, i.e., skills that allow, even under unfavourable conditions, build and deploy behaviour favourable to oneself and to the own environment that surrounds it. Several young people said in this regard:

> …If I catch this disease, I have to accept it and move forward and now take care of myself and take care of other people…(male, 23 years old)
> …I don't know how people negatively prefer to infect everyone and don't care about anything, don't care about anything else. In my case I'm not like that. I prefer to take care of myself and take care of the person by my side, my… (male, 24 years old)
> … in a relationship, but I already know that I have to take care of myself, but I would do anything for the other person, because I wouldn't like to do to someone else what they did to me…(male, 17 year old)

In terms of negative behaviour, coping resources, young peoples, before the revelation of HIV conducted as main action hide your diagnosis, appealing to different strategies to be able to keep it secret from family, no close friends or work colleagues.

On the other hand, interviewees highlight the importance of Social support in HRQOL, i.e., if the young man has an affective network and contention that help the coping with the condition. Most of the parents of the study subjects were unaware of the diagnosis and young people received, not just emotional support, but also instrumental:

> …my family's giving me all the support I need when I feel bad. When I'm sick they're always watching out for me; and my friends, whenever I need them, they also there for me…(male, 24 years old)
> They try to give me psychological support, try to be with me telling me not to give in, controlling that I'm following the treatment, see now they were going to come with me, but they couldn't, they're calling me and so… They are supportive in this regard, to help me get well…(male, 24 years old)

In other cases, they only knew one diagnosis of parents or siblings and the other was unaware of the analysis. One of the young commented in this regard:

> …Not emotionally, because… we're different… My mom is cool (says it with disappointment) we clash… since I was a kid, with my mom; his departure, I've felt much rejection against my mom…(male, 24 years old)

Friends are a very strong and important support in nearly all teens analysed, especially confidential type. In one case a young man concerned have a friend who also lived with HIV he did have empathy and confidence to share disease:

> ..They talk about it, that is not a disease that can be spread by kissing, embracing, all that… (male, 24 year sold)…
> I feel a little better informed, a little more content, because the suffering and good done by this whole issue of social networks, and all that. He meets people….learns different, different stories about people, you know…(male, 23 year old)

In young concerned fear homosexual practices, friends with similar sexual preferences occupy the role of surrogate family in the absence of support from family, especially parents who generate behaviours of rejection by the choice of the sexuality of children. The interviewed young people, who work, noted that social support of co-workers there is no since they are unaware of the disease.

Finally, emphasis is placed on young people with HIV feel emotionally against the disease and if you have changed something in their life, it is either negative or positive, i.e. to what extent feel satisfaction with life despite living with HIV.

Thus, the majority of young people with HIV manifest feel good emotionally at the time of the interviews against the disease, after crossing the different stages of mourning and that change little life that were doing. Some young people were pronounced:

> …in spite of everything, I'm trying to smile, not to let myself fall because it's a normal disease, one can have a normal life, always taking care of the other person. I'm well, calm… Well, all in all. I'm trying to push on like other people…(male, 24 years old)
> Emotionally well, because I don't put up a barrier a barrier, er… as they say… when… treatment that the disease does not affect my head, I try to think it's part of my life and contro lmyself and go on with my normal life…(male, 24 years old)
> Emotionally I feel quite well, normal and, for me, normal is pretty good…(smiles nervously) I'm doing pretty well at the University, I feel livelier…(male, 17 years old)

However, despite the acceptance of the condition, they referred some positive and negative aspects of living with HIV. Few young men expressed positive aspects with respect to disease. General outlined that the disease served them as an instance of learning for life, and in turn, also help to better understand people living with HIV and have no prejudices about them.

On the negative aspects is where the subjects expressed greater concerns. Young men reported to have uneasiness at the time maintaining sexual practices with current partner or initiate new relationships with others for fear of rejection of those couples. Another aspect mentioned by them was the concern of some young people by the desire to have children. Young people pointed out in this regard:

> …for, er, if I have a couple I have to say although, er, I suppose that that couple'll still want to be with me, or breaking off the relationship, you somehow have to say…(male, 24 years).
> I said my life is over, as we say, everything… no longer the same relations, I'll be one sick person, as they say… the first thing they say, you have a disease… you're going to sick all your life, and sometimes it's ugly to feel…(male, 23 years old)
> If I believe it would be difficult for me to get a boyfriend, but not for fear of telling her I'm HIV positive, but because I'm not prepared…(male, 24 years old)

> …as it's beginning to change… that already from now on if you want to be with someone, again I am afraid to be with someone new or want to get to know someone…(male, 24 years old)

Another aspect related to the mentioned above is the concern of some young peoples is about the fatherhood. One young people said:

> Because if I can't have any children, do you understand me… say if I want to I have to be well, but… If 'm not I'm going to get something else… and that's what I don't want. That directly me I am only and it is… not… to ruin someone else's life, do you understand me… or to get someone to like me and I directly think not… because it's already happened to me…(male, 23 years old)

On the other hand, also referred to as something negative, employment problems, since they think that they may have difficulties in income when the employer applies for routine blood tests and seropositivity is revealed to HIV in the results. In this respect a young man said:

> They closed doors on me, as for example, I wanted to see if I could get into the police force and that kind of thing that you aspire sometime or you've ever wanted…because they always ask for these… ask for these health analysis… Good shops and stuff, I also know that I won't be able to…Sooner or later when they want to have my papers in order it will happen to me that, that's going to come out that… (male, 22 years old)

In turn, the generation of family conflicts are glimpsed from diagnosis. By the way a young man expressed:

> Well, at first nothing went well… my family moved away, turned away from me, most of my family, I expected another reaction from my family… and no, they walked out on me, all of them… can get or I can… they don't understand that there are methods to avoid contagion, but as they are all boys and I might infect them the door are closed…(female, 19 years old)

Among the positive aspects young people perceived of living with HIV perceived it as an instance of learning in life and have no prejudice with other subjects:

> Nowadays, I see people in a different different way, I manage to understand other people, I'm not prejudiced, but at the same time we are also biased, even with myself and if I can't do this because I have this disease, and maybe if I can do it, mostly because of prejudice and my low self-esteem… (male. 22 years old)

6.5 Conclusions

In this qualitative study interviewed young people expressed, from a psycho-social aspect of HRQOL, emotionally feel good with a positive impact in the diagnosis of HIV and a global vision in life favourably with appropriate psychological and social well-being. In regards to social support, it should be noted that participants had adequate support, both emotional and instrumental, friends and parents had minor pictures depressive, as well as a better perception of quality of life since they used effective defeats resources to cope with the condition. One must understand then, that HIV/AIDS is not only a mere disease from biological, if it is not a psychosocial phenomenon in a given socio-historical-cultural context.

This research evidence of some progress in several ways since it becomes a source of theoretical, methodological and practical knowledge of reference in research on HIV/AIDS. First, it generates an acquisition of other knowledge from the social sciences, not only personal but also professional level. This occurs by a subjective interaction between the interviewer and the vulnerable population so discriminated against and stigmatized by society. Secondly, the approach of the QoL in subjects with HIV with qualitative methods is imperative to understand and interpret the subjective aspects of the individual, and thus have a better general understanding of the experience of the subject with the condition, since it is currently a controllable chronic disease in the long run.

Finally, the results presented in this study emphasize the need for a therapeutic approach integrated between infectiologists physicians, mental health services and social assistance, as it is considered the person who lives with HIV/AIDS as a complex phenomenon, requiring a comprehensive and multidisciplinary management this will make more rational decisions to the of the subject who lives with HIV and perform in this way, interventions that can cause greater impact and effectiveness in public health programmes

While there are some limitations of the study, as the greater predominance of males with homosexual preferences and the amount of subjects interviewed, this study is only a new look of a research integrating the individual with HIV to get not only a greater survival of the subject, but a better quality of life and have hope in the future to carry an everyday normal interference-free and full of satisfaction. Without any doubt, HIV/AIDS is a complex constellation of psychosocial, stigma and discrimination alterations that affect family, working and social life of the subjects and becomes unavoidable will be current studies is directed towards qualitative research to better understand the socio-cultural determinants of the process health—care in these subjects.

References

Ardila, R. (2003). Quality of life: An inclusive definition. *Revista Latinoamericana de Psicología, 35*(2), 161–164.

Arita, B. (2005). Homeostatic theory of well-being and life satisfaction. *Psicología y Salud, 15*(1), 121–126.

Arjona, J., & Guerrero, S. (2004). A study on the styles and coping strategies and their relationship with the variable adaptation in high school adolescents. *Psicología Científica*. http://www/Psicologiacientifica.com/publicaciones/biblioteca/articulos/ar-ar-jona01.htm. Accessed 10 April 2012.

Ayres, J., et al. (2006). Risco, vulnerablidade e praticas de prevencao e promocao da saúde. In G. Campos et al. (Eds.), *Tratado de saúde coletiva* (pp. 375–418). Sao Paulo: Hucitec.

Bergner, M. (1989). Quality of life, health status, and clinical research. *Medical Care, 27*(3), 148–156.

Bradburn, N. (1969). The structure of psychological well-being. *On Psychological Well-Bein* (pp. 1–5). Chicago: Aldine publishing company.

Brannon, L., & Feist, J. (2001). *Health Psychology.* (pp. 15–90). Madrid: Paraninfo.

Braun, V., & Clarke, V. (2006). Using thematic analysis in psychology. *Qualitative Research in Psychology, 3*(2), 77–101. doi:10.1191/1478088706qp063oa.

Cantú Guzmán, R., Álvarez Bermúdez, R., & Torres López, E. (2012). Psychosocial impact in HIV-AIDS patients in Monterrey, Mexico. *Psicología y Salud, 22*(2), 163–172.
Cardona-Arias, J. (2010). Social representations of health- related quality of life in people suffering from HIV/AIDS in Medellin, Colombia. *Revista de Salud Pública, 12*(5), 765–776.
Chesney, M. (2003). Coping effectiveness training for men living with HIV: Results from a randomized clinical trial testing a group based intervention. *Psychosomatic Medicine, 65,* 1038–1046.
Cuadra, H., & Florenzano, R. (2003). Subjective well-being: Towards a positive psychology. *Revista de Psicología de la Universidad de Chile, 12*(1), 83–96.
Diener, E. (1984). Subjective well-being. *Psychological Bulletin, 95*(3), 542–575.
Diener, E. (1994). Subjective well-being. Psychosocial intervention. *Revista sobre igualdad y calidad de vida, 3*(8), 67–113.
Diener, E., Suh, E., Lucas, R., Smith, H. (1999). Subjetive well-being: Three decades of progress. *Psychological Bulletin, 125*(2), 276–302.
Fernández, J., Hernández, R., & Siegrist, J. (2001). Profile of quality of life for chronically ill (PQLCI): A method for evaluating well-being and functional impairment in clinical practice. *Atención Primaria, 28*(10), 680–689.
Fierro, A. (1997). Stress, coping and adaptation. In M.I. Hombrados (Ed.). *Stress and Heath* (pp. 11–37). Valencia: Promolibros.
Font, A. (1990). *Coping Strategies, Adaptation and Quality of Life.* II Congress official of psychologists, Area 5: Health psychology. Book of communications (pp. 90–96). Madrid: Publication's COP.
Foreman, M., Lyra, P., & Breinbauer, C. (2003). *Understanding and Responding to Stigma and Discrimination on HIV/AIDS in the Health Sector.* Pan American Health Organization/World Health Organization. http://www1.paho.org/spanish/AD/FCH/AI/Stigma_report_spanish.pdf. Accessed 10 June 2010.
García-Viniegras, C., & González, I. (2000). Psychological well-being, its relationship with other social categories. *Revista Cubana de Medicina Integral, 16*(6), 586–592.
Jones, D., Manzelli, H., & Pecheny, M. (2004). Daily life of people who living with HIV/AIDS and/or Hepatitis C: An application a grounded theory to health. http://www.facso.uchile.cl/publicaciones/moebio/19/manzelli.htm. Accessed 15 June 2012.
Kubler-Ross, E. (1969). *On Death and Dying.* New York: Macmillan.
Kuczewskiahe, M. (2004). Re-Reading On Death & Dying: What Elisabeth Kubler-Ross can teach clinical bioethics. *American Journal of Bioethics, 4*(4), W18–W23. doi:10.1080/15265160490908031.
Lazarus, R. (1988). Coping as mediator of emotions. *Journal of Personality and Social Psychology, 54*(3), 466–475.
Lertora, J., & Foster, M. (2008). Adverse reactions and interactions of the antiretroviral drugs. In Benetucci, J (3rd Ed.). *AIDS and associated Diseases: Diagnosis, clinic and treatment* (pp. 746–747). Buenos Aires: FUNDAI.
Liberalesso, A. (2002). Subjective well-being in adulthood and old age: toward a positive psychology in Latin America. *Revista Latinoamericana de Psicología, 34*(1–2), 55–74.
Moreno Jiménez, B., & Kern, E. (2005). Health related quality of life in childhood and organ transplantation: A review of the literature. *Revista Colombiana de Psicología,* (14), 46–52.
National Programme of Fight against Human Retrovirus, AIDS and STDs. (2011). Resource document. Newsletter on HIV/AIDS in Argentina N°. 28, Year XIV. http://www.msal.gov.ar/sida/boletines.html. Accessed 15 June 2012.
Patrick, D., & Erickson, P. (1988). What constitutes quality of life? Concepts and dimensions. *Clinical Nutrition, 7*(2), 53–63.
Patton, M. (1990). *Qualitative evaluation and research methods.* 2nd ed. (pp. 298–306). Newbury Park: Sage Publications.
Pecheny, M., Binstock, G., Manzelli, H., Hiller, R., Bruno, M. (2012). Characterization of women newly diagnosed with HIV in Argentina. Institute Gino Germani, University of Buenos Aires, Center for population studies and Ministry of Health. Final Report of research. http://www.onusida-latina.org/es/argentina-2/316-caracterizacion-de-las-mujeres-recientemente-diagnosticadas-vih-en-argentina.html. Accessed 12 June 2012.

Schwartzmann, L. (2003). Health-related quality of life: Conceptual aspects. *Ciencia y. Enfermería, 9*(2), 9–21.
Shumaker, S., & Naughtozn, M. (1995). The international assessment of health-related quality of life: A theoretical perspective. In S. A. Shumaker & R. A. Berzon (Eds.). *The international assessment of health-related quality of life: Theory, translation, measurement and analysis* (pp. 3–10). Oxford: Rapid Communications of Oxford.
Taylor, S., & Bogdan, R. (2000). *Introduction to qualitative research methods: The search of meanings*. Barcelona: Paidos.
Tonon, G. (2009). La entrevista semi-estrucutrada como técnica de investigación. In G. Tonon (comp). *Reflexiones Latinoamericanas sobre Investigación Cualitativa*. (pp. 56–75). San justo, Buenos Aires: Editorial Prometo libros-UNLAM.
Tonon, G. (2012). *Como analizar los datos en estudios cualitativos*. Documento de trabajo para el curso Introducción a la integración de metodologías, cuarta edición. Washington. INDES-IADB.
UNAIDS. (2009). *Report on the Global AIDS Epidemic*. Resource document. UNAIDS (Joint United Nations Programme on HIV/AIDS. http://www.unaids.org/es/dataanalysis/knowyourepidemic/epidemiologypublications. Accessed 10 Feb 2012.
Vinaccia, S., Quiceno, M., Gómez, A., & Montoya, L. (2007). Health related quality of life in patients with a diagnosis of mild hypertension. *Revista Diversitas: Perspectivas en Psicología, 3*(2), 203–211.
WHOQoL Group. (1995). The World Health Organization Quality of Life Assessment (WHOQoL). Position paper from the World Health Organization. *Social Science & Medicine, 41*, 1403–1409.

Chapter 7
Children's Quality of Life in the Caribbean: A Qualitative Study

María Dilia Mieles-Barrera and Graciela Tonon

7.1 Introduction: The Methodological Challenges Involved in the Study of Children's Quality of Life From a Qualitative View

The study of quality of life is a serious issue, considering the constant individual and general concern that has historically existed, in the long quest for gratifying forms of existence for human beings.

The concept has acquired great relevance in contemporary theoretical discussions in the fields of philosophy, economy, political science, sociology, and psychology, regarding the preoccupation about people's expectations, potential activities, freedom, justice, recognition, personal fulfillment, individual and collective prosperity, the influence of the daily life context, the establishment and personal experience of subjectivity, and human development as a whole, among other aspects. Likewise, it is considered a central theme of public policies regarding people's access to possessions and services, which includes the rules and actions oriented to resolve and find answers to multiple needs, interests and preferences of the groups and individual

The present article invites reflection, through the selection of relevant aspects of the methodological process developed in the doctoral thesis by María Dilia Mieles Barrera: *Quality of life of young middle-class boys and girls: case study carried out in Santa Marta, Tourist Cultural and Historic District, Colombia*, directed by Dra. Graciela Tonon.

M. D. Mieles-Barrera (✉)
Universidad del Magdalena, Santa Marta, Colombia
e-mail: mariadilia61@gmail.com

G. Tonon
UNICOM, Faculty of Social Sciences, Universidad Nacional de Lomas de Zamora, Lomas de Zamora, Argentina
e-mail: gracielatonon@hotmail.com

CICS, Faculty of Social Sciences, Universidad de Palermo, Ciudad Autónoma de Buenos Aires, Argentina

G. Tonon (ed.), *Qualitative Studies in Quality of Life*,
Social Indicators Research Series 55, DOI 10.1007/978-3-319-13779-7_7

persons that form a society, and to create instruments to make a practical assessment of the conditions which may produce satisfaction or dissatisfaction.

Thus, the assessment of quality of life becomes one of the most important indicators of human development in a society, for it attaches significance to the people's daily experiences, beyond the conditions labeled as "adequate" by experts (Casas 1996). The exploration of life experiences reveals deficiencies and potentialities, as well as the relationship between the individual and the social spheres—the latter being vital to the field of public policies, for it calls for prevention and promotion with an inter-disciplinary, inter-program, and inter-sector focus which will promote quality of life and lay the foundations for a positive social change. According to Tonon (2006), the studies on quality of life offer a new theoretical outlook oriented to working on potentialities rather than deficiencies, with a psychosocial anchorage in the community which includes an analysis of the socio-political context.

Thus, embracing the knowledge on quality of life involves an attempt at understanding, in complex detail, the way in which people's lives are affected by external conditions (economic, cultural, socio-political, educational, environmental, among others) which may either favor or hinder their freedom, the display of their capacities, and their chances of being actors –in other words, the perspectives of human development. Furthermore, it involves the study of the bearing these and other aspects (related to life projects, values, emotional ties, aspirations, interests, wishes, and personal biographies), have on people's perception, as well as the satisfaction or dissatisfaction they experience in the various aspects of their own lives, expressed in statements, and positive and negative emotional states present in their daily lives—as a manifestation of their subjectivity. (Mieles and Tonon 2012).

These circumstances give the concept of quality of life an interpretive character, and turn it into great potential for the comprehension of the lives of individual people and of groups of humans in certain contexts, as well as a reference in the assessment of daily experiences. In this perspective, the research on quality of life has been oriented towards the shaping of basic dimensions founded on people's valuation of what they consider essential to the fulfillment of an existence that will allow the display and enjoyment of all their human dimensions. In fact, when asked about their quality of life, it is noticeable that the latter represents something different to each subject: material issues are more relevant to some, while others regard them as the least of their priorities, since they privilege the satisfaction of being surrounded by their loved ones; occasionally, it is related to happiness or, alternatively with achieving some sort of balance between aspirations and achievements—the unattained being always in sight, thus investing quality of life with a strongly temporal character which transcends the present (De Pablos et al. 2009). These personal perceptions are, in turn, permeated by cultural and psychological patterns, social structures, demographic characteristics (age, gender, religious beliefs, among others) which have an incidence on the diverse valuations people make of themselves and of the public and private institutions, in the contexts they live in (Lora 2008; Ferris 2006).

Quality of life is considered a dynamic, multidimensional, multi-disciplinary concept, indirectly measurable and universal. (Setién 1993; Allison et al. 1997;

Campbell et al. 1976). Its dynamic character is related to its constant evolution and re-conceptualization; it is multi-dimensional for it comprises the multiple facets and dimensions in the development of people's daily lives; it is multi-disciplinary because it requires the approach of its contents from the point of view of a diversity of concepts and theories originated in sciences such as psychology, economy, medicine, political science, ecology, sociology, and anthropology, among others; it is indirectly measurable for it may only be explored through the accounts people offer of themselves; and it is universal considering that, in spite of its multiple approaches, it has been a source of concern to people and whole societies from the beginning of time.

The acknowledgement of this complexity, the same complexity that characterizes the human beings whose quality of life is under study, has allowed for reflective work regarding research approaches and methodologies, seeking to advance towards a conception of the person as a whole, and to find an answer to our need "to live rather than survive, which requires another kind of knowledge, a comprehensive and intimate knowledge which, far from placing us at a distance, will bring us into close personal contact with our object of study" (Santos 2009, p. 53).

It is worth mentioning that, in the course of 82 years—since the first allusion was made to this concept by Pigou—diverse instruments for the measuring and assessment of quality of life were devised, most of them constructed from a quantitative epistemological point of view. These endeavors have given invaluable fruits in the design of public policies which have contributed to the improvement of the quality of life of citizens all over the world—though failing to account for the daily lives and sense of welfare constructed by the people thus calling for the inclusion of a qualitative perspective, as stated by Casas and Bello (2012).

In embracing the knowledge of quality of life, we are attempting to understand- in a complex manner- the way in which people's lives are marked out by external economic, cultural, socio-political, educational, environmental conditions, to mention a few, which may favor or hinder the enjoyment of their liberties, the display of their capacities, and their scope of action, considered as perspectives of their overall development. We are, likewise, devoted to the study of the incidence of these and other aspects related to a life project, values, emotional ties, expectations, interests, desires and individual biographies, on the perception people have of their own lives and their satisfaction or dissatisfaction in different contexts of their lives, expressed in the form of opinions and positive and negative emotional states, as a manifestation of their subjectivities.

The development of qualitative studies implies "the recovery of subjectivity as a space for the construction of human life, the vindication of daily life as the basic scenario for the understanding of the socio-cultural and historical reality, as well as inter-subjectivity and consensus as vehicles to the acquisition of valid knowledge on human reality" (Guardián-Fernández 2007, p. 112).

Moreover, qualitative research as proposed by Taylor and Bogdan (1994) is characterized by being: inductive, more related to discovery and findings than to proof or verification; holistic, for it assumes the situation or scenario from a total perspective, as an integral whole, responding to an inherent logics of organization, operation and signification; inter-active and reflective, for its researchers are sensitive to the effects they may cause on the persons participating in the study; free, for no visions or perspectives are pre-imposed; open, for no antagonistic data gathering or analysis are excluded due to their valuable perspectives—all scenarios and persons are worthy of study; humanistic, seeking different means of access to privacy, to personal experiences, detecting perceptions, concepts and actions of the protagonists; rigorous, for the researchers must resolve the problems of validity and trust through exhaustiveness (detailed and deep analysis), and through inter-subjective consensus (shared interpretations and meanings).

In this perspective, when we focus our research on comprehension/interpretation, we are acknowledging the discovery of new and better states of being and relating with others and/or finding more potentialities than deficiencies in the world (Ricoeur 2003). We, likewise, make reference to "dialogic events in which the speakers run similar risks, and which produce a change in them; they understand each other so long as they are understood within a third horizon they cannot dispose of, but rather are disposed by" (Vattimo 1991, p. 61). Moreover, we refer to the "interpretive character of all forms of knowledge and to the fact that all forms of human understanding are based on a previous comprehension, i.e. on its possibility" (Herrera 2009, p. 159). Thus, it is important to highlight that comprehension is vital to existence and the scenario of human experience, which explains why social sciences have been reflecting on the comprehensive-interpretive character of their work, since the interpretive turn that took place in the 60's (Gadamer 1997).

Apart from the need to move forward towards the consideration of new forms of research, the studies on quality of life should also transcend the adult look for, although it is a highly popular concept which has been studied in different populations and fields of application, the studies on quality of life in young boys and girls have, in most cases, considered the boy or girl as a mere object of study; for it is the adults—parents, teachers, baby-sitters, or siblings—who voice those children's reality, ignorant of the political sense of this concept which implies the participation of the subjects involved (Casas 1998). Studies have, likewise, been developed by using scales, questionnaires, or surveys, with all the inconveniencies that they involve when it comes to accounting for the sense and perception that young boys and girls construct day by day, and their special susceptibility to give the researcher the "desired" answer, intimidated by the adult's "power" or by the situation of being assessed by a strange person in a strange context. (Cummins and Lau 2004).

In this respect, it should be considered that the studies embracing the relationship quality of life-infancy and adolescence are relatively recent. Taking an interest in these people's lives implies an advance in the comprehension of this population group, independently from the figures which reflect demographic characteristics—school attendance, morbid-mortality, nutrition, risks—thus making it crucial to include their own perspective in the concrete assessment of their living conditions. This new outlook may be situated in the late 1980's, as expressed by Huebner (2004) who, in his careful study, reports 30 research studies developed between 1980 and 2003, centered in the assessment of satisfaction in the lives of children and adolescents in developed countries.

Research work on the quality of life of children and adolescents began with the use of scales, and has developed steadily for three decades through the construction and validation of new scales, questionnaires, and surveys. This tradition, which has succeeded in obtaining a closer look into the lives of children and young people, still shows certain limitations, for it does not account for the experiences and perceptions that children construct on a daily basis, and overlooks their special susceptibility in giving the researchers the "desired" answer, intimidated by the adults' power or the fact of being assessed by an unknown person in an unfamiliar environment (Cummins and Lau 2004). Likewise, in the "studies on population welfare, it has been demonstrated that the answers to the different scales do not coincide with the typical statistic normality curve (Gaussian bell curve), most people's answers tend to be above the neutral point of any bipolar scale" (Casas and Bello 2012, p. 28), which evidences the existence of a slant that may distort positive and negative aspects of people's lives, a situation which may be accentuated when working with boys and girls due to their difficulty in quantifying their perceptions. Regarding this question, Casas and Bello (2012, p. 22) have stated: " we are conscious that, in the future, a more qualitative focus is pending; this will allow us to achieve a deeper comprehension of what boys and girls actually understand by welfare". This paper aims at making a contribution to the abovementioned challenge.

Twenty-four years after the enforcement of the International Declaration of Children's Rights, we are still a long way away from putting them into practice in the daily lives of boys and girls, as part of their subjective constitution as rightful subjects. Research on quality of life is closely related to the fulfillment and comprehension of these rights and to the consideration of children as active citizens and members of the social structure—participation being regarded as inherent of the political significance of this concept. This implies a creative construction of spaces and work forms which may propitiate the actual participation of boys and girls in the assessment of their own satisfaction or dissatisfaction, and the construction of alternatives which might boost their full development as human beings.

7.2 Remember Children's "Place" in Social Sciences Research

It is important to consider that the consideration of childhood merely as an "object of study" has not been only an omission in the research on quality of life, it has been a generalized tendency in the social sciences due to the dominating conceptions regarding children's lack of capacity to construct an inherent sense of their lives and the surrounding global and local circumstances, which would enable them to participate in the public sphere, and even "make use of their sound reason".

Hirschfeld (2002), referring to anthropology, points out that this absence of children as subjects of research responds to an impoverished view of cultural learning which overestimates the role played by adults and underestimates the children's contribution to cultural reproduction, together with lack of awareness regarding the scope and force of child culture.

Likewise, in the field of economy, children (boys and girls) usually appear in statistics as figures which conceal the reality they are faced with in their daily lives, and the abysmal inequalities and injustices they undergo. From the sociological perspective, there has been a similar omission regarding the studies carried out with young boys and girls, for there has been a tendency to confuse them with pre-social beings or incomplete social agents, thus leading to underestimation of their role as active constructors of their surrounding social space, as well as of the their internalized interpretations of the way social life operates, i.e. "children are merely considered from the perspective of reproduction of the social order" (Neustadter 1989 p. 200). Ambert (1986), further points out that the absence of children in sociology is tied up with the factors which have excluded women and their gender, i.e. a masculine bias which attaches little importance to child-care, and still less to the activities carried out by children.

Authors such as James and Prout (1997) put forth that the root of the problem is not so much in the omission as in the silence surrounding it. In fact, anthropology had an early interest in the study of child-breeding practices, considering them vehicles of the transmission of culture (Mead 1930) yet, even these studies gave little attention to childhood itself, as well as to the active influence boys and girls exert on their raising processes.

Nevertheless, this tendency has been recently reverted gradually, as aforementioned, due to the interpretive turn in social sciences during the 60s, which allowed the acknowledgement of greater agency in the social subjects, as well as an aroused interest in the conforming of subjectivities. There are several outstanding papers which make a systematic analysis of the considerations of childhood as a socially constructed historical category, and are concerned with their own right to the understanding of the ideas, activities, and daily experiences of children (Saporiti and Sgritta 1990; Caputo 1995; Stephens 1998; Nunes 1999; Gaitán 1999, 2006a, b; Hirschfeld 2002; Cohn 2005; Enriz 2006; Tassinari 2007; García y Hecht 2009; among others). As is pointed out by James and Prout (1997), as members of the social structure, boys and girls are social subjects actively involved in the construction of their own lives, the lives of those who surround them, and of the societies they live in.

In fact, researches with children have shown that the latter tend to be more mature, more rebellious, or more active in their own process of socialization than we have expected, "we have no evidence of studies that may prove that children are more immature or "childish " than may be expected" (Fine and Sandstrom 1988, p. 72). Testimonies such as these give way to a new paradigm on infancy which, though variable in content, may be characterized as such, in-so-far as it includes a series of typical characteristics such as:

(a) it propounds that boys and girls should be subjects of study per se; (b) that they should further be considered observation units; (c) they should be allowed to voice their own experiences; (d) childhood should be contemplated as part of a given social structure; (e) boys and girls should be studied from a dimension in the present, not only as future adults; (f) childhood should be contemplated as an inter-generational perspective (Brannen and O'Brien 1996). James and Prout (1997) have added to the preceding, (g) childhood should be characterized as a social construction or as a structural and cultural component of society (without denying its biological and natural character); (h) there should be an acknowledgement of the existent relationship between childhood and other sociological categories such as gender or social classes; (i) boys and girls should be considered active agents in the construction of their social lives; (j) qualitative methods should be rendered proper for the study in question; and, finally, (k) the presence of a "double hermeneutics" is required in order to relate this new paradigm to the task of reconstruction of childhood in modern societies (Rodríguez 2007).

This new outlook on childhood recognizes children's potential agency, normalizing them as subjects of research in relation to adults. Still, it must be admitted that children are not comparable to adults, as subjects of research. In most cases, this peculiarity is expressed in the form of three great challenges: (a) those derived from their own cognitive and discursive capacities, (b) the unavoidable question that the researchers should take up an asymmetrical position before the children, owing to their condition as adults, (c) the consideration of the child population as a preserved or protected group (Rodríguez 2006).

Fuhs (1999, quoted by Rodríguez 2006) slightly amplifies the question of asymmetry or generation gap as instrumental in research with children. According to this author, this is a problem which may branch off in the following ways:

- The generational axis turns out to be impossible to bridge, since it takes a bearing on all theoretical or methodological initiatives. Even though research may be focused "from the point of view of childhood" it, in fact, only offers an adult reconstruction of the children's perspective (Honnig 1999, quoted by Rodríguez 2006).
- On the other hand, the assertion of the children's capacities as social agents ("agency" of the young ones) should not lead us to overlook the fact that children live their childhood in a network of adult social relations which exert a significant influence over their socialization processes and their personal development.
- Direct contact with children is not possible for researchers, for it depends on the issuing of duly authorized permits in virtue of a system of child protection which is, in turn, anchored to a generational axis. Those circumstances will, very often, trigger the possible interference of adult figures in the research process—something "less probable" when working with adults. In that respect, it is vital to consider that adults are also influenced by other adults of their acquaintance when taking part in research process and that their answers are, in many cases, circumscribed to their personal or social interests.
- To conclude, we must not underestimate the way in which a researcher's own childhood memories may affect the research practice, for they may leak into the analysis of the particle of reality they are studying. The problem is that adults have already gone through childhood and, therefore, believe themselves to possess a vaster knowledge on the subject than they actually have.

All of the aforementioned exposition on the implications of doing research with children of both sexes is sure to be common knowledge to researchers; yet little has been said regarding the actual ways of approaching this question, i.e. the types of research, techniques, or instruments used. Perhaps it may be considered that there is an ample variety of techniques, yet when it comes to putting them into practice—in other words, the types of research, techniques or instruments that ought to be used—there is little information on the subject. The variety of techniques may be considerable, still, a mere adaptation of techniques would be insufficient, for boys and girls are worthy of particular considerations.

According to Rodríguez (2007) to a great extent, the difficulties already implied may be resolved by orienting the research towards the convention of children's rights, considering the three "P's": provision (offer the participants adequate conditions and the necessary resources that will put them at their ease); protection (always avoid unnecessary risks), and participation (allow them to be heard).

7.3 The Project

Recognition of the active role played by boys and girls within a social structure, of their capacity to reflect upon their own lives, the consideration of their closest and their more global environments, of their right to participate, and that their perceptions, expectations, and wishes be taken into account in the construction of public policies or other projects related to their lives; the need to generate knowledge about the population of children in a city which has traditionally rendered them invisible; the urgent need to overcome the conception of boys and girls as projected to the future "when they become grown-ups", rather than attending to their present need for welfare and integral development; in fact, the consideration of the concept of quality of life as an organizing principle oriented to the improvement of the present society, will allow the construction of the research project "Quality of life in middle-class boys and girls from the city of Santa Marta".

This project is an approximation to the understanding of the dimensions and aspects related to the quality of life of middle-class boys and girls between 7 and 10 years old residing in the city of Santa Marta, Tourist, Cultural, and Historic District (Colombia); as a pioneer project in this city, it attempts to respond to new epistemological and methodological proposals of the social sciences, moving away from the tendency that traditional studies have on this topic by giving it a qualitative approach which seeks to make progress in the comprehension of the sense and significance boys and girls confer to their quality of life in their daily existence.

At this point, the reasons for the study of quality of life in boys and girls may be clear, but the decision of studying children who specifically belong to the middle-class in this city, was not taken at random. These children, like so many others, feel the need to be heard and regarded as visible, yet most of the participations and research is oriented towards children of a lower socio-economic status and, even though this treatment is no more than fair, there are powerful arguments in favor of assigning a leading role to the middle-class. In the first place, this social class is considered to comprise between 40 and 60 % of the population (Minujín 2008), likewise, this population plays a fundamental role on the generation of income, consumerism, and the eliciting of public opinion. On the other hand, it is a population which has of late been undergoing a process of impoverishment and diversification as a result of the macro-economic policies derived from the neoliberal focus, which have reverted the experience of progress and growth in this population in the XX century (Minujín 2008).

Consistent with our purpose of dealing with positive and subjective aspects of QL, and promoting participation in our study, we have adopted the qualitative approach, the case study being our methodological design, since it allows us to probe into certain aspects which might not be accessible through other methods for, quoting Stake (1998), the case study is the study of the peculiarity and the complexity of a singular case, in order to be able to understand its activity in major circumstances. Out of the three modes described by Stake (1998), This research responds to the *instrumental* type, for a particular case is examined in order to contribute ideas to the tackling of a problem, or to refine a theory, and is therefore deeply probed into, its contents examined, its ordinary activities detailed with a perspective of clarifying the problem in question. The case may or may not be regarded as typical of other cases, its choice responds to the expectation of making progress in the understanding of theoretical and practical interests beyond the specific case.

The study was developed in four phases or momentum:

In the first place, the case was constituted. In this first phase, contact was made with seven educational institutions in the city, situated in different sections, and whose population of students mainly consisted of boys and girls belonging to strata three and four[1]; school-heads' and teachers' permission was obtained for the presentation of the project to boys and girls in order to determine their degree of interest in the research; a conversation was held with those who displayed interest, in order to probe into their motivation and capacities regarding oral and written skills, followed by an interview with their parents with the object of updating them on the project and obtaining their express consent. Thus, a case was formed, as an intentional sample (Hammersley and Atkinson 2001), consisting of six boys and six girls (12 in all), who fully complied with the pre-established criteria for their inclusion: that they should belong to the middle-classes (socio-economic strata three and four), interested in taking part in the research, and certain oral and writing skills.

In its second phase, which took up the greatest amount of research time, (approximately 6 months), the field work and analysis of the information were carried out. These two processes were connected at all times, i.e. the process of analysis gradually determined the field work, in other words, the latter was not pre-established but was constructed on the basis of the need for further probing, which naturally came up whenever a better understanding of the subjects and the object of the research were required to assess QL.

Considering the reduced number of components in the group of subjects under study, and with the purpose of conferring greater force to the information obtained

---

[1] Article 102 from Act 142 passed in1994,in which six socio-economic strata are defined for Colombia: 1, low-low; 2,low; 3,low-middle; 4,middle; 5,high-middle; 6, high.

through it, three focal groups were formed with boys and girls who shared the features of the initial group (15 boys and 15 girls), with whom we socialized, discussed, and complemented the information obtained during the research process.

This latter process was likewise submitted to rigorous analysis and comprehension which allowed the consolidation of the categories of analysis that constituted the results of the research.

7.4 Participation as One of the Principles of Field Work

Before carrying out a detailed development regarding the working techniques for the field work contained in the research model for the study of QL that we are putting forth, and which results from the aforementioned study, it is important to consider the underlying principle of this design, and the engine of each of the strategies and phases of the research: "participation".

In order to describe the role of participation in this research model, it is necessary to establish the concept of participation in the context of childhood. According to the Committee for Children's Rights and, according to UNICEF, participation is a key principle, a "facilitating" right, which means that its fulfillment is instrumental to the fulfillment of all the other rights. It is not just a means for an end, or a simple "process": it is a civil and political right for all children and is, therefore, an end itself. Thus, UNICEF considers that participation must be respected not as a mere aim, but also as a strategy to fulfill other aims. (Rojas 1998).

Certain criteria have been established in the research, in order to guarantee the exercise of this right, thus:

- During the research process, the only feasible information to be taken into account in the comprehension of the quality of life of boys and girls should be provided by them, in other words, adult informers have been excluded from the entire design.
- The children's participation in the research was their own decision, they were provided with all the necessary information for that purpose, moreover, their decision was corroborated by their parents' consent.
- Apart from facilitating the boys' and girls' free expression, each and every one of the techniques used in collecting the information implied a promotion and training in the skills required for their participation, thus enabling them to communicate their ideas and feelings with greater fluency.
- The participation of boys and girls was not only taken into account in the process of collecting information, but they were also consulted during the process of comprehension and wording of the final report thus validating, or not, the interpretations of the research group.

Doubtlessly, the consideration of these aspects has given way to one of the most important products in the research process, i.e. the act of transcending mere inquiry in order to make progress in its transformation; thus, participation in a research not only creates background reference to create strategies for the solution to problems, but the research process itself also produces positive changes among the participants. Hence, during the development of the field work it became evident how the boys and girls improved their capacity to express themselves, developed critical thinking by expressing very sensible thoughts about issues in their own lives, school, family, city, personal recognition, etc., and generated ties of friendship, solidarity, and cooperation with their mates of both sexes.

A determining element and permanent challenge in the achievement of this kind of results as part of a research process is to succeed in maintaining the boys' and girls' motivation during the course of the research. Meeting this challenge required the consideration of certain vital aspects, such as:

- Provision; in other words, the boys and girls were guaranteed adequate welfare conditions, which was achieved by offering the parents the transfer of the children to the venue in secure and comfortable means of transport, providing the latter with healthy food and beverages during each day's field work, and taking them to places they would consider interesting and appropriate for the development of the planned activities.
- The creativity displayed in the course of the research in the development of the field work: design of work-shops, round tables, daily activities, consulting the participants about their interests, and taking into account the capacities shown and yet to be developed.
- Empathy between researchers and participants, i.e. the capacity of a person to stand in another's place, and thus be able to understand his point of view, his reactions, feelings (Eisenberg 2000), which is evidenced in the growing friendship that developed in the course of the research process, the joy that arose from each encounter, and the affection and fraternity which has united the group and which still lasts.

In general lines, as expressed by Apud (s.f), the development of child participation implies children and adults learning to provide each other with feedback, which is the best way of expressing their mutual acknowledgement as rightful subjects.

7.5 Methods and Techniques

Different techniques were used: ludic-reflective workshop, round table, personal diary, semi-structured interview, and focal group. Each of these techniques will, herein, be explained in detail.

Ludic-reflective workshops in this research, is conceived as a collective space constructed in order to allow the development of certain abilities through personal experience rather than mere transmission. It involves learning through games, which it gratifying for knowledge is acquired in a concrete and practical way, while carrying out an activity related to the formation required through a methodology of participation. It further promotes the development of various aspects of knowledge:

cognitive, operational, relational (learn how to listen, plan with others, accept the opinion of others, take collective decisions, summarize, tell the difference between relevant and non-relevant information…). It is based on the participants' experience, moreover it is an integrating activity which unites intellectual and affective processes, is centered in problems and interests common to the group, and requires active participation of the group members. Diverse techniques may be used, especially debating. (Careaga et al. 2006). Workshops have played a very important role in the development of the field work for this research, since they guaranteed the boys' and girls' participation and motivation, due to the fact that they allowed a display of creativity on the part of the research team. Four workshops were carried out to explore different aspects of children's daily lives. The first one was called "Getting to know myself", and its object was to recognize boys' and girls' appreciations and perceptions about themselves and about the way they are perceived by others. The second one, called "How I express my emotions and feelings", aimed at encouraging the participants to express their most frequent emotions and feelings, and to identify situations and behaviors associated to them. The third workshop, "A day in my family's life" sought to probe into the way boys and girls live through certain situations, emotions, and feelings in their daily lives with their families and to explore relationships and how the family is composed. The fourth one called "The city I live in" explored the boys' and girls' perceptions of their city and the life they lead in it. No doubt, workshops play a major role in the purpose of transcending mere enquiry—for though it may appear not to be as efficient as an interview or a focal group when it comes to collecting volumes of information and saving time—it allows us to make progress in achieving the very aim of every research, namely, transformation which, for the purposes of this research, has been reflected in the boys' and girls' growing capacities to participate, express their ideas and thoughts, share with others, get to know themselves better, reflect upon their city, their families, their feelings and emotions, thus assuming themselves as agents of their own daily lives.

In spite of being inscribed within the discursive genre, round table is conceived as a valid research instrument for working with children, in the sense that it creates pleasant collective spaces with an atmosphere of freedom in which they socialize their productions (written and graphic narratives), the participants' opinions and beliefs, always respecting the privacy of the information as well as the individual capacities and differences. In the research experience on children's quality of life this technique was used in order to collect information obviously derived from reflections, discussions, disagreements, or agreements related to aspects, common to all participants. Four round tables were held. The first one, "My school", sought to obtain the opinions and appraisals that boys and girls had of their school, their routines, their spaces, social relations, tasks, rewards, punishment, pleasant and unpleasant aspects, among other issues. This turned out to be the one with the highest degree of participation and the information obtained was vital to the comprehension of the school as a scenario which permeates a large part of the children's lives, constituting a fundamental aspect in the perception of their quality of life. The second round table explored "The leisure-time activities", and it allowed us to identify the games, recreation, most frequented places, persons they share with, among other aspects. Finally, the last two tables sought to collect information on "*gender and culture*" and "*children's commonest problems in the city*". Their purpose was to attempt to understand what it means to boys and girls to belong to a certain gender or culture; and to identify their opinions and perceptions regarding issues that affect them in the local context. Though this technique plays an important part in the research design, it was not simple to achieve the ultimate aim of the round table i.e. promoting discussion by raising arguments, for boys and girls are not used to debating and speaking freely in public, which explains the option of their presentation as television programs in which each member was a qualified guest; or rehearsal in small groups, previous to the public expositions.

The personal diary is a technique which allows an approximation to the participants' subjective view or representation of their lives as well as of the outer world, in general. The fact that it is a free narrative of the participants', it offers a closer observation of facts and makes it more reliable, for it guarantees a more accurate connection between the facts written in the diary and the cognitive structures of their authors, at the time when they are being recorded. This implies that a prolonged use of the diary may succeed in reflecting, not only the subjective vision of a particular moment, but also globally embrace the time elapsed while the narrations were being made. In our research experience on quality of life in children, participant boys and girls were asked to keep personal diaries for which purpose they were handed a note-book, in which to make a daily record of their different activities, routines, personal experiences, feelings, and thoughts, either in writing or through drawings. The information obtained from these diaries has been extremely valuable in order to become acquainted with their different daily situations related to meals, use of their spare time, school routines, relationships with friends and with their close and extended family circles, their perception of their homes and home facilities, among other things. It was, likewise relevant in order to capture major events and circumstances which might have been overlooked by using other techniques, such as for instance some pleasant or unpleasant event, their preferences in music, fashion, their hobbies, entertainment, rewards and punishment at home, their daily feelings and emotions, to mention a few situations. Yet however useful they have been to the research process, diaries showed some limitations: in the first place, it was difficult to induce the children to acquire the habit of making daily entries—taking into account that adults were asked not to interfere with the process—which explains why, at this age, children's habits and responsibilities are planned by their parents. On the other hand, these boys and girls found it very hard to have a view of themselves, maybe because the educational system and the social context they are immersed in offers them few opportunities to express their opinions, their feelings, causing this practice to become some kind of "homework", a circumstance which was eventually overcome in the course of the research process. Furthermore, some boys and girls manifested "aversion to writing" for they were compelled to practice cursive handwriting at school, to a certain degree of perfection, which was quite difficult for them, while they found script much easier. In this case, they were allowed to either write or draw freely in their diaries.

Owing to the major role we intended to assign to the subjectivity of the participant boys and girls as a fundamental dimension of QL—as well as the importance of considering phenomena within the context in which they occur—the semi-structured interview has acquired great relevance, the research interview being regarded as a fundamental space for the subjects' encounters to allow the disclosure of their subjectivities (Tonon 2009). Quoting Alonso (1999, p. 228) through the gathering of a set of private information, the semi-structured interview aims at the construction of the social sense of the individual behavior of the interviewed subject, or that of his reference group; it thus allows access to a communicative portion of reality in which the spoken word is the main "vehicling" vector of a personalized, biographical, and un-transferrable experience. These interviews were individual and approached aspects of the subjects' private lives, family, school, among other topics, and probed into de different issues tackled through other techniques, namely life in the city, education, health, environment, security, fulfillment of rights, social recognition, use of leisure time, relations with the TIC, etc., attempting to reach higher levels of comprehension of the different dimensions already studied. Owing to the great amount of peculiarities to be tackled, the aforementioned interviews were held in several sessions, anticipating the fact that the boys and girls might feel too exhausted to keep up the empathy required for their free expression.

The focal group technique, according to Korman (1978, quoted by Aigneren 2002, p. 2) is "The gathering of a group of individuals, selected by the researchers to discuss and elaborate, from their personal experience, a theme or social fact which is the research object". This technique becomes an actual interchange of experiences since, when the subjects interviewed perceive that their interviewer has had a similar personal experience, or possesses information on the issue in question, they usually have a positive reaction; furthermore, this communicational situation boosts their interest. The characteristics of the focal group lead to the decision to apply this technique in the final phase of the field work and—after a preliminary analysis of the collected information, in order to complement it—achieve an adequate saturation of the themes and sub-themes thus enlarging the comprehensions reached, so far. Three focal groups were organized in different educational institutions, constituted by 30 boys and girls (ten for each group, five boys and five girls), selected according to the criteria established for the research. These spaces have sought to create an appropriate environment for discussions on themes which had not been sufficiently explored—such as gender and culture—in order to reach better understanding of the significance that being a member of a certain sex or culture has to the boys and girls under study; or, in turn, the exercise of their rights, social recognition, and participation in the public sphere. Apart from the discussion of themes that called for greater enlargement, questions related to the interpretive hypotheses of the research group were included, such as themes related to school and family for, though there was enough information on those issues, it was deemed important to count on the opinions of other boys and girls, in order to avoid misinterpretations. Apart from constituting a space for child participation, the focal groups played an important role in the processes which lend scientific rigor to the qualitative research, as is the case of triangulation and saturation—the former being regarded as the combination of different methods of information gathering, or of data sources within the same study. According to Taylor and Bogdan (1994), triangulation is a form of protection from the researchers' biases and of submitting the informers' accounts to a reciprocal control. Moreover, other criteria were applied to strengthen the qualitative research, namely: credibility, the possibility of confirmation, saturation, contextual significance, the existence of recurrent patterns, and the possible transference to similar cases (Leininger 2003), thus excelling the criteria of reliability and soundness inherent of the quantitative approach. The participant boys and girls enjoyed each and every one of the activities developed in the course of the research, for the latter always involved dynamics and free games that allowed the children to interact more confidently, have fun, and explore new spaces—something uncommon in their everyday lives. In their own words "*they felt freer and taken into account*"; "*they did not want the research to end, even if they had to get up early on Saturdays*", i.e. the day appointed for the field work.

7.6 Thematic Analysis as an Alternative for the Processing of Information

The analysis of information, or data processing, plays a major role in the scientific results obtained from it, regardless of the type of research used. From a qualitative research approach, we might define analysis as the process through which we transcend the information in order to gain access to comprehension/interpretation of the phenomenon under study; it is the process through which the researcher expands the data beyond the descriptive narrative. However, this definition may seem too broad, which has led different authors to put forth alternative proposals, yet failing to achieve consensus either on the meaning of this term, or of its techniques and strategies.

In spite of this lack of consensus regarding the analysis of information and its procedures, it is clear that it is a rigorous process which must be consistent with the epistemological-methodological focus of research, as well as with its aims, the context in which the research is developed, the participant subjects, and the resources that support its process.

The aforementioned has led us to the choice of thematic analysis as the procedure to analyze the information gathered in the research on quality of life in boys and girls, since this research fits the social phenomenological proposition made by Alfred Schutz (1967), regarded as a comprehensive and interpretive theory of social activity which explores subjective experience in the everyday world of people who are deemed to possess "common sense". This proposition considers that people living in this everyday world are capable of giving significance to a situation; thus, it is the subjective significance of the experience that constitutes the focus of study. Schutz (1973) proposed three essential postulates to be followed during the research process:

- The postulate of logic consistency: the researcher must establish the utmost clarity in the conceptual and methodological background and in the methodology applied which must, in turn, follow the principles of formal logics.
- The postulate of subjective interpretation: the model must be based on the subjective significance that the "actors" confer to their actions, the nature of the data being the actual experience expressed by the participants in the study—whether past, present, or anticipatory—and these data must be recorded and transcribed in text.
- The postulate of adequacy: there should be coherence between the typified constructions made by the researcher and those found in the common sense experience; the model must be recognized and comprehended by the "actors" in everyday life.

These postulates are conceived from a thematic analysis, defined as a method for the processing of information in qualitative research, which allows the identification, organization, and detailed analysis, as well as the report of patterns or themes based on a careful reading and re-reading of the information obtained, in order to infer the results leading to the adequate comprehension/interpretation of the phenomenon under study. (Braun and Clarke 2006). Identifying, establishing, and reporting on themes and structures, allows the researcher to reveal, not only the experiences, signification, and realities of the subjects, but also to examine the circumstances in which those events realities, signification, and experiences are a product of the discourse of society.

The analysis of information in this research was carried out taking into account the six phases of thematic analysis (Braun and Clarke 2006), namely: (1) familiarization with the data, (2) generation of categories or initial codes, (3) research of themes, (4)theme revision, (5) definition and denomination of themes, (6) production and final report.

Phase 1: Familiarization with the data (information).

This first phase, parallel with the field work, consisted in the literal transcription of the information obtained, and identification of the elements of the preliminary analysis, all of which was the result of the reading and re-reading of the information. The transcriptions were numbered according to the order in which the information was obtained and, as in the former case, conventions were applied in order to protect the identity of the subjects.

Phase 2: Generation of initial codes.

Once the familiarization with the data was achieved, the codifying process began. It consists in organizing the information into groups of similar significance, which requires the fragmentation of the information into short quotes which are, in turn, codified. The work involved two types of coding: theoretical and inductive, i.e. some codes were previously established as a result of the familiarization with the theory, while new codes came up during the process of analysis of the information.

Phase 3: Research of themes.

Once the information was classified in codes, we proceeded to carry out a research of themes, in other words, to generate broader categories under which to group the codes, thus giving sense and structure to the information.

Phase 4: Theme revision.

Since the process of analysis is not linear, some exercises were carried out with the aim of recoding the information, a necessary task considering the extent of the themes and the need to limit the contents in order to avoid digressions.

Phase 5: Definition and denomination of themes.

Once defined, the themes were categorized to allow a global interpretation of the research theme.

Phase 6: Editing of the final report.

The writing of the report was carried out through a process of interpretive triangulation in which the object of study was gradually constructed; in other words, the comprehension of the boys' and girls' quality of life voiced by three actors: the research subjects, represented in the textual quotes; the researchers, through their descriptions and interpretations; and the theoretical and investigative research bases, all of which allowed the comprehension of the collected information within a more global context.

7.7 The Most Significant Results

Approaching quality of life, in the light of this research, implies a more integral and complex outlook on childhood, for it considers aspects of their daily lives, and is not only concerned with the causes that lead to welfare and happiness in boys and girls but also with those deriving in their discomfort and pain. This knowledge should be oriented to visualize the circumstances surrounding children's lives—taking into account the successes that enrich and strengthen them, together with the inequities and injustices that affect them. The aim is to generate a new individual and collective awareness of the reality experienced, yearned, planned, desired, enjoyed, and endured by boys and girls, today—regarding the fulfillment and exercise of rights and the need to improve quality of life as vital elements in the construction of a society where the imperatives of justice, autonomy, liberty, dignity and equality of opportunity, are possible for every human being.

The process developed with boys and girls has corroborated the fact that in their daily lives, interrelating with their peers as well as adults, they internalize and construct significance in their lives as well as in the reality of which they are part, by giving shape to meanings, challenges, practices which constitute them as unique, unrepeatable, different, singular human beings (subjectivity). On the other hand, their opportunity to interact makes boys and girls aware of what they have in common, which allows for dialogue, deliberation, self-knowledge, and recognition as subjects carrying a discourse and capable of transforming action—issues which are ignored or disregarded in family circles, schools and social circles, thus accentuating the individual and collective position of inferiority, dependence, or incapacity of boys and girls. The results of this research shed light on children's enormous potential to attend to their own lives, reflect upon them and produce knowledge which will aim at improving the conditions in which they construct their own biographies.

This research reveals that boys and girls relate their quality of life with: living conditions, family, friends, school, public life, rights, use of technology, and global satisfaction. These themes make allusion to the two dimensions through which this concept may be studied: objective and subjective, articulated in daily experience.

The objective dimension has been traditionally more often considered in the assessment of quality of life; it refers to material possessions and service a person may have access to, and is characterized by the fact that the information it offers may be corroborated by external agents. When making allusion to this dimension, the boys and girls under study showed a clear comprehension of the economic and labor situation of their parents, since they assume it as a determiner of their living conditions (food, housing, education, recreation, among others), and as a conditioning factor in the construction of their projection of the future.

In spite of the evident preoccupations of the middle classes to guarantee a worthy existence for their families, and of their great efforts to cope with basic needs, more than half the population of mothers and fathers of boys and girls participating in the research show signs of labor vulnerability and instability which derive in the persistence of problems related to health (common recurrent illnesses); nutrition (unhealthy menus, frequent consumption of junk-food or fast-food); habitation (not owning a house); quality of the education received (the latter being generally considered low, according to State testing); and recreation (short periods, deteriorated and insecure recreation spaces, or complete lack of them). This brings on negative consequences for the human development and welfare perception of children experiencing situations of inequality and uncertainty. On the other hand, a more encouraging situation is experienced, in some respects, by children whose parents have succeeded in achieving labor stability and more stable incomes.

Likewise, there is a similar concern about the conditions which must be guaranteed by the State—such as, security, enjoyment of recreation spaces, playing and interacting with other children, health and environment—for the latter show serious deficiencies in a city which the children perceive as adverse, since they are forced to remain prisoners in their own homes, behind the railings surrounding their homes and screens, unable to carry out physical activities, and forced into an interaction restricted to the members of their families and the school community, for the prevailing situation outside their homes is considered threatening.

The subjective dimension, seldom approached in the studies on quality of life yet deeply explored in this study, is understood as the result of the global balance people make of their vital opportunities; of the course of the events they must confront; and of the emotional experience derived from it. On account of these peculiarities, it possesses a strong incidence on the satisfaction or dissatisfaction experienced in their daily lives and in the significance people give to their own lives and to the environments in which they develop.

Though the following list does not necessarily point to a certain hierarchical order of precedence, the boys and girls under study perceive their welfare as:

- The love, care, attention, and company of their parents and other members of their families.

- The support they receive from their parents or other people when complying with their school tasks.
- Their parents' economic and labor stability.
- Time for playing and sharing with their friends.
- Acknowledgement of their families, school and town.
- Obtaining high grades and taking part in cultural, sports, or artistic activities at school.
- Enjoying school breaks.
- Kind relationships and fair treatment on the part of their teachers.
- Having a good relationship with their school-mates.
- Outings, not only to shopping malls, or visiting their families, but also to recreation places; contact with nature (the beach, the riverside), among other places.
- Owning a house and having their personal space in it.
- Material possessions such as clothes, toys, school things, etc.
- Having access to technology (television, computer, video-games).
- Not being ill.
- Being satisfied with their physical appearance, weight, height.
- Experiencing values such as respect, sharing, responsibility, and helping others.
- Having someone in whom to entrust their most intimate experiences.
- Dissatisfaction is associated to the following:
- Quarrels among their parents on issues related to child-support among others.
- The absence and lack of support on the non-cohabitating parent.
- The death of someone close.
- Insecurity, slovenliness, disorder, and traffic problems in their cities.
- The lack of public spaces for recreation, sports' practice and cultural activities.
- Problematic situations undergone by boys and girls in the city.
- Punishment and ill-treatment received from their parents or teachers.
- Conflicting situations or bullying on the part of their classmates.
- Their parents' economic and labor difficulties.
- Not being owners of their houses.
- Being ignored by local authorities or by other significant adults, such as politicians or teachers.
- Having insufficient opportunities for recreation, playing or taking part in interesting activities.
- Their lack of participation in decision-making related to their family lives, their schools, and their city.
- Unfavorable conditions at school, lack of hygiene, reduced spaces, short recesses.
- Being unable to participate in community groups or activities.
- Boredom derived from having nothing to do and being cooped up at home for too long.
- Moments of loneliness experienced in the course of their daily lives.
- The low quality education they receive and the un-dynamic and uninteresting strategies adopted by their teachers.
- Having few friends and little time to share with them.
- Feeling sick.

The above list of aspects, regarded by boys and girls as indicators of satisfaction and dissatisfaction, involve values, hopes, assessments, preferences, and needs, especially related to their family, school, and social and physical environment.

The relationship with their families is a source of affection, security, company, help, recreation, and satisfaction of needs—so long as the family atmosphere is favorable; otherwise, it becomes a significant source of suffering and frustration (quarrel between parents, absence of the non-cohabiting parent, long absences of the parents from home owing to work, solitude, boredom, etc.). These situations—with a clear bearing on the construction of the children's personality, identity, comprehension and appreciation of the different aspects of the human relationships—have deep implications in the formation of their subjectivity, considering the role played by parents as significant models in the construction of filial relationships.

Through the relationships with their peers, children experience social roles, learn to control their aggressiveness, settle conflicts, earn respect and friendship, learn to acknowledge diversity and become conscious of the needs and feelings of others. Thus, on the one hand, limitations in their interaction with their peers in the acts of sharing and playing or, on the other hand, being the target of aggressiveness have serious repercussions on the children's personal, moral and social development.

The school—conceived as a privileged place for the strengthening and display of people's capabilities, as well as a space for the citizens' formation for public life—is showing deficiency in the eyes of boys and girls who feel trapped in routine, in the exercise of different forms of violence and despotic relationships which hinder participation and the exercise of their rights. This leads to the neglect of potential talent; the meager development of citizens' values and principles such as justice, autonomy, and liberty; and to a perception of the school as related to duty and obligation rather than to pleasure. The value they find in it lies in that it is a meeting place with their peers where they may have access to knowledge which will, in turn, allow them to make progress at higher levels of education and eventually, to obtain a position in the labor field.

The city, as a wider social and physical environment, far from becoming a place of encounter and interchange as well as enjoyment of its natural beauty, has become a hostile place, lacking in hospitality, contaminated, violent and chaotic, with leaders who show indifference and negligence towards a large portion of citizens—boys and girls—whom nobody has taken into consideration in the development plans, in the generation of opportunities to develop their potential talents, or in the construction of spaces and forms of gratifying and more harmonious cohabitation. Still, there is a glimmer of hope since, in the last two years, reference has been made to turning Santa Marta into a city which aspires to place boys and girls in the foreground of attention—at least in the development Plan: *Equidad para todos, primeros los niños y las niñas/Equity for everyone, boys and girls first* (Alcaldía de Santa Marta 2012).

Another theme emerging from research, which permeates children's lives, is their long daily exposure to television, computer and video-game screens as a means of occupying their leisure time, chances of recreation, and even company. Thus, together with quality formative games, they also gain Access to violent, low quality video-games which offer a crude aspect of reality. Likewise, through these media, boys and girls become gullible to advertising which, by exposing them to consumerist pressure, turns them into consumer- persuaders of their parents. Many of these situations occur in an environment where dialogue and reflection with adults is absent. It seems as though fathers/mothers were only concerned with their sons/daughters being busy, oblivious of the consequences this might have in their development as human beings—considering that, though some research has been done on those themes, there are no conclusive theories regarding their incidence on cognitive, affect, and social aspects. However, there is greater certainty regarding the side-effects of sedentary lives and consumption of unhealthy food.

Our research show signs that children have difficulty in relation with (a) body or physical health: (adequate health, nutrition, and habitation); (b)physical integrity: the capability to move freely from one place to another; feel protected against violent attacks or domestic violence; (c) senses, imagination, and thought: receive education which will allow them to develop their capacities in an atmosphere of freedom to express their likes and beliefs; be able to enjoy pleasant experiences whilst avoiding unnecessary pain; (d) emotions: capability of loving themselves and others, of being included in the diverse forms of human association; (e) practical reason: make a critical reflection when planning their own lives; (f) affiliation: the capacity to live with and for others, to acknowledge and show interest in other human beings, to participate in a diversity of social interactions, to stand in the other's place, to be respected not discriminated; (g) other species: the capacity to live a close and respectful relationship with animals, plants, and other species in the natural world; (h) play: the capacity to laugh, play and enjoy recreational activities; (i) control over their own environment: the capacity to actually participate in political decisions, have the right to political participation, and to be protected by freedom of expression and association.

The wide knowledge obtained, directly and feasibly, in this research through the diverse accounts of the participant boys and girls, offers a broad and genuine understanding of the perception they have of their lives, and has allowed us to focus our attention both on the satisfaction and dissatisfaction they experience. This offers important clues to more global public policies of promotion and prevention, both coherent and efficacious, which should be promoted by the States; but it also proposes challenges in the transformation of child-raising practices, school life, and living conditions in the city—for it is precisely during childhood that the foundations of a good quality of life are laid, by developing their capacities, creating opportunities for valuable functioning, and turning them into agents of their own life projects.

Listening to boys/girls, taking their thoughts into consideration "here and now", acknowledging them as protagonists—in keeping with the political sense of the concept of quality of life—not only lead to the achievement of a facilitating right (the right to participate), but also to contribute information on the fulfillment of the rest of the rights contemplated in the Convention. Children's welfare, their quality of life, must no longer be considered a future aim, or an altruistic concession made by adults, it is a right inherent of their condition of human beings, which must be closely contemplated at a family, school, and community level, and become a priority in the field of public policies, which should be oriented to a fairer and more equitable treatment of childhood.

In order to contribute to these purposes it is necessary to make widespread the information obtained in the diverse studies, with the object of sensitizing fathers/mothers, teachers, public opinion, authorities and public representatives, thus urging them to assume responsibilities and take the necessary decisions to guarantee the children's right to construct the rest of their lives on firm bases, considering the present global crisis.

Since a good or bad quality of life is associated to interrelated social, economic, political, cultural, environmental, and educational phenomena, it turns out to be multi-cause, and is therefore impossible to tackle with partial or isolated proposals; this implies the need for policies, programs, projects, and inter-disciplinarian strategies, inter-program and inter-sector coordination in order to incite the participation of civilians, the private and public sectors in the achievement of common objectives.

The middle-classes, to which the boys and girls in the research study belong, though decisive in the development of all countries—for they generate income, consumption, and opinion—require public policies which take into consideration their peculiarities and vulnerabilities in overcoming crucial problems related to work, health, education, recreation. In a society with inequalities in terms of income distribution, human development, and broadening of *capabilities*, the vigorous incorporation or the middle-classes to the country's development process, guarantees better opportunities for their off-spring (with the consequent enlargement of this segment of society), greater collective prosperity, thus enabling the construction of citizenship, the exercise of rights and actual participation in public spaces—vital to the lives of young boys and girls—with the perspective of broadening and consolidating a more democratic society.

In the sphere of research and participation in childhood issues, it is necessary to overcome stereotyped visions and beliefs deeply rooted in adults, for they set up barriers which obstruct the outlook on different and often unexpected situations positively or negatively assessed by children, due to the fact that they are regarded through the eyes of adult power or authority, very frequently overlooking their own gratifying or painful childhood experiences, which are easily set behind. In this respect, curiosity, attention, sensitivity, and simplicity are greatly required in adults and, above all, the conviction that boys and girls have a lot to say and offer. Thus, it is imperative to encourage them to wish, invent, to make propositions and contributions.

Another contribution of this thesis paper is the "visibilization" of the city's infant population by recognizing them as its major actors and giving way to the construction of work forms which allowed boys and girls to internalize their own discourse on quality of life, thus generating an impact in the formulation of public policies in favor of childhood.

The development of studies on boys and girls contributes to empower them as research subjects *per se*, in the perspective of overcoming theoretical and methodological vacuums evidenced by the social sciences regarding child population. Research makes us conscious of the need for broader studies, the design of more sensitive research instruments and techniques, the inclusion of boys and girls as actors in every phase of the process, and the need to develop in them greater research capacities in order to make their dialogues with adults more fruitful.

The abovementioned requires the researchers to have an open and pleasant interchange regarding the construction of theoretical and conceptual backgrounds, based on research developed with boys and girls—who will account for themselves in the present social context—thus considering them permanent members of the social structure and highlighting the significance they attribute to their own lives, through the consideration of coexistence in diverse stages of infancy.

It should be underlined, in this matter, that research on child population does not require the creation of outrageous or complex methodologies; the point is to acknowledge people's lives and social realities as complex and diverse, therefore calling for a plural epistemological and methodological study inherent of social sciences, dispensing with dogmatism and improvisation, faithful to scientific rigor, with the aim of constructing a wide, profound, and truthful knowledge of the person or group considered as research subject.

This research work shows that the boys and girls under study have taken their participation very seriously, showing themselves spontaneous and honest in their semi-structured interviews, participating in focal groups and in work-shops, writing and drawing in their diaries, thus allowing observation and participation in their activities and natural dialogue with the researchers. That is possible when the proper conditions and atmosphere are created to that effect and, above all, when genuine importance is attached to their right to participate and credibility of their contributions.

Research on boys and girls is a gratifying and exhilarating task, though not without difficulties, not only in the research process proper, but also in practical matters such as the difficulties derived from obtaining consent, putting limits to the incidence of adults, taking care of emotional and physical integrity, protecting the right to intimacy and confidentiality. Hence, the ethical considerations which must rule all research work involving human beings should be considered before, during, and after the research; furthermore, considering the factors of vulnerability present in the children's lives and the responsibility we must embrace, as adults, in order to avoid any sort of risk.

It is, likewise, important to be aware of the differences between the boys and girls and the adults carrying out the research work. Thus, vigilance and reflection should pervade the whole process, on account of the preconceptions, memories, or prejudices present in the interaction, which may distort the procedure and the collected information. Moreover, it is vital to acknowledge the fact that, though relationships based on fraternity and trust may be established, there are ethical and role limitations which invariably influence the process and the collected information.

7.8 Final Reflection

Quality of life assessment is one of the major indicators of human development in a society for it attaches importance to people's life experiences, apart from the conditions defined as "adequate" by the experts. The exploration of life experiences sheds light on deficiencies and potentialities as well as on the relation between the individual and social spheres—vital in the field of public policies, which involve a closer consideration of prevention and promotion from an inter-discipline, inter-program, and inter-sector focus that may promote quality of life and lay solid foundations for a positive social change.

By uniting the perspectives of human development and quality of life, boys and girls are conceived as subjects of permanent potential change, with the right to develop their capacities and abilities to the fullest, thus becoming entitled to the utmost enjoyment of their essential rights and liberties. Development is conceived as a permanent process which enhances welfare and quality of life, in justice and equality.

Research with boys and girls makes sense and acquires importance insofar as it helps to empower them as subjects entitled to the exercise of rights, and generates knowledge that contributes to the transformation of parental and social practices which have a negative effect on their existence; and furthermore creates more gratifying and enriching life environments, thus encouraging the development of their capacities and their condition as agents.

This requires an open and pleasant academic dialogue on the construction of renewed theoretical and conceptual backgrounds based on the research carried out with boys and girls—together with the construction of new methodologies and research techniques that may define them in the present contexts—regarding them as permanent members of the social structure and highlighting the significance they attribute to their own lives, by considering the coexistence of diverse infancies.

This production of knowledge and methodologies enriches the social sciences by integrating this traditionally "invilibilized" population, and shows the need to develop inter-disciplinarian work in order to shed light on the complexities of infancy and generate public recognition of boys and girls as protagonists in research processes.

Nevertheless, it should be pointed out that the research on child population does not require the invention of outrageous or complex methodologies; it simply calls for recognition of the lives and social realities of people, regarded as complex and diverse realities, who ought to be studied within the epistemological and methodological plurality that characterizes the social sciences, leaving dogmatism and improvisation aside, being true to scientific rigor, and in the perspective of constructing a comprehensive, profound and faithful knowledge of a person or group taken as a research subject.

On the other hand, it is necessary to become conscious of the differences between the boys and girls and the adults doing the research, which requires the whole process to be characterized by permanent vigilance and reflection, since there are preconceptions, memories, prejudice, that may be present in the interaction and thus distort the procedure and the collected information. It is likewise vital to admit that, though fraternal, trustworthy relationships may be established, there are ethical and role limitations which invariably influence the process as well as the collected information.

This research work has corroborated that boys and girls take their participation very seriously, giving spontaneous and honest answers in the semi-structured interviews, participating in focal groups, work-shops and round tables, writing and drawing in their diaries, allowing observation and participation in their activities, and holding natural conversations with the researchers. This is possible when the proper atmosphere and conditions are created to enable this and, above all, when genuine importance is given to their right to participate, as well as to the credibility of their contributions.

Doing research on boys and girls is an exciting and gratifying task, not without difficulties both in the process proper, and in the difficulties resulting from obtaining consent, limiting the adults' incidence, protecting the children's emotional and physical integrity, as well as their right to intimacy and confidentiality. Thus, the ethical considerations which should rule all research work involving human beings must be taken into account previous, during, after the research; more so, considering the diverse factors of vulnerability which are present in the lives of the children and our responsibility, as adults, to avoid any kind of risk.

The research on the quality of life of boys and girls from the perspective adopted in this research paper is coherent with the political significance that this concept has acquired, for it calls for the participation of those involved and a deep probing into the objective and subjective conditions that have a bearing on individual welfare or dissatisfaction. Children's welfare, their happiness and their harmonious development are no longer a challenge for the future, they are a challenge of the present which we as adults should understand and assume not only from the consideration of their rights, but also through a necessary transformation of our relationship with boys and girls which involves an acknowledgement of their capacities and potentialities as well as of the diverse problems that affect their lives. The research work on quality of life may contribute knowledge and comprehension of what boys and girls expect and require from their families, school, government, and society as a whole.

It is essential to continue to make progress in the development of research work that may reflect the daily lives, living conditions, activities, human relations, behavior, and subjective construction of boys and girls—to mention a few issues—acknowledging them as research subjects *per se*, in the perspective of overcoming the theoretical and methodological voids evidenced within the social sciences, as far as children's role in society is concerned.

This calls for an open and friendly academic dialogue surrounding the construction of new theoretical and conceptual backgrounds based on research developed with boys and girls, and the construction of new research methodologies and techniques to account for their place in the present contexts, considering them permanent members of the social structure, and privileging the significance that they give to their own lives, considering the coexistence of diversity in childhood.

This production of knowledge and methodologies enriches the social sciences by integrating this population—which has been traditionally "invisibilized"—and evidences the need to develop inter-disciplinarian work that may expound on the complexity of childhood, and generate the empowerment and public recognition of boys and girls as protagonists of the research processes.

References

Aigneren, M. (2002). La técnica de recolección de información mediante los grupos focales. *CEO, Revista Electrónica, 7.* Retrieved from http://aprende enlinea.udea.edu.co/revistas/index.php/ceo/article/viewFile/1611/1264. Accessed 8 April 2014.

Alcaldía de Santa Marta (2012). Plan de desarrollo Equidad para todos: primero los niños y las niñas 2012–2015. Retrieved from http://www.santamarta-magdalena.gov.co/planeacion.shtml?apc=plPlan%20de%20Desarrollo%20Municipal-1-&x=1741071. Accessed 6 April 2014.

Allison, P. J., Locker, D. Y., & Feine, J. S. (1997). Quality of life: A dynamic construct. *Social Science and Medicine, 45*(2), 221–230.

Alonso, L. (1999). Sujeto y discurso: El lugar de la entrevista abierta en las prácticas de la sociología cualitativa. In J. M. Delgado & J. Gutierrez (Eds.), *Métodos y técnicas cualitativas de investigación en ciencias socials* (pp. 225–239). Madrid: Editorial Síntesis.

Ambert, A. M. (1986). Sociology of sociology: The place of children in North American sociology. In P. Adler & P. A. Adler (Eds.), *Sociological studies in child development* (pp. 11–31). Greenwich: JAI Press.

Apud, A. (s.f.). Participación Infantil. Enrédate con UNICEF. Retrieved from http://www.ciudadesamigas.org/doc_download.php?id=20. Accessed 23 Aug 2012

Brannen, J., & O'brien, M. (1996). *Children in families: Resarch and policy.* London: Falmer Press.

Braun, V., & Clarke, V. (2006). Using thematic analysis in psychology. *Qualitative Research in Psychology, 3*(2), 77-101. doi:10.1191/1478088706qp063oa. http://www.tandfonline.com/doi/abs/10.1191/1478088706qp063oa#.U34D-SiTIbw. Accessed 26 March 2012.

Campbell, A., Converse, P., & Rodgers, W. (1976). *The quality of american life: Perceptions, evaluations, and satisfactions.* New York: Russell Sage Foundation.

Caputo, V. (1995). Anthropology's silent 'others'. A consideration of some conceptual and methodological issues for the study of young people and children's cultures. In V. A. Talai & H. Wulff (Eds.), *Young people Cultures: A cross cultural perspective.* London: Routledge.

Careaga, A., Sica, R., Cirillo, A., & Da Luz, S. (2006). *Aportes para diseñar e implementar un taller.* http://www.dem.fmed.edu.uy/Unidad%20Psicopedagógica/Documentos/Fundamentacion_talleres.pdf. Accessed 4 April 2012.

Casas, F. (1996). *Bienestar social: una introducción psicosociológica.* Barcelona: Editorial PPU.

Casas, F. (1998). *Infancia: perspectivas psicosociales.* Barcelona: Paidos.

Casas, F., & Bello, A. (coords.) (2012). *Calidad de vida y bienestar infantil subjetivo en España. ¿Qué afecta al bienestar de niños y niñas españoles de 1° de ESO?* Madrid: Unicef.

Cohn, C. (2005). *Antropologia da Criança.* Rio de Janeiro: Jorge Zahar Editor.

Cummins, R., & Lau, A. (2004). *Personal Wellbeing Index—Pre-School (PWI-PS)* (2nd Ed.). Melbourne: Deakin University.

De Pablos J. C., Gómez, Y., & Pascual, N. (2009). El dominio sobre lo cotidiano: La búsqueda de la calidad de vida. *Reis, 86,* 55-78. Retrieved from *dialnet.unirioja.es/servlet/dcfichero_articulo?codigo=759786.* Accessed 5 April 2014.

Eisenberg, N. (2000). Emotion, regulation, and moral development. *Annual Review of Psychology, 51,* 665–697.

Enriz, N. (2006). *¿De qué chicos hablamos?* In Congreso Argentino de Antropología Social, VIII, 19–22 septiembre 2006. Universidad Nacional de Salta, Argentina.

Ferris, A. (2006). A theory of social structure and quaility of life. *Applied Research in Quality of Live, 1,* 117–123. Springer. Dordretch, Heilderberg, New York, London.

Fine, G. A., & Sandstrom, K. L. (1988). *Knowing children: Participant observation with minors.* Newbury Park: Sage.

Fuhs, B. (1999) «Die Generationenproblematik in der Kindheitsdforshcung», en: Honing, M-S et al. (Hrsg.) *Aus der Perspektive von Kindern? Zur Methodologieder Kindheitsforschung,* München, Juventa-Verlag. *[The Problem of Generations in the Research of Childhood].*

Gadamer, H. (1997). *Verdad y método. Vol. I.* Salamanca: Ediciones Sígueme.

Gaitán, L. (1999). *El espacio social de la infancia. Los niños en el Estado de Bienestar.* Madrid: Comunidad de Madrid.

Gaitán, L. (2006a). La nueva sociología de la infancia. Aportaciones de una mirada distinta. *Política y sociedad, 43*(1), 9–26.

Gaitán, L. (2006b). El bienestar social de la infancia y los derechos de los niños. *Política y sociedad, 43*(1), 63–80.

García, M., & Hecht, A. C. (2009). Los niños como interlocutores en la investigación antropológica. Consideraciones a partir de un taller de memoria con niños y niñas indígenas. *Tellus, 17,* 163–186.

Guardián-Fernández, A. (2007). *El paradigma cualitativo en la investigación socioeducativa.* Colección Investigación y Desarrollo Ejecutivo Regional (IDER). Coordinación Educativa y Cultural Centroamericana (CECC) y Agencia Española de Cooperación Internacional (AECI). San José, Costa Rica.

Hammersley, M., & Atkinson, P. (2001). *Etnografía. Métodos de investigación.* Barcelona: Paidós.

Herrera, J. D. (2009). *La comprensión de lo social. Horizonte hermenéutico de las ciencias sociales* (1st Ed.). Bogotá: CINDE.

Hirschfeld, L. (2002). Why don't anthropologists like children? *American Anthropologist, 104*(2), 611–627.

Honing, M.-S. et al. (Hrsg.). (1999). *Aus der Perspektive von Kindern? Zur Methodologie der Kindheitsforschung,* München, Juventa-Verlag.

Huebner, E. S. (2004). Research on assessment of life satisfaction of children and adolescents. *Social Indicators Research, 66*(1-2), 3–33.

James, A., & Prout, A. (Eds.). (1997). *Constructing and reconstructing childhood: Contemporany issues in the sociological study of childhood.* London: Routledge falmer Press.

Korman, A. (1978). *Psícología de la industria y de las organizaciones.* Madrid: Marova.

Leininger, M. (2003). Criterios de evaluación y crítica de los estudios de investigación cualitativa. In J. M. Morse (Ed.), *Asuntos críticos en los métodos de investigación cualitativa* (E. Zimmerman, Trad., pp. 114–137). Medellín: Universidad de Antioquia.

Lora, E. (Coord). (2008). *Calidad de vida más allá de los hechos.* Washington D.C.: Banco Interamericano de Desarrollo BID-Fondo de Cultura Económica.

Mead, M. (1930). *Growing up in New Guinea.* New York: William Morrow.

Mieles, M. D., & Tonon, G. (2012). *Calidad de vida de niños y niñas de sectores medios de la sociedad: estudio de caso en Santa Marta, Distrito Turístico Cultural e Histórico, Colombia.* Tesis doctoral inédita. Manizales: CINDE, Universidad de Manizales.

Minujín, A. (2008). *Vulnerabilidad y resiliencia de la clase media en América Latina. Programa de graduados en asuntos internacionales.* New York: The New School.

Neustadter, R. (1989). The politics of growing up: The status of childhood in modem social thought. *Current Perspective in Social Theory, 9,* 199–221.

Nunes, A. (1999). *A sociedade das crianças A'uwë-Xavante.* Por uma antropologia da criança. Instituo de Innovaçao Educacional, Ministério da Educaçao, Lisboa.

Ricoeur, P. (2003). *Sí mismo como otro.* México: Siglo XXI.

Rodríguez, I. (2006). Redefiniendo el trabajo metodológico cualitativo con niños: el uso de la entrevista de grupo aplicada al estudio de la tecnología. *Empiria Revista de metodología de ciencias socials,* (12), 65–88.

Rodríguez, I. (2007). *Para una sociología de la infancia.* Monografías (No. 245). Madrid: CIS, Centro de investigaciones sociológicas.

Rojas, H. (1998). Promoviendo la participación de niñas, niños, adolescentes y jóvenes: Las experiencias de Aquitania y CORABASTOS, Colombia. En: Abegglen, B. y Benes, B. (Comp.). *La participación de niños y adolescentes en el contexto de la Convención sobre los derechos del niño: visiones y perspectivas.* Actas del seminario, Bogotá 7-8 de diciembre de 1998, 77–84. Bogotá: UNICEF.

Santos, B. (2009). *Una epistemología del sur: la reinvención del conocimiento y emancipación social.* Editor José Guadalupe Gandarilla Salgado. México: CLACSO-Siglo XXI editores.

Saporiti, A., & Sgritta, G. (1990). *Childhood as a Social Phenomenon: National Report* (Vol. 2). Italy: European Centre.

Schutz, A. (1967). *The phenomenology of the social world* [Trans.: G. Walsh & F. Lehnert]. Evanston: North Western University Press. (Trabajo original publicado en 1932).

Schutz, A. (1973). *Collected papers II: The problem of social reality.* La Haya: Martinus Nijhoff.
Setién, M. L. (1993). *Indicadores sociales de calidad de vida: Un sistema de medición aplicado al País Vasco.* Monografías (No. 133). Madrid: CIS, Centro de Investigaciones Sociológicas.
Stake, R. (1998). *Investigación con estudio de casos.* Madrid: Ediciones Morata, S.L.
Stephens, S. (1998). Challenges of developing an ethnography of children and childhood. *American Anthropologist, 100*(2), 530–531.
Tassinari, A. (2007). Concepçoes indígenas de infância no Brasil. *Tellus, 13,* 11–25.
Taylor, S. J., & Bogdan, R. (1994). *Introducción a los métodos cualitativos de investigación. La búsqueda de significados.* Barcelona: Paidós.
Tonon, G. (Ed.). (2006). *Juventud y protagonismo ciudadano.* Buenos Aires: Espacio Editorial.
Tonon, G. (Ed.). (2009). *Reflexiones latinoamericanas sobre investigación cualitativa.* Buenos Aires: San Justo. (Prometeo libros- UNLAM).
Vattimo, G. (1991). *Ética de la interpretación.* Barcelona: Paidós.

Chapter 8
Qualitative Studies of Young People's Quality of Life in Urban and Rural Areas

Lucia Zanabria Ruiz

8.1 Satisfaction with Life in the Community

The study of life satisfaction in the community has been developing since the 1980 s, showing a display from the twenty-first century.

Whorton and Moore (1984) in their study *Summative scales for measuring community satisfaction* developed a welfare measure based on six dimensions community. The dimensions were chosen from a wider range of issues related to the community, a panel of experts who are actively involved in EU research and implementation of technical assistance to communities whole. These dimensions included: concern about crime, concerns about the availability of jobs, concerns about access to adequate health care; concern about available housing, satisfaction with public education, and community satisfaction.

Zumbo and Michalos (1998) conducted a study entitled *Quality of life in Jasper Alberta*—Canada, which explored and explained the beliefs and attitudes of citizens' satisfaction in a wide variety of aspects of their community and their lives. This extensive research employed open-ended questions about the best and worst things about living in Jasper, and that would change things to improve the quality of life. Health, hospitals and clinics, recreational opportunities, social services, shopping centers, personal courage, sanitation and taxes, child care, services for the elderly and disabled. In the present study the following indicators were taken into account waste disposal, finance, home and neighborhood, work, government, educational opportunities and relationships.

This chapter arises from the author's doctoral thesis entitled: *Satisfaction with life in the community, a study of young people in urban and rural communities*, for which she obtained a Ph.D. in Psychology from the Universidad de Palermo, Argentina. The thesis was directed by Dra.Graciela Tonon.

L. Zanabria Ruiz (✉)
CICS Faculty of Social Sciences, Universidad de Palermo,
Ciudad Autónoma de Buenos Aires, Argentina
e-mail: luciazrf217@hotmail.com

G. Tonon (ed.), *Qualitative Studies in Quality of Life*,
Social Indicators Research Series 55, DOI 10.1007/978-3-319-13779-7_8

Sirgy and Cornwell (2001), the study *Further validation of the Sirgy et al.'s measure of quality of life* community. They proposed a measure of the quality of community life (QOL). This measure reflects satisfaction with services based on the way these services contribute to the overall community satisfaction and satisfaction with life in general community. Whereas satisfaction with the services provided by the government (police, fire, library, etc.), with business services (banking/ savings, insurance, department stores, etc.), with nonprofit services (assistance abuse drugs and alcohol, crisis intervention, religious services, etc.) and satisfaction with other aspects of the community and the quality of the environment, the change in the natural landscape, the cost of living, crime, relationships with people, neighborhood and housing.

Later Sirgy (2001) have performed a study method *Measurement and evaluation of the quality of life of the community*, based on the theoretical concept which states that the satisfaction of the members of a community in relation to public service individual (police, fire protection, rescue services and libraries), business services (banks and savings, insurance, and trade) and non-profit services (care services for drug addicts, the crisis intervention and religious) influence mood overall satisfaction with the community (general community satisfaction). The author suggests that the overall community satisfaction, with satisfaction with other relevant areas of life (work, family, leisure, etc.) influences overall life satisfaction, and use the theory Bottom-up-spillover, firmly established theory in the investigation of quality of life to explain the theoretical concepts

Christakopoulou et al. (2001) in their research, entitled *The community well-being questionnaire: theoretical context and initial assessment of its reliability and validity*, developed a community welfare measure, based on a review of the research literature regarding the antecedents and consequences of satisfaction of the community. The authors identified six dimensions that captures the concept of welfare of the community: a good place to live (the degree of satisfaction of residents with housing and environmental conditions), a social community (the residents feel there is a sense of community, formal and informal social networks within the area provide access to resources, social support, moral, and assistance in dealing with problems of life), an economic community (the relative strength of the local economy, the relative appeal of commercial areas), a political community (degree to which residents are involved in receiving information about future developments in the area and the degree of participation in decision -making regarding with local development projects), a community that provides residents personal space (sense of belonging compared to live there) and a community that is part of a larger geographical entity (perception that the community is linked economically and socially with access to a larger urban area that provides access to the facilities and services which are beyond the local community).

Tonon, since 2002, has conducted research with young people, using different questionnaires considered, the level of satisfaction with life as a whole, the level of satisfaction with being part of the community, the level of perception of neighborhood safety, the evaluation of life and having a life project.

Royuela et al. (2003) developed a model study of the quality of life in the community based on three pillars: advancement opportunities (leads to the study of the possibilities of social mobility of individuals, the possibilities of improving infrastructure and equipment of housing opportunities and promotions for subjects in the employment and education) level, the existence of social inequalities, and the study of living conditions in the community (housing, equipment and building structure; public transit, educational services, schools for education, libraries, health care system, hospitals, clinics and nursing homes, private practices, community care health, pharmacy, environment and climate, cultural centers, cinemas, theaters, houses of culture, libraries, art galleries, museums, spaces for the enjoyment of leisure and sports, clubs, sports fields, gymnasiums, squares.

Another relevant study about quality of life indictors are included in *the Guidelines for National Indicators of Subjective Well- Being and Ill -Being,* conducted by Diener in 2005 in the Journal of Happiness Studies, considering: health care, public health, social services, parks and recreation, work life, transportation, family, and the environment.

Sirgy et al. (2008) developed a study that argued that satisfaction with community services plays an important role in community well-being, understand as overall satisfaction with the community, the perception of quality of life in the community and perceived quality of life. The hypothesis was that the level of satisfaction with the community in which the subjects was determined largely by government services it will provide businesses that can be developed and non-profit services. The axes analyzed were: satisfaction with: housing, education, local government, health care, the possibility of finding employment, public safety, the existence of places to religious worship, the existence and availability of shopping, public transportation, the existence of places to enjoy leisure time. The study also showed that satisfaction with the community led people to commit to it and that greater satisfaction with community services (eg. police) and the conditions of life in the community (eg. ethnic relations), potentiated greater satisfaction with life in the community (Sirgy et al. 2008).

In the research *Developing a Measure of Community Well -Being Base on Perceptions of Impact in Various Life Domains* conducted by Sirgy et al. (2009) in Flint, Michigan, United States, the authors proposed a new measure of community well-developed based on the notion that residents have concerning their perception of their quality of life, the impact of community services and conditions in various areas of life (fourteen specified areas: welfare social, leisure and recreation, health, safety, family and home, politics, spirituality, neighborhood, environment, transport, education, work, economy and consumer satisfaction). These perceptions influence the general level residents on the welfare of the community, their commitment to the community, and satisfaction with life in general.

The level of satisfaction with life in the community of a person is a report of how he/she considers the level of life satisfaction in community-dwelling. Likewise refer to construct raised by Tonon (2010) positive community when being part of it, allows its members to develop a good life or at least a better life if they inhabit another community, and argues that situations forwarded to feel satisfied in the community would be: in public safety, social services, interaction among neighbors, infrastructure and equipment, public transportation, ability to work, enjoy leisure time, possibility of meeting in public spaces with community members to exchange ideas and discuss common problems and concerns.

Sirgy and Cornwell (2001) indicate that satisfaction with community services and community conditions predict a significant portion of the variance in satisfaction with the community, the authors suggest that satisfaction with the community was a predictor of satisfaction with life, the premise was that it is functionally relates satisfaction with all areas of life.

In a study conducted by Sirgy et al. (2008) on how to influence the community services on the quality of life for residents, revealed that satisfaction with community services tend to have an impact on the welfare of the community directly or through life satisfaction in several areas, education, health, availability of labor, government, public safety, transport and shopping. Importantly, almost all of these indicators were used in this investigation except for shopping.

Royuela et al. (2003) presented the Quality of Life Index (CQLI) applied to 314 municipalities in the province of Barcelona (Spain) during the 90s. The CQLI considers three main components of quality of life: (a) individual opportunities of progress in terms of wealth, work, education, health, (b) opportunities for mobility, social balance index that considers social, whether sexual inequality, migration, housing, access to services for seniors (c) conditions of life of the community, considers housing, public transit, educational services, health care, environment, culture and local taxes. Yet it is an instrument to be used by local policy makers as it presents an overview of the quality of life in local communities and focused on each dimension of the same vision.

The results of the study conducted by Tonon (2005) on quality of life of young people showed that the level of satisfaction of being a member of the community has an average of 6.04 which is below the overall average obtained in other studies this trend is also observed in other countries. Only 17.8 % of participants reported participating in an organization or community institution. The author said that actually the participation of young people is more connected to virtual communities than to the socio- geographical spaces in which they live.

With the foregoing and in accordance with Tonon (2009) one of the objectives of democratic societies is to promote the good life of citizens, thereby achieving a society in which people feel happy, healthy, able to have a high level of welfare. That is why public policy should make you feel happier and more committed to the lives of citizens, so could not think targeting public policies, only to grow the economy, being necessary to enhance the lives of local communities. It is in this sense that the present investigation seeks to recognize dimensions that promote life satisfaction in community for young people that live in different types of communities.

8.2 Urban and Rural

8.2.1 The Neighborhood as Urban Community

In methodological terms, the definition of urban and rural has not been without problems, since it is complex compatibility criteria of different types (numeric, political-administrative, landscape, functional, etc.) and, in general, the researchers there has been a heated debate on the definition of both terms.

The world not so long ago was primarily rural, the industrial revolution brought about by the emergence of technological development, created favorable economic conditions that profoundly affected the configuration of cities, significantly increasing its size. The changes throughout the twentieth century, generated a set of changes in transport, production, organization, and migration accelerated in the urban centers, generating some urban revolution, as a result of the above paper of cities in the direction of the economy, politics, culture became stronger; ran parallel giving a quantitative growth of cities and urban centers of different order, hence the development is part of the most visible transformations and deepest of modern society, rapidly in the twentieth century, urban centers are turning into places whose demographic weight is dominant. One hundred years ago 9% of the world population lived in cities, and by the end of the last century and beginning of this, 50% of people living in an urban environment, in the case of Latin America has experienced strong population growth in recent decades, a process associated with severe and uncontrolled urbanization between 1995 and 2009, the total population of the region increased from 472 to 575 million people, representing an increase of 103 million (CEPAL (2008).

The traits most often been considered to characterize the urban reality are essentially the size and population density, construction, life lines, road networks, non-farm activity, higher education (compared with the rural environment), more specialization of labor and mode of life, as well as certain social characteristics, such as the heterogeneity, urban culture and the degree of social interaction of urban areas.

Urban areas include large concentrated masses that are not interested, at least immediately, by obtaining raw materials, food, textile and general comfort, but are linked to the transport industries, the trade and the education of the population, the state administration or simply to live in the city. The general characteristics of urban communities include social density, spatial density, different degrees of pollution and are pollution by different means of transport as well as its volume, visual, auditory, olfactory pollution, high levels of educational endowments, sanitation cultural infrastructure, sports, parks, public spaces, social connections, entertainment, etc.

Urban communities are the set of individuals organized and established in the same territory, for its size and shape, development of cities. For methodological purposes of the investigation, the term urban community is taken, similar to the neighborhood given by Buraglia (1999) who defines it as an identifiable unit planning, an organized system of relationships at a certain scale of the city and the seat of a particular urban community and relates this communicability features, sociability, sustainability, variety, recursion, rooting, security control, tolerance, solidarity and prospecting. The neighborhood is a space familiar to the subjects involved known social and cultural practices and, by the same author and from a socio- spatial position, the neighborhood is container components such as territory, centrality, social facilities and common references, the neighborhood treated as coordinator between the various scales of urban social life, family life integrator, spatial reference, identity generator, coordinator between various degrees of privacy and inclusive social networks of solidarity and support.

About the location, Saraví (2004) states that this can be understood as that portion of the public space in general (anonymous for everyone) where creeps slowly particularized private space due to their everyday practical use. As a result of this closeness and immediacy, the neighborhood public space assumes a particular relevance in the experiences and lives of those involved (the neighbors), and can be attributed a direct effect on the local community to the extent that gives rise to various practices of sociability, in fact, the public space is fundamental to the very existence of the community ingredient, but its effects on the community as a whole and neighbors in particular, can be positive or negative (in terms of an advantage or a disadvantage).

8.2.2 The Rural Community

At present the rural areas cannot be considered independently, but high interdependence relationship with urban space, relationship materialized through migration, displacement for service provisioning, food, education or uses should be established recreational, residential, and strong changes that wins the rural economy today by multiple sectors and diversified, producing a rural—urban continuum (Espindola 2002). This dynamic has led to a reconceptualization of rural areas in the scientific community called "new rurality" in which it is no longer possible to refer to the backward versus modern, or at agricultural versus industrial.

Actually numerous features exist showing multidirectional process of linking urban and rural, in this case the strong boundaries between urban and rural are blurred and require a more dynamic concept of rural young people definition, so some authors emphasize its heterogeneity, according to various characteristics of each geography where articulate differently the local culture itself and the strong influence of global culture (Romero 2003). Added to that, Camos (1995) reports that rurality, in advanced industrial societies is undoubtedly heterogeneous and changing, there is a homogeneous rural world: the difference between coastal towns, mountain villages and towns of the interior is very important, but above all, each located rurality consists of many children, adults, young people, immigrants, neo-rurals (revalued people, rural areas), tourist homes which receive live and have very different attitudes of the rural world around them.

In relation to psychology, the emphasis of study and research occurred in urban populations, leaving out rural, especially the specifics of the populations living in these areas, it is therefore important to recognize the profound differences between life contexts.

In 2010, Mexico published in the journal *Contributions from Psychology and Sociology at Rurality* (Rojo 2010), it issues facing psychosocial analysis of subjective well-being and quality are addressed life in rural Mexico and Brazil, the conceptual problems of the new paradigm of rurality and the factors associated with social capital raises. In the conclusions on life satisfaction, it is found strongly related to social support networks, following this association levels and finally the expectations of education, in the same order of importance as food. In a study conducted by Browne (2004) found that the social group in which the individual is determined by your state of health and quality of life. The rural area averages presented in all assessments of quality of life including: general health, vitality, mental health, general physical functioning scale and, by tapping low only in social functioning. There seems to be agreement that the low level of community participation in family groups and generates a perception of poor social functioning (Browne 2004; Chamblas and Godoy 2007; Mikkelsen and Velázquez 2010).

In the case of Argentina, most of its economy revolves around agricultural production. The concept of rurality currently used in the country, was coined in nineteenth-century, and the main measure of rural -urban differentiation is a threshold determining the size of agglomerated population (number of inhabitants per city). We have generalized the consideration of the rural and sparsely populated spaces or localized in concentrations of no more than 2500 inhabitants, this approach provides an approximate and useful reference for empirical research, which was considered in this investigation.

On rural concept, we can say that it is a socially and historically specific construction, which defines a portion of territory different from other (eg urban), with certain attributes, physical, geographical, administrative, political, demographic characteristics and economic functions and social. It can be defined as a socioeconomic institution in a geographical area with four basic components: a territory that works as a source of natural resources and raw materials, receiver and support economic activities, a population, based on a certain cultural pattern, practice activities very various production, consumption and social relationship, forming a complex socio-economic fabric, a set of settlements that relate to each other and to the outside through the exchange of people, goods and information through channels relationship, a set of public institutions and private organization and co- operation of the system, operating within a certain legal framework (Ramos and Romero 1993, cited in Perez 2001). Rojo and Martínez (2010) describe the rural social space as a network of social relations characterized by a set of features (particular but not exclusive) among them, a particular relationship with the land and nature as a resource, proximity, given by the coexistence around a common space, a high frequency of interactions and exchanges made possible by neighborhood relations, the relative stability over time of associative links, and overlapping relationships and kinship, which tend to narrow ties such as personalized treatment.

The more or less pronounced presence of these features is associated with the production of two types of main effects that grant some autonomy and specificity to rural social space, the first of these effects is given by the production of what Coleman (1990) calls the phenomenon of closure (closure) office, which has a special strength in the contexts of sociability own rural areas, this effect in thick lines denote the emergence of reciprocal control in social interactions that occurs as a result of the multiplication obligations and expectations that are established among close circles of people based on their interdependence, bounded territorial dimension of rural communities, clearly favors this type of closure. Second, a type of effect that is expressed in a low density of social relations in the rural area feature commonly represented by the dominance of strong ties (close with a great emotional charge involved and producers trust networks appears) over weak ties (distant, impersonal and networking opportunities producer) (Durston 2000).

8.3 Methodology

8.3.1 Design

We developed a qualitative study with young people. The qualitative approach involves an interpretive approach to the world, seeking to make sense of or interpret phenomena in terms of meanings people give them (Denzin and Lincoln 2005). The main objective in qualitative research is the understanding of the phenomena, the internal relations capture investigating the intentionality of actions. In qualitative research designs have a pop character as it is constructed as it progresses in the research process and therefore often assume via an inductive approach, starting from a concrete reality and specific data and then theorize (Vieytes 2004).

8.3.2 Sample

The total sample was 30 selected young people, males and females, between 18 and 25 years old. 15 live in the rural community and 15 in the urban community. The process to select them was organized according to the snowball technique (Taylor and Bogdan 1998) by the natural social networks, friends, relatives, personal contacts, etc. The selection criteria was the age (between 18 and 25 years) and being residents over 3 years in the community. Then the principle of belonging (Morse and Field 1995), which is derived from the identification and consideration of participants who can make greater contributions to research according to the theoretical requirements of the study was applied.

Key informants were chosen in the same way taking into account the criteria set by Morse (1988) who said that the best informants are those who have the knowledge and experience on the subject and willing to answer an interview they must also have the ability to reflect and articulate, time for questioning and should be ready to participate in the study.

8.3.3 Data Collection

8.3.3.1 Technique

For data collection the semi -structured interview, considered by Tonon (2009) as an encounter between subject and as a technique that enables reading, comprehension and analysis of subjects, contexts, social situations, being the generator once used situations and events communication.

8.3.3.1.1 Themes

Through research technique (semi -structured interview), the investigative work has been organized around themes of reflection and from guiding questions (script) in order to generate an interactive process circular and incremental. The script was constructed taking into account the objectives of the investigation but is not organized in a sequential structure since what matters is that the respondents produce information about each of the topics considered.

The list of axes and/or questions about this study verified that the same information has been collected from each of the interviewees. The axes have built the script seek to recognize and define dimensions and measures that promote life satisfaction in perceived community young people from different communities.

The thematic axes are:

1. Spaces of public action
2. Environment
3. Social Opportunities: work, education and health
4. Public services in the community
5. Community safety
6. Social organizations in the community
7. Belonging, identification and trust
8. Social support, participation and collaboration
9. Equity and equality in the community
10. Solidarity in the community
11. Spirituality and Religiosity in the community
12. Celebrating festivities or social activities in the community
13. The best of living in the community

8.3.3.2 Data Logging

A recorder and audio tape audio file assigned to each interview, a sheet with the script of the interview, notebook, pen, a computer for transcribing were used for data logging, interviews Word 2010 document, the same were printed in A4 format to start with the analysis. The researcher personally takes the interviews with each of the participants, consent agreement and acceptance by young people with permission to use the information was obtained.

8.3.3.3 Validity

Castillo and Vasquez (2003) state that there are some criteria for assessing the quality and scientific rigor of qualitative studies, these are, credibility, confirm ability and transferability. Credibility is achieved when the study findings are recognized as true or certain by research participants and those who have experienced or been in contact with the phenomenon investigated. Confirm ability neutrality refers to the interpretation or analysis of data, which is achieved when another researcher can follow the path followed by the original researcher and reach similar findings. Transferability is the ability to apply the results to other settings or groups.

For this research, in order to bring to the credibility and support that what is reported is consistent with the reality studied, the interviews were recorded and then the art of counter—check or feedback to informants was used. This requires that participants become to verify if the researcher understood things right. This is to say that the participants verify the accuracy of reproduction by the researcher of the information provided in interviews and constructions or interpretations made by the researcher, through reproduction, summary or paraphrase (Yanow and Schwartz-Shea 2006). Thus respondents could correct, expand and/or delete information in this process there was no change or correction by minors.

8.3.4 Data Analysis

8.3.4.1 Thematic Analysis

It is an analysis method used to encode qualitative information that allows the construction of social meanings. In this study thematic analysis is used in the version of Braun and Clarke (2006), this allows the researcher to analyze, identify and report issues and structures, and can thus reveal both experiences as the meanings and realities of the subject, and examine the ways in which events, realities, meanings and experiences are the effects of the discourse of a society. The authors argue that the thematic analysis has the flexibility to be used with a wide range of theoretical frameworks. Hence the relevance of the conceptual framework of the research and some assumptions of the researcher explained clearly.

8.3.4.1.1 Phase 1: Familiarizing Yourself with Your Data

This phase involves transcribing, reading and rereading the material and annotation of generating ideas. In the study, the researcher starts taking interviews and transcribed them immediately after (as the same were taken). The transcript is given through the computer program Microsoft Office Word 2010, for each recorded audio of the interview. The aim of this quick transcript is not losing any relevant detail that is left in the memory of the researcher. On this theme, Krista (2010, cited in Tonon 2012) notes that those researchers who decided to make them the transcriptions of their fieldwork, take a decision that is more ethical, prudent and allows new opportunities for analysis.

It is important to note that at all times the confidentiality of respondents to this key (initials of their names) and numbers (in order of interview), gender, age and the community to which they belong is used ensured. Subsequently already completed all interviews with their respective transcription the researcher had to detailed and repeated reading of the information, whether printed transcripts, personal notes recorded during the process and those arising thereafter. In this way we sought to enhance familiarity with the data, some initial insights about the topics were generated, also began to see the first possible categories to be developed later.

In each interview the following elements were identified:

a) The name of the interviewee (using the initials of his name), are used to identify each respondent when the appointment in the written report of the final results of the investigation.
b) The number of order in which the interviews took, this helps to easily locate and take notes as appropriate.
c) Age and gender of the respondent
d) Community to which belongs: Urban—Rural

Subsequently, the pages of each interview as well as the lines of the printed interview continuously throughout the text are numbered. This allows faster identifying data extracts during analysis of the interviews. It also allows the reader to locate context of gender, age and community, compared to the quotations of the words of the interviewees with whom the results are illustrated.

Results such as: .... (SS, female, 23 years, Urban C.)

8.3.4.1.2 Phase 2: Generating Initial Codes

This phase involves the encoding of the interesting features of the data consistently throughout the data set, collecting data relevant to each code (Braun and Clarke 2006). In the present investigation is meant by code segment or more basic information or raw data can be considered as significant in relation to the topic under study (Boyaztis 1998) element. The way of coding is used to link the data with the ideas on that data. In qualitative studies the goal is to rearrange fracture data into categories that facilitate internal comparison in each category and between categories, allowing the development of theoretical concepts (Maxwell 1996, cited in Tonon 2012).

Braun and Clarke (2006) raise a number of guidelines to follow in this phase, which were used in the first place the greatest possible amount of information patterns were coded, secondly, he joined in each code sufficient information to not lose sight of the context, thirdly, it was felt that a single abstract data can be encoded more than once. At this stage the researcher worked with each of the separate interviews began by identifying the interview paragraphs corresponding to each thematic area of study: spaces of public action, environment, social opportunities: jobs, education and health; public services, safety, social organizations, belonging, identification and trust, support, participation and collaboration, equity and equality, solidarity, spirituality, religiosity, holiday celebrations, the best of community living. Subsequently worked with paragraphs of each particular axis, marking them all code, performed the above, all the data obtained for each interview in a Word file with a table of two columns they turned, in the first were placed the initial codes identified for each axis and the second line number to determine the location of each initial code identified in the interview, and thus as an initial code mentioned at the beginning could be found in various positions, as shown in Table 8.1.

Table 8.1 Sample prepared in the initial code generation

Interview 2MA Urban C. codes	Number of row
General characteristics of the community *Axis I: spaces of public action*	
Several plazas, shopping, bingo halls, bars	3, 4, 14
Cultural centers with free events	7, 8
Restaurants, cafes, clubs	10, 16
Axis II: Environment	
Important transportation	21, 22
Dirty and dangerous center area for many people and the presence of brothels	24, 26
Immigrants came downtown area	20, 21
Axis III: social opportunities	
Health	
S. Good hospital and medical	33, 38
Public hospital missing inputs, few turns	35, 36, 39
Education	
Primary and secondary public garden and private	42, 48
Priority is given to people in the neighborhood, accessible	50, 51
Work	
Not very active, we are far from the center	31, 32
The mall generates work	33
Axis IV: Public services in the community	
They are normal as elsewhere	53
They work well, electricity, gas, water, garbage collection	56, 60, 61
Axis V: community safety	
Advancing insecurity (everywhere)	62
Do not walk alone at night in the center	64
Because my neighborhood, I feel re quiet	66
Here all greet, friendly attitude	71, 73
Axis VI: Social organizations in the community	
Retirement centers and cultural neighbors	74
Neighborhood club activities	76
Bingos organized by neighbors	8
Specific features of the community *Axis VII: Belonging, identification and trust*	
Many identification with the neighborhood	85
If there is a sense of identification and belonging	89
Lot identification Football Club	88
I love my neighborhood and I identify trusted	87, 66
Axis VIII: social support, participation and collaboration	
Collaborative movement	91

Table 8.1 (continued)

Interview 2MA Urban C. codes	Number of row
New Year Festival, people like to get together	92, 93
It was lost before it had more neighborhood meeting	95, 96
Axis IX: equity and equality in the community	
Overall a middle-class neighborhood	98
Middle class, not much difference	98, 99
Justice is like everywhere	100
Axis X: solidarity in the community	
Donate some houses innermost	103, 104
I know many caring people	105
Support people feel	107
Axis XI: spirituality and Religiosity in the community	
Quite open in this sense	110
There is a general of the Catholic religion	110
It's everything I see another cult trial	115
Axis XII: Celebrating festivities or social activities in the community	
Corso and murga carnivals/ new year	118, 119, 120
Several social activities	8, 9
Axis XIII: the best of community living	
Tranquility feel comfortable in the known	122
Neighborhood atmosphere, friendly people	126, 70

Then the researcher made the tables and armed then, proceeded to find that in every interview they are included all codes axle. The final 30 files (one for each interview), with 13 tables each file corresponding to the axis 13 of the script of the interview was obtained. Counting each table with two columns one for the identified initial code and the other for location in the interview. Each table holds the number of lines as the initial code is identified. Each file includes the initials of the name of the respondent as well as gender, age and community.

8.3.4.1.3 Phase 3: Searching for Themes

It relates to interleaving codes possible topics gathering all data relevant to each potential theme (Braun and Clarke 2006). One theme that captures something relevant information relating to the research question, representing a response rate is considered structured or meaning. Also as a part of the information found at least describes and organizes information, and performs maximum aspects of a phenomenon (Boyatzys 1998).

This phase proceeded to build 30 tables in total (including the two communities), a table for each thematic area (that is 13), but the axis III Social opportunities, includes three issues, work, education and health, so they were 30. Within each table codes all interviews within the same axis is included. In these tables the codes were transcribed, even when they were repeated, without differentiating the interview and where they come from, resulting in a long list of codes. Subsequently ordered and grouped according to topics that cover or prospects looking to establish relationships between codes and themes to generate a first organizing thematic map of topics and subtopics. Colors were used to group the codes associated with the same theme. In Table 8.2, a sample of codes grouped into potential issues in reference to the environment of the rural community sample.

At this stage some initial codes can reach large form themes, or may form subthemes, and other discarded be, however may occur topics that do not fit candidates main themes, for them the authors advise using a broad subject called several. At this level is already beginning to have a sense of the importance of individual issues, but at this stage not abandoned anything, this is perhaps the biggest part of the thematic analysis and reflection and flexibility needed by the researcher for not including codes on a similar topic or otherwise not open to a multitude of issues that can be part of one.

8.3.4.1.4 Phase 4: Reviewing Themes

In this phase re- codification and discovery of new threads is done, being necessary to define the limits of the search to not be exceeded. When there are potential issues,

Table 8.2 Extract grouped into potential issues in reference to the environment in the rural community codes

Axis II: Environment	
Code	*Potential themes*
Air and noise	Without contamination
It is a well nice, quiet	Without contamination
It's clean, too clean	Without contamination
No pollution or noise	Without contamination
Good air quality	Without contamination
And I think if there is contamination	Contamination
The trash is burned and pollutes the air	Contamination
This better than other cities	Without contamination
Pretty neat, if the air	Without contamination
It's too quiet, peaceful	Without contamination
It is not heavily polluted	Without contamination
When you turn the dump contaminated	Contamination
I see by now well	Without contamination
Pretty neat	Without contamination
It is very clean all the air is well	Without contamination

continuously refining issues. At this stage it becomes clear whether any of the candidate topics are not really, whether there are insufficient data to support or are very different, or could two topics merge into one or more topics broken down into data. Regard Patton (1990) notes that each topic is considered in relation to its internal homogeneity and external heterogeneity. So in this process was essential that each item possesses consistency and that was easily identifiable. This phase includes two levels (Braun and Clarke 2006) and refined the review in the first was necessary to read all the extracts collected for each subject and see if they seem to form a coherent pattern, exceeding this level, the following involves a process similarly, but in connection with the complete data set. As in the previous phase of the investigator the flexibility required to debug themes.

8.3.4.1.5 Phase 5: Defining and Naming Themes

This phase requires a clear definition and the names of each item submitted for analysis. It starts when you are satisfied with the thematic map of the data obtained in the previous phase, this is necessary to consider the themes in itself and in relation to other themes. The names of the subjects should be concise, establishing the essential, not very large or complex, should give the reader a sense of what the topic is about. This phase required a thorough analysis searching for the scheme that best reflects the perceptions of young people.

8.3.4.1.6 Phase 6: Producing the Final Report

This phase begins when the subjects were taken full analysis and writing, (Tonon 2012) thus generating an analytical narrative that goes beyond complying information not as a mere summation of data. Braun and Clarke (2006) recommend that what is sought is to tell the story of the data obtained convincingly about the validity of the analysis. This requires that the analysis provides a concise, coherent, and logical, without repetitions and interesting description, covering every theme itself and flirting with each other, adding to its extracts information showing the various items provided by young people (in this case).

Among the evaluation criteria to establish the consistency of thematic analysis are identified: the potential usefulness of the code and research findings that allow the project to be replicated, the fact that different researchers, working on the same data, detect the same issues, the possibility that one researcher made a similar observation at two different times or different scenarios, two researchers working with the same information by encoding each by double – side code, and can then compare their codes with each other.

8.4 Analysis of Results

8.4.1 Urban Community

Young people in the community perceive various areas of public action; outdoor public spaces, highly accessible where you can find and interact freely and spontaneously. With which, you can confirm the existence of third places (Oldenburg 1989), taking the characteristics of informal meetings are voluntary and spaces frequented regularly present, fun, good company and conversation. They positively affect the subjective experience of belonging to a larger community, becoming a cohesive element that gives rise to the development of sense of community, allowing social interaction, sharing stories and common experiences, relationships and emotional connection between the members to recognize the identity, common destinations (Sánchez 1996) and territorial roots.

They identified the young, two geographical areas defined in relation to the environment, the center portion having damage caused by humans; key elements that support your vision about are important transportation generating lots of people daily, noise accumulation waste, etc. This is an indicator but a negative influence on satisfaction with life in the community, in the case of the young people interviewed, their daily life is given in the residential area which has no such characteristics.

Regarding Social Opportunities, young people interviewed perceive that there are social opportunities and access to them in their community, the above states through the results: specifically the issue of health, young people express that their community has services accessible public health perceive a hospital especially as important and representative of their community, recognizing the quality of health, but consider that there are deficiencies in the health sector (saturation of patients seeking treatment for immigrants, shortage of supplies and tools, lack of staff, etc.). In turn consider the poor services provided are not in relation to the community itself but in relation to the general situation of the country in this regard differ young people act good doctors and poor infrastructure hospital

In the education area, perceptions of young people are positive, have various learning centers; public and private, primary and secondary levels are easily accessible, with access for residents of the community and in turn provide a good service, some young people point to the absence of higher-level educational services in their community.

On work, the young people interviewed perceive that there are job opportunities and access to them in their communities, point to a growing community of new construction at the creation and opening of several businesses, which shows an increase in jobs, the comparison made with previous years, likewise often consider obtaining a job of personal will and not aware of the situation of the country, thus reflecting optimism in relation to work.

Young asserts that utilities (electricity, water, gas, garbage collection) are there in your community satisfied continuously and uniformly regulate the needs of the citizens, the perceived general and efficient level and recognize that the quality of thereof, are related to the services provided throughout the great city that is part of your community.

On the safety theme, although young people identify two distinct geographical areas in your community center a related area, described as insecure with the existence of crime, on the other hand, perceived as safe residential area. However, in further analysis, dominated perceptions of insecurity in the community that relate to the risks that come rising, get hurt or worse getting killed by a result of assault, robbery or rape. Relate such uncertainty as a feature macro level, installed in society, in the current situation and feel that is has been increasing.

Young people identify various social organizations in the community; said many of them are formed on the initiative of the neighbors, not the state. Overall existing organizations seek to solve their own community needs, help children, workshops for seniors and as is the quirky and interesting football club community representative case, that beyond the sporting aspect, supports different activities, settling into real support networks and community containment.

Young perceive that there is sense of belonging, identification and trust in your community and appreciates the significant place in the community soccer club in the development of the same in this regard we note that neighborhoods with high sense of community made more social activities with their neighbors (the club being a generator of it) and show a greater quality of life, in this sense Tonon (2009) reports that community membership, contains not only a sense of rootedness, but involves a sense of responsibility and loyalty, as is explicit in the interviews.

Young people perceived low social support, participation and collaboration. To be sure young people understand what this axis as the social support of the entire community, especially of older generations that they, in interviews identified the predominant model adult individualism of modern society and observe in their own community, why that this is also an important issue for them, they have very present in their daily activities and about performing from their places to edit at some point, have the willingness and motivation to support, participate and collaborate.

From the perspective of young people, we can say that there are attitudes of fairness and equality, which leads us to also review previous axes, as equal opportunities to start educational cycles and paths, and employment, equal opportunities to access the good material, participation in the public space and health, support networks. See in the community as predominantly middle class, without great contrasts, which are more similarities than differences, equality and balance.

Regarding solidarity in the community, young people perceive in their community, as there are help centers and volunteering and events are held to support different causes, centers to provide help to others, highlighting the role of the Church and Maya Jariego (2005), describes when he says that people are turning to a variety of reasons to explain their voluntary actions, among which is one of the most common religious faith. In the case of the young people interviewed can be identified among the most common reasons, personal satisfaction and political option for active citizenship (which also says the same author), allowing to develop ways to collaborate with others, willingness to participate, serve, value work, commitments and in relation to the virtues that are promoted, justice, humanity and transcendence. The results in all the interviews allow us to say that there is freedom of worship and religious expression in the community, having respect for different religions and religious practices.

Young people perceive social activities and festivities are held in the community, although they believe are still few recognize that are increasing and that on several occasions they themselves that encourage and conduct.

Finally, mostly young people value their community, the friendliness of the people who are involved in the essence of neighborhood they express about Michalos (1993) argues that this outcome (friendly people) is what most people in almost every city in the world consider as the best to live in their communities. And also appreciate the quiet, still young for an issue of paramount importance is however necessary to clarify that relate with the residential area, as they mention essence of neighborhood that even perceive and appreciate (affective evaluation) in the area residential, where young people live their daily lives, separating it from the downtown area.

Young people' perceptions of satisfaction with life in urban community (Summary)

Codes	Sub-themes	Themes
General characteristics of the community *Axis I: spaces of public action*		
Restaurants, cafes, clubs	Different places to meet	Various areas of public action in the community
Plaza, bars, cafes, pizzerias		
Plaza, a cultural center, parks, football clubs		
Several plazas, shopping, bingo halls, bars		
Axis II environment		
Dirty and dangerous center area for many people and the presence of brothels	Downtown area: pollution, conglomerate, dangerous, immigrants, trains and bus terminal	In general attitudes prevalent contamination in the community
Centro, dirty, noisy		
The downtown area is a mess, traffic, people cars, dirt		
Station-area center is terrible		
Middle Area immigrants came		
And here's all good no problem	Residential District: no contamination, clean, safe, without immigrants	
What is the neighborhood if (clean)		
Towards better neighborhood within the		
Axis III: social opportunities		
Hospital S. very good and doctors		Health-Hospital S. good, but there are good medical infrastructure deficiencies
There are many diagnostic centers		
Easy access, supplies, public health has good doctors		

Codes	Sub-themes	Themes
There are more jobs than in other years		Work-Existence of Labor job opportunities in the community
Many stores that are opening		
It's growing Liniers at work		
Signs are seen, people are needed, many businesses are personal		
Raising awareness young first job		
Very good, very comfortable, you comply		Education-A good general level of educational services in the community. Foul higher level of education.
Gardens, primary and secondary public and private		
Public and private schools, you get basic		
Access brothers and neighborhood priority		
Missing universities, west zone is forgotten		
Codes	*Sub-themes*	*Themes*
Axis IV: public services in the community		
I see quite well, electricity, water, gas	Electricity, water, gas, waste collection, public transport good service	A good general level of public services in the community
Light garbage collection, water, gas well		
Infinite number of collective		
All services reach all		
They work all right if		
Services are being met		
Axis V: community safety		
I suffered my family has suffered assaults	Downtown area: insecurity, crime	Dominated perceptions of insecurity in the community in the downtown area
Divided into two parts crime center		
Mas pickpocketing in the downtown area, shopping		
Walking at night through the dangerous passages		
Far from the low center insecurity	Residential district: safe	
The residential part well, I see no great		
Because my neighborhood, I feel re quiet		
I had a problem in 10 years		
Axis VI: social organizations in the community		
Chess Organizations neighborhood taekwondo, painting, building societies	Various social organizations	Existence of social organizations in the community
Cultural centers for senior citizens and neighbors		
It helps the football club		
Cultural center (workshops)		

Codes	Sub-themes	Themes
Specific features of the communityAxis VII: Belonging, identification and trust		
Football Club captures the sense of belonging	Belonging, identification and trust	There is a sense of belonging and confidence in identifying community
I love my neighborhood and I identify trusted		
I feel quite comfortable, quiet, I identified if		
I'm glad my neighborhood		
Axis VIII: social support, participation and collaboration		
I do not see support	Low social support participation and collaboration	Attitudes predominate little social support, collaboration and community involvement
Very little, miss more uniting people		
Everyone thinks of himself not only here		
You start to see a little more drive	Social support, participation and collaboration	
No, if the Club would not be, it would be much less than it is		
New Year Festival, people like to meet		
Axis IX: equity and equality in the community		
It is a balanced neighborhood (economically)	Equity and equality	Predominant attitudes of fairness and equality in the community
It is almost his great average middle class		
A typical middle-class neighborhood		
No, not a part is very poor	Inequality	
The difference is very marked		
Some have a good life, economic and social		
Axis X: solidarity in the community		
Churches useful if you are well	Solidarity	Solidarity in the community
Dining and church to volunteer		
It's about helping the other between neighboring community		
Axis XI: spirituality and religiosity in the community		
There are several churches, I see places	Existence of various churches and conducting religious activities	There is freedom of worship and religious expression
Being atheist went to a Catholic school, either		
Religious Activities of all kinds		
In the district gets one pants comes out walks, does not want to do		
If there are respected religious freedom		

Codes	Sub-themes	Themes
Axis XII: celebrating festivities or social activities in the community		
Summers, murga in the square	Various celebrations	Celebrate festivals and community activities
Murgas, rock, christmas, new year		
Related to football, anniversary		
Feature, organize and celebrate in the square, I do not think of it in other neighborhoods		
Axis XIII: the best of community living		
'People/ kindness	Quiet, friendly people, mobility, football club	Friendly people and quiet are the best of the community
Tranquility (essence of neighborhood)		
Miscellaneous: Transportation, Club Soccer, and friends		

8.4.2 Rural Community

Young people see in the community, the Hall sports as the only public action space, but this is not permanently open to the public only when activities are performed either sports and/ or social, which is why we can say that the residents do not have spaces for public action and third places.

Young people agreed identified as a positive feature of their community, no contamination at a general level, the issue of the environment to the young people as part of their national life context (continuous contact with nature).

The community has a health center public free access, but has shortcomings of human and material resources, in cases of emergencies depend on surrounding communities with the highest population density. This directly influences the satisfaction with life in their community, as regards Sirgy et al. (2008) when they point out, the effect it has on quality of life, satisfaction with health care in the community, the greater is the success of the health system in their own community, the greater the satisfaction with the health system and the greater the satisfaction with personal and family health.

Young people perceive that basic education caters to the population, so does the access is open and free, yet lack in the community the opportunity to continue with higher education and/ or technical, generating its absence, forced migration, this is mostly seen when finishing high school, young people who want and can perform these studies leave their homes (migrate), often permanently by the lack of facilities that provide these capabilities, these results are consistent with those found in the work of Caputo (2002) and Román (2003) on rural Argentina really is relevant to note that migration is considered as one of the central issues related to rural young people (Caputo 2002; Román 2003; Kessler 2005; Dirven 2003; Durston 2000).

Employment is one of the issues that is of interest to young people, taking into account the life cycle traverse, they perceive serious problems that brings the lack of job opportunities and sources of employment, generating voltages (greater degree than their peers urban), as noted by Kessler (2005) between migrating or staying, between local and global identities, between seeking to study or work to survive; during interviews is perceived in them, anxiety and frustration, not only from having to and leave their land and families, but because it directly affects the identity (with themselves, with their habitat), self-concept, self-efficacy and the enormous uncertainty involved from a place you do not know if they found what they are looking for (purposes changes, opportunities, hopes, personal fulfillment, among many others), and the situation is further complicated if one takes into account the level of education they have (given the distance with their urban counterparts) and because their experiences are very different from skills demanded by urban or suburban markets work (Caputo 2000)

They perceive waste collection services, electricity services and police services as satisfactory. On the issue of drinking water, its lack is perceived as a serious problem in your community that creates conditions unsuitable life.

Young people perceive safety in their community and the tranquility characteristic related to their community, almost no crimes committed, you can move freely and with confidence throughout the community at all times.

Important valuation represents the Scout group for young people in the community is appreciated, involved young people aged 13 to about 25 years, this group allows them their own space, as it promotes interaction, support, responsibility, solidarity, entertainment within their activities can travel to other places thereby establish new links, there are also many children and young people from other nearby villages are mobilized to attend its meetings. We can say that next to the church group, are the most numerous in terms of young people participation and acceptance, with the above noted that young people perceive the presence of social organizations in your community that provide various forms of support for habitants.

The results show that young people perceive that there is a sense of belonging, identification and trust, most analyzed interviews show a deep appreciation for their community (emotional and affective valuation connection), identify with it and trust, agreeing with those reported by Tajfel (1984) on the social identity, as that part of an individual's self-concept which derives from his knowledge of belonging to a social group, together with the evaluative and emotional meaning associated with it. Therefore, in accordance with Maya Jariego (2009), identification with the community regarding the saved community satisfaction, promotes relations with neighbors and enhances the perception of control over the environment.

The results confirm that young people perceive attitudes of social support, participation and collaboration in the community. These results relate to the social and solidarity organizations as social interaction with members of these constitutes a potential source of support, being obtainable resources, information, support, resulting in a feeling of belonging and integration to the wider community, which impacts on personal and social well-being, this axis appreciates the need for strengths and virtues for development and justice, humanity and courage. This axis ratio is most evident in the case of rural communities compared to urban, because in it, while social interaction is absent in public and/ or third places, if there is a recognition of who is who among the people, a common feature in rural areas, allowing more quickly identify as social organizations, eg impact on participation and social support.

Predominant attitudes of fairness and equality in the community, young people cannot find or social situations, or where economic differences are marked, being a rural community facilitates the visibility and awareness of all inhabitants, not perceived injustices same as for opportunities and access to education, health and work with the community that counts.

We can say that young people perceive their community solidarity, because there are help centers, initiatives to support people in difficult times: as seen in the urban community, the churches play a vital role in the collaboration, solidarity and helping others, we also include the Scout group again as an organization that promotes solidarity, the importance of the Scout group in the young, it may lie in what Durston (1998) calls intergenerational solidarity and its relevance to rural life this becomes the mutual aid among young people that builds in their daily relationships is often essential, while households are characterized by not being democratic or give much independence to young people.

As in the case of the urban community, the results in all the interviews allow us to say that there is freedom of worship and religious expression in the community, showing respect for different religions and religious practices.

From the perception of young people, the community celebrates festivals and performs various social activities during the interviews it was observed that are social, sporting and folkloric activities, which generate more enthusiasm in young people, most of them performed in the Hall sports

The vast majority of the stories say final issue tranquility, deriving from the security community, this coincides with studies on rural communities, which given the characteristics of these contexts characteristics these issues are representative and highly valued by inhabitants.

Young people's perceptions of satisfaction with life in rural community (Summary)

Codes	Sub-themes	Themes
General characteristics of the community *Axis I: spaces of public action*		
There are very few places here	Few places to meet	Importance of Sports Hall, as the only public space community action
No places like		
But elsewhere as well as to meet no		
Are quite limited places there		
A party, an event, but in the sports hall	SportsHall	
Salon sports, where events are the place most people concur		
Sports hall, is the only thing		
Here the only place in the sports hall		

Codes	Sub-themes	Themes
Axis II Environment		
Good air quality	Without contamination	The contamination not as community property
Is too good here		
Fairly clean		
I consider good		
Overall is good, clean		
Axis III: social opportunities		
You do need doctors (specialties)		Health-free access and free. Deficiencies of human and material resources, depend on another city
Missing things (instruments, drugs)		
No doctors on call		
Emergency deliveries or take you to another city		
We, the garden, primary and secondary (good)		Education Free and open-access, supplies. Lack of higher level, generates forced migration
Covers, does not lack anyone come (come from other towns)		
Be nice to have a tertiary (college, careers)		
After high school to go, you have to go outside		
Would be nice to stay here to study more comfort for them		
No work (very poor)		Work absence of employment opportunities, lack of jobs, generates forced migration. More opportunities for men
People go out to find work,		
If you have no education, you do not manage		
The man have more chance of getting a job than women		
Companies, factories (no negative impact drinking water) is required		
Survive-it odd jobs (short papers), masonry, hunting, guest houses, and/ or social state plans		
Codes	*Sub-themes*	*Themes*
Axis IV: public services in the community		
We do not have running water (potable)	Without drinking water or natural gas	Lack of potable water and natural gas Waste collection services and good electricity
Water, have no bad affects in summer		
Natural-Gas have not only carafe		
-Transportation (only middle distance) to nearby towns and cities		
Electricity works well		
Garbage collection without problems Police Service, either	Waste collection and good police service	
Axis V: community safety		
Quiet nothing happens, honest people	Security	Security as community property
Rarely stolen, you can ride quiet		
You leave out things nobody grabs		
No danger of anything		
There are not criminals, murder, rape, drugs are not the shots		

Codes	Sub-themes	Themes
Axis VI: social organizations in the community		
Caritas, Catholic and Evangelical church, scouts, explorers	Social organizations	Existence of social organizations in the community
There are some associations that are always together		
Caritas, the nuns help much		
The municipality also helps a lot		
Specific features of the community *Axis VII: belonging, identification and trust*		
Yes, I'm born and raised here, I like	Belonging, identification and trust	There is a sense of belonging and confidence in identifying community
I think it would not change my community		
Until now opening possibilities, study here, work will not have to go		
If given the choice I choose a thousand times		
I am part, I want it (your community)		
Axis VIII: social support, participation and collaboration		
Pretty good people involved	Social support Participation and collaboration	Predominant attitudes of social support, collaboration and community involvement
There is a lot of support from them		
Most latches involved		
If you sometimes could support more	Low social support participation and collaboration	
No, very few people involved only when there are activities		
Axis IX: equity and equality in the community		
Today all equitable	Equity and equality	Predominate attitudes on gender equity and equality in the community
If I believe that if there is equality		
Everything is good, no equality, justice can be		
There are contrasts do not have all the same	Inequality, inequity	
Equal-no, no discrimination		
If you're poor you nasty looks		
Axis X: solidarity in the community		
Is supportive if	Solidarity	Solidarity in the community
There was a fire, helped a lot		
If you think that if people outside you will receive will aid, opportunities		
To donate to the school or church		
To help may be the hospital, municipality		
Axis XI: spirituality and Religiosity in the community		
Perform religious activities Masses	Performing religious activities	There is freedom of worship and religious expression
They have meetings, go on retreat		
Celebrate festivities		
Any express his feelings	Freedom of religious expression	
Yes, I have my evangelical religion is respected		
There is freedom, non-discrimination		

Codes	Sub-themes	Themes
Axis XII: Celebrating festivities or social activities in the community		
Fairs and social parties, domas (2 times per year)	Celebration	Celebrating holidays and/ or activities
Dance in the sports/ football		
San Pedro, Mother's Day, Flag Day		
Jineteadas, people engage		
Axis XIII: the best of community living		
Tranquility	Tranquility	Tranquility offered by the community
It is quiet, we all know each		
Quiet, safe living		
Peace, peace, security		
Tranquility, we are not exposed to hazards		

8.4.3 Results of the Two Communities.

General characteristics of the community		
Sub-dimension	*Urban C*	*Rural C*
Spaces of public action	Diverse spaces	Only hall sports space
Environment	Pollution focused in the downtown area	Without contamination
Social Opportunities health	Public services and public health	Deficiencies of human and material resources
Education	Education opportunities	Basic education supplies, lack colleges, migration generates
Work	Career opportunities	Lack of employment opportunities, generates migration
Public services	Efficient	No water or gas service
Community safety	Insecurity focused in the downtown area	Security
Social organizations	Existence of various organizations	Existence of social organizations
Specific features of the community		
Belonging, identification and trust	There is a sense of belonging, identification and trust	There is a sense of belonging, identification and trust
Social support, participation and collaboration	Low social support, participation and collaboration	Social support, participation and collaboration
Equity and equality	Equity and equality is perceived	Equity and equality is perceived
Solidarity	Solidarity is perceived	Solidarity is perceived

General characteristics of the community		
Spirituality and Religiosity	Freedom of religion and religious expression	Freedom of religion and religious expression
Celebrating festivities or social activities	Festivities are celebrated and social activities take place	Festivities are celebrated and social activities take place
The best of community living	Friendly people	Tranquillity

8.5 Conclusions

In qualitative studies, the researcher has a challenge, the mission of capturing the world of people under study in the best way, ie subjectivity, emotions, the ways in describing and experiencing events, the ways they apprehend reality; requiring this active listening, reflection, relationship of empathy and constant evaluation to describe these processes.

In this research, the methodology used and favored place allowed everyday life of young people as a basic research stage in different contexts of life, both rural and urban was essential. What allowed the understanding of the meaning and significance that young people give satisfaction with life in their communities (key in the study of quality of life issues), in the case of rural areas, they perceived little satisfaction with community life derived from material deprivation (social welfare), in the case of urban areas, they perceived satisfaction with life in their community.

The methodological proposal of thematic analysis by Braun and Clarke (2006) is a rigorous, systematic and efficient way to process qualitative information, as demanded clarity on the conceptual framework, it relies on the subjective meaning that young actors have in the action, also their experience was expressed in the study, these were captured and transcribed as text, and the consistency between subjects who demanded that the researcher builds and experience brought by young people were implied in this research.

The proposal notes that the authors highlights the continuous work the researcher followed with the data and showed that the process was carried out for understanding and interpretation the satisfaction with life young people feel in the communities where they live (rural/urban). Thus the thematic analysis is widely recommended in qualitative studies on quality of life in different populations and contexts.

References

Boyatzis, R. E. (1998). *Transforming qualitative information; thematic analysis and code development*. Thousand Oaks: Sage.

Braun, V., & Clarke, V. (2006). Using thematic analysis in psychology. *Qualitative Research in Psychology, 3*, 77–101 (Edward Arnold Publishers).

Browne, F. (2004). Calidad de vida y entorno social en dos comunas de la zona central de Chile. *Pharos, 11*(002), 119–150.

Buraglia, D. (1999). El barrio, desde una perspectiva socio-espacial. Hacia una redefinición del concepto. http://www.barriotaller.org.co/el.htm. Accessed 22 Feb 2012.

Camos, S. (1995). Ruralidad y calidad de vida: Una propuesta conceptual. *Intervención Psicosocial, 4*(12), 7–16. http://www.copmadrid.org/webcopm/publicaciones/social/1995/vol3/arti1.htm. Accessed 12 Dec 2011.

Caputo, L. (2000). Identidades trastocadas de la Juventud Rural en contexto de exclusión. Ensayando una reflexión sobre la juventud campesina paraguaya. Biblioteca Virtual, CLACSO. http://bibliotecavirtual.clacso.org.ar/Paraguay/base-is/20120911115138/Doc102.pdf. Accesed 21 Feb 2012.

Caputo, L. (2002). Informe de Situación juventud rural argentina. 2000. Ministerio de Desarrollo Social y Medio Ambiente, Dirección Nacional de Juventud. Bs. As.

Castillo, E., & Vásquez, M. (2003). El rigor metodológico en la investigación cualitativa. *Revista Colombia Médica, 34*(3), 164–167.

CEPAL (2008). Juventud y cohesión social en Iberoamérica: un modelo para armar. Naciones Unidas. http://www.oij.org/file_upload/publicationsItems/document/doc1255080249.pdf. Accessed 15 April 2012.

Christakopoulou, S., Dawson, J., & Gari, A. (2001). The community well-being questionnaire: Theoretical context and initial assessment of its reliability and validity. *Social Indicators Research, 56*(3), 321–345.

Coleman, J. (1990). *Foundations of social theory*. Cambridge: Belknap Press.

Denzin, N., & Lincoln, Y. (Eds.). (2005). *Handbook of qualitative research*. Londres: Sage.

Diener, E. (2005) Guidelines for national indicators of subjective well-being and ill-being. *Applied Research in Quality of Life, 1*, 151–157.

Dirven, M. (2003). Algunos datos y reflexiones en torno al rejuvenecimiento de la población en los territorios rurales. Instituto Interamericano de Cooperación para la agricultura http://www.fidamerica.org/admin/docdescargas/centrodoc/centrodoc_411.pdf. Accessed 17 Apr 2012.

Durston, J. (1998). Juventud y Desarrollo Rural: Marco Conceptual y Contextual. Naciones Unidas. Comisión Económica para América Latina y el Caribe CEPAL. Serie Políticas Sociales 28. Santigo de Chile.

Durston, J. (2000). Juventud rural y desarrollo en América Latina: Estereotipos y realidades. In D. Solum (Ed.), *Adolescencia y juventud en América Latina*. San José de Costa Rica.

Espíndola, H. D. (2002). Nuevo enfoque en políticas públicas de juventud rural. Documento presentado en Seminario Internacional, La revalorización de los grupos prioritarios en el medio rural. México. www.sagarpa.gob.mx. Accessed 5 April 2012.

Godoy, A., & Chamblás, I. (2007). Calidad de vida y política habitacional. La realidad de los sin techo propio: familias beneficiarias de viviendas sociales sin deuda en la provincia de Concepción-Chile. *Revista del centro de investigación, 7*(28), 133–148.

Kessler, G. (2005). Estado del arte de la investigación sobre juventud rural en América Latina. Instituto Internacional de Planeamiento de la Educación. IIPE—UNESCO Sede Buenos Aires. http://www.relajur.org/tema%20del%20mes/Tema%20del%20Mes%20Enero.pdf. Accessed 17 Oct 2011.

Maya Jariego, I. (2004). Sentido de comunidad y potenciación comunitaria. *Apuntes de Psicología, 22*(2), 187–211 (Colegio Oficial de Psicología de Andalucía Occidental-Universidad de Sevilla). Maya Jariego, I. (2004) Sentido de comunidad y potenciación comunitaria. *Apuntes de Psicología, 22*(2), 187–211 (Colegio Oficial de Psicología de Andalucía Occidental-Universidad de Sevilla).

Maya Jariego, I. (2005). Ponencia: Voluntariado, innovación y comunidad. 3 Congreso Andaluz de Voluntariado. http://evoluntas.files.wordpress.com/2006/08/iiicavimj.pdf. Accessed 9 Sept 2011.

Maya-Jariego, I. (2009). Mallas de paisanaje: el entramado de relaciones de los inmigrantes. Revista REDES. http://revistes.uab.cat/redes/article/view/385/256. Accessed 18 Oct 2011.

Michalos, A. (1993). Global report on student well-being. *Employment, Finances, Housing and Transportation* (Vol.3). New York: Springer-Verlag.

Michalos, A., & Zumbo, B. (1999). Public services and the quality of life. *Social Indicators Research, 48,* 125–156.

Mikkelsen, C. y Velázquez, G. (2010). Comparación entre los índices de calidad de vida. La población rural del partido de General Pueyrredón 2001-207. *Revista de Geografía, Norte Grande.* V 45, pp. 97–118.

Morse, J. (1988). Strategies for sampling. En M.J. Morse (Ed.), *Qualitative Nursing Research* (pp. 117–132). Rockville, MD: Aspen.

Morse, J., & Field, P. (1995). *Qualitative research methods health professionals* (2nd ed.). Thousand Oaks: Sage.

Oldenburg, R. (1989). *The great good place.* New York: Marlowe.

Patton, M. (1990). *Qualitative evaluation and research methods* (2nd ed.). Newbury Park: Sage.

Perez, E. (2001). Una nueva ruralidad en América Latina. La crisis del modelo de crecimiento y las nuevas funciones del medio rural, Ramos y Romero 1993. Buenos Aires: CLACSO. http://biblioteca.clacso.edu.ar/clacso/gt/20100929125458/giarraca.pdf. Accessed 23 Jan 2012.

Rojo Pérez, N. (2002). La investigación cualitativa. Aplicaciones en Salud. In V. Bayarre, M. E. Astraín, G. Díaz, & L. Fernández (Eds.), *La Investigación en Salud.* La Habana: MINSAP, ENSAP.

Rojo-Martínez, G. E. (2010). Desarrollo forestal y ruralidad. In E. Rojo, A. Vera, & R. Martínez (Eds.), Aportes desde la Psicología y Sociología de la Ruralidad. Universidad Autónoma Indígena de México. http://www.uaim.edu.mx/Documentos/AportesRuralidad.pdf. Accessed 11 June 2012.

Román, M. (2003). *Los jóvenes rurales en Argentina.* Elementos para una estrategia de desarrollo rural. SAGPyA-PROINDER, Serie de Estudios e Investigaciones 4, Buenos Aires.

Romero, J. (2003). Metodología de investigación para el abordaje del sector juvenil rural. Universidad de la Republica Uruguay UDELAR - RIJUR. http://www.iica.org.uy. Accessed 24 Jan 2012.

Royuela, V., Suriñach, J., & Reyes, M. (2003). Measuring quality of life in small areas over different periods of time. *Social Indicators Research, 64*(1), 51–74.

Sánchez Vidal, A. (1996). *Psicología Comunitaria. Bases conceptuales y métodos de intervención.* Barcelona: PPU. Pp.46.

Saravi, G. (2004). Segregación urbana y espacio público: Los jóvenes en enclaves de pobreza estructural. Revista de la CEPAL 83. http://www.eclac.org/publicaciones/xml/8/19418/lcg2231e-Saravi.pdf. Accessed 24 Aug 2011.

Sirgy, M. J. (2001). Medición y método de evaluación de la calidad de vida en la comunidad. *Intervención Psicosocial, 10*(1), 71–84. http://www.copmadrid.org/webcopm/publicaciones/social/68008.pdf. Accessed 3 Oct 2011.

Sirgy, M. J., & Cornwell, T. (2001). Further validation of the Sirgy et al.'s measure of community quality of life. *Social Indicators Research, 56*(12), 5–143.

Sirgy, M. J., & Cornwell, T. (2002). How neighborhood features affect quality of life. *Social Indicators Research, 59*(1), 79–102.

Sirgy, M. J., Gao, T., & Young, R. F. (2008). How residents' satisfaction with community services influence quality of life (QOL) outcomes? *Applied Research in Quality of Life, 3*(2), 81–106.

Sirgy, M. J., Widgery, R., Lee, D. J., & Yu, G. B. (2009). Developing a measure of community well-being based on perceptions of impact in various life domains. *Social Indicators Research, 96,* 295–311.

Tajfel, H. (1984). *Grupos humanos y categorías sociales: estudios de Psicología Social.* Barcelona. Herder.

Taylor, S. J., & Bogdan, R. (1998). *Introducción a los métodos cualitativos de investigación. La búsqueda de significados.* Buenos Aires: Paidós.

Tonon, G. (2005). Apreciaciones teóricas del estudio de la calidad de vida en Argentina. *Hologramatica, Año II, 1*(2), 27–49. www.unlz.edu.ar/sociales/hologramatica/hologramatica2-V1_pp41-49.pdf. Accessed 19 May 2011.

Tonon, G. (2008). *Desigualdades sociales y oportunidades ciudadanas.* Buenos Aires: Espacio Editorial.

Tonon, G. (2009). La entrevista semi-estructurada como técnica de investigación. In G. Tonon (Ed.), *Reflexiones latinoamericanas sobre investigación cualitativa* (pp. 46–68). San Justo: Prometeo-UNLAM.

Tonon, G. (Ed.). (2010). Comprender las relaciones: calidad de vida, comunidad, niñez y desarrollo en América Latina. In *Colección Cuadernos de estudio de la Facultad de Ciencias Sociales*. Lomas de Zamora: UNLZ.

Tonon, G. (2012). Como analizar los datos en estudios cualitativos. In *Documento de trabajo para el curso Introducción a la integración de metodologías, cuarta edición*. Washington, DC: INDES–BID.

Vieytes, R. (2004). *Metodología de la investigación en organizaciones, mercado y sociedad*. Buenos Aires: De las Ciencias.

Whorton, J., & Moore, A. (1984). Summative scales for measuring community satisfaction. *Social Indicators Research, 15,* 297–307.

Yanow, D. and Schwartz-Shea, P. (Eds.). (2006). Interpretation and Method: Empirical Research Methods and the Interpretive Turn, Armonk, NY: M.E. Sharpe. Published, 2006.

Zanabria Ruiz, L. (2013). Satisfaction with life in the community, a study of young people in urban and rural communities. Doctoral Thesis in Psychology (in-edit). Argentina: Universidad de Palermo.

Zumbo, B. D., & Michalos, A. C. (1998). Quality of life in Jasper, Alberta. *Social Indicators Research, 49*(2), 121–145.

Chapter 9
Young People's Rural Quality of Life in the Colombian Andes: A Qualitative Study Using Triangulation

Antonio José López López

9.1 Invisibilization of Young People Living in Rural Areas

This section aims at approaching the problems resulting from the young people's invisibilization or negative visibilization in the rural context in the high Colombian Andean mountains[1]. This is a situation that affects the quality of their lives, not only before any wrong actions by the State, resulting from an approach in which the youngsters are considered as objects of protective actions aiming at social welfare, but before the fact that said actions and their results can contribute to the construction of their perceptions about themselves. This section also refers to how these actions are supposed to develop in order to reach what these youngsters consider a good standard of rural life for themselves, for their families, their community and for the rural environment where they live.

Effective the validity of its political Constitution of 1991, Colombia has been recognized as a social juridical state in the form of a unitarian, democratic, participative and pluralistic state, on the basis of respect for human dignity, the solidarity among its people and the prevalence of general interest, the Colombian Andean high-mountain young peoples; that is to say, those belonging to the farming economy, among others, are not consulted about their perception about the quality of life and the way how the rural dynamics of their environment contributes or obstacles the obtaining of what they consider a good rural life or a good rural quality of life. These predicaments oblige, from one perspective, to approach the comprehension

[1] The Colombian Rural Andean Zone is considered as that one consisting of the high-mountains and traditional-farming production sectors located in the Colombian Andean mass of mountains. The term high-mountain refers to those sectors over 2,700 m above sea level, and the traditional farming production to that area derived from the passive and inadequate adoption of the agrarian model of the Green Revolution, which is very different from the industrialized commercial production resulting from the active adoption of this method.

A. J. López López (✉)
MEN. Colciencias, Bogotá, Colombia
e-mail: ajoselop33@hotmail.com

G. Tonon (ed.), *Qualitative Studies in Quality of Life*,
Social Indicators Research Series 55, DOI 10.1007/978-3-319-13779-7_9

consisting of how these young peoples construct, along with their daily activities, their meanings about the "rural quality of life". From another other perspective, they refer to the judgment about the practical importance of qualitative research methods and the methodological triangulation in order to approach the quality of life of the rural young peoples in the study context, the main reason for this reflection.

In the Latin American sphere, young peoples living in rural areas are seldom taken as valid social actors to be consulted by the planners, decision makers and administrators in rural development programs that, finally, aim at improving their social welfare conditions. This situation is different in the various bands of young people living in rural areas who are provided with better attention (Becerra 2001; Kessler 2005). It is a fact that reflects a scarce attainment of human rights represented fundamentally in a few or invalid voice rights in making family and community decisions and in controlling the resources (Durston 2002). The origin of this lack of recognition could be explained by the fact that most part of literature about the history of childhood and young people, that has been written from the perspective of social sciences, has been made from a Western reality, which entails a certain ethnocentric bias with reference to the conceptualization of young people and obviously of rural young people and of the rural quality of life. Accordingly, both the studies on indigenous peoples and those on farming and urban families, "tended to see their study subjects as indigenous, farmers, settlers, men, women, capitalists, workers, but not as children and less, as young peoples" (Feixa and González 2006, p. 177).

Nevertheless, socio-cultural research studies are identified where, without explicitating a generational posture, the consideration of young peoples who move from apathy to protest and social complaint remains implicit in their results and recommendations. This is the case of the "Andes Farmers" authored by the Colombian sociologist Orlando Fals Borda (1961) where he defines how the apathy *ethos* generated by traumatic experiences in the Andean rural community during the Conquest, the Colony and the Republic, is a factor that mentally and socially impoverishes the community members. Such ethos is kept by means of the formative training of adolescents within the adults' apathy molds, a situation which slowly becomes modified due to "progressive rationalism" as a consequence from modernization. The Andean rural community acquires, effective that time, an adequate sense of social injustice "which generates a resignation transition to dissatisfaction and gives birth to social conflicts in Colombia, Mexico, Bolivia, Argentina and Guatemala, among others (Fals Borda 1961, p. 303).

From 1985, with the proclamation of the International Young people Year by the United Nations, it has been possible to identify socio-cultural studies that evidence how the formative training detected by Fals Borda characterizes the prevalence of a training which lacks the impulse to an effective participation of the rural young people in the decisions affecting their lives and their quality of life. This scarce participation is evidenced in the administrative and academic functions of rural educational institutions, in the lack of spaces to share general and specific information about themselves and their rural environment, and in the "minimal socio-community link with other entities working on rural juvenile aspects" (Quiroga 2002, pp. 98–108). Besides, the social conflicts identified by Fals Borda are also present in the modernization processes of countries such as Chile, thus accompanying a juvenile identity configuration in the rural sector, which ranges from a weak ascription tensed by the vital cycle, goes through a generational identity and arrives, at the end of the decade of the 80s, at "the foundation of juvenile cultures" (González 2004, pp. 643–653).

Research studies on young people carried out in Latin America from 2000, with reference to factors influencing social welfare, agree in their findings and main conclusions: (1) coexisting sectorial policies aiming at young people[2] and specifically young people-oriented policies, which are dislocated and redundant; (2) lack of specific programs to reduce the deficit in service coverage and inequities concerning the gender and ethnic conditions of belonging to rural zones; (3) the presence of the paradox that considers the youngsters as the central actors of development, at the same time that the rural young people becomes invisibilized (Bango 2000, pp. 19–21; Hopenhayn et al. 2004, p. 36; Kessler 2005, p. 5). These studies[3] identify approaches on young people where its beginning is assumed, from a natural condition, in the physiological puberty, and ends, from the perspective of a psychological condition, when there is maturity to assume adult responsibilities and when society recognizes that adult status, which evidences its perception as "a cultural universal, a natural phase of human development which would be found in all societies and historical moments" (Feixa and González 2006, p. 172).

In the Colombian sphere it is also possible to evidence the traditional trend to visibilize the urban zone in the development policies much more than the rural zone. This is due to the fact that social welfare is considered inferior, among other reasons, because the dispersed rural area presents bigger deficiencies in domestic infrastructure, the families are large and undergo a lot of lacks; besides, boys, girls and young peoples, who "are more than 50% of the population and the most vulnerable elements of the society (…) when reproducing their parents' situation", little by little revert this situation on those who work and decrease their economic independence (Bonilla et al. 2004, p. 97).

On the other hand, "Young people" is identified as a social category that emerges in the research studies carried out in the Colombian urban context no matter the reiterated mentioning of the "urban-rural" category in most research studies about

[2] The Sectorial Policies with an intentionality towards young people are assumed in this paper as those formulated from 1950 in the Latin American countries, which without explicitating their goals towards this population sector, display a clear intention, by the State, to satisfy what its agents consider young people needs or to solve societal problems which have been considered as related to the young people action.

[3] The results from these research studies can be consulted in the following texts: "Young people Policies in Latin America: evaluation and reformulation" (Bango 2000), with the bases for the formulation of these policies in the context of regional challenges and opportunities at the beginning of the XXI century; "Young people in Latin America. Trends and urgencies" (Hopenhayn et al. 2004) with a diagnosis of the Young people situation through the review of young people policies in Latin America, taking as a reference the approaches on rights and integral citizenship, and in "State of the art of research on rural young people in Latin America" (Kessler 2005), where the approaches, themes and conclusions from the research studies carried out in Latin America are described.

any topic on young people. This category centers around the urban matter, being this a fact that has been described not only as a verification of the localities referred to in the texts but also as a set of juvenile existential conditions in the cities. The rural dimension, mentioned in the research studies, centers around the scarcity of opportunities for academic and labor training for the young peoples living in the countryside, which makes them prone to join armed groups or to devote themselves to illegal activities. The research studies investigate, first, about the link of the rural young people with the guerrilla, with paramilitaries or with activities related to illegal crops, and about the impact of such activities on their biographies. Second, they investigate about the flows and connections between the rural and urban spheres which express themselves, for example, "through the appropriation that these young peoples make rural practices, meanings and objects taken from the urban world" (Escobar et al. 2004, p. 191).

In the course of the last forty years there has been an orientation onto different conceptions about young people. As a matter of fact, from the 1980s to the year 2000, "young people" has been perceived as a homogeneous reality; the juvenile period has been defined by its "adult" referent and by its transitory state; youngsters have been considered a problem or "risk that must be corrected", whose socialization agents are the family, the school and the public institutions. The State has been conceived as the protector for which the young peoples are the receptors of social assistance and, of course, as the object of undifferentiated sectorial policies which tend to, as it has been explicitated, the betterment of the quality of life (Sarmiento 2004). Effective the year 2000, "young people" has been conceived as a new stage of life endowed with enough and proper elements that make it autonomous. The juvenile period loses its centrality from the "adult" statute before the complexity and heterogeneity of the juvenile reality; the young people is seen as a "strategic factor for development" and as a potentiality that has to be promoted. Their socialization agents are the market, the mass media, the new technologies and their own spaces; the State is conceived as a State that agrees with civil society and with young peoples in their quality of subjects of rights, in the process of constructing young people policies which promote and stimulate their integral training aiming at their empowerment, conditions which "stay just on the books" (Sarmiento 2004, pp. 128–134).

In general, it is possible to state that the results from research studies that evaluate the decisions and actions of the State towards the "young people" in Colombia express the urgent need to modify, not only what is stated in the books but in the reality. These studies express the urgent need to modify those stereotypes and stigmatizations that identify the young peoples belonging to urban popular, marginalized and rural sectors of the high Andean mountain as passive, helpless and apathetic to social reflection, and which consider them as related to problems, predisposed to delinquency and sluggishness, lacking judgment and autonomy and as being in permanent risk which can be corrected (Serrano et al. 2002, p. 76; Escobar et al. 2004, pp. 219, 227). This need implies the task of visibilizing positively, among others, the young peoples belonging to high-mountain sectors in the Colombian Andean zone.

Rural young people has been visibilized from the year 2000 in the State actions and decisions, in aspects which do not take into account their active and effective participation even though they affect the young peoples' lives. They are actions resulting from sectorial policies with an intentionality towards young people and associated to the mandatory military service, the creation of the figure of farmer-soldier, the offering of rewards for denouncing the presence of "sectors out of the law" in the rural zone, the manual eradication of illegal crops in natural parks with all deriving consequences, and their link, free or forced, to migration, to the guerrilla, to paramilitarism or to drug dealing.

In the last ten years, rural young peoples visibilize themselves in the "false positives"[4], as they have been called by the mass media, which are simply the execution of rural young peoples, farmers and aborigines by members of the police force or the army and by the urban popular sectors. These young peoples are presented to the mass media as "guerrilleros killed in action" or as "important achievements of the police force or army", in the course, mainly, of the so-called policy of democratic security. Its goal is to "obtain illegal results without delegitimizing the institutional actor; thus, violating the war rules by making use of a fiction that will allow to legitimize crime as a response to other aggressive violence, that is, as "legitimate defense" (CINEP 2013, p. 7).

9.2 The Research Context

The geographical space identified as the Colombian Andean high mountains is part of what has been called the "Andean Mass"; one of the nine continental spaces[5] of the territorial mosaic of South America, constituted by the longest mountain chain in the world, with 7500 km which go from the Antartic continent to the Caribbean space, with a width of 320 km. Its highest peak is in Aconcagua, which reaches

[4] According to the Center for Research and Popular Education (CINEP), one of the most important research centers in Colombia, between August 14, 2006 and June 16, 2007, the so-called "false positives" happened in 22 states of the 32 which form the country. Meta was the most affected state: "From this part of the country we knew about 24 cases with 39 victims, authored by troops belonging to the 12 Mobile Brigade, 21 Vargas Battalion, 4 Mobile Brigade and José Joaquín París Battalion of the National Army (CINEP 2007, p. 1). Recently, Todd Howland, agent of the High Commissioner's Office for Human Rights of the United Nations in Bogota stated that "We did not receive information about this type of violation in 2012, but the Public Prosecutor's Office has information about almost 5,000 victims of this phenomenon; there are antecedents of several years and there are very few sentences at present. Then, it is important that Colombia do more with reference to this problem of false positives" (CINEP 2013, p. 7).

[5] The Continental Spaces are big regions with arcifinious or natural limits that are shared by various countries.They are characterized by being different and stable, not only with reference to their physical, topographic, ecological and landscape configurations, but also with reference to the idiosyncrasy of every human group inhabiting the region.The continental spaces in South America are as follows: Amazonia, Orinoquia, Marabina Basin, Andean Mass, Caribbean Space, Pacific Space, Brazilian Massif, Chaco-Pampa and Patagonia Cone (Mendoza 2000, p. 40).

6950 m above sea level and hosts old ethnic archetypes which yield a vast cultural variety (Mendoza 2000, p. 44). The Andean Mass encompasses three different physiographic zones: a humid zone that goes from the Mérida Cordillera in Venezuela to the northern part of Peru; a semi-arid zone that includes the Central Andes of Peru and Bolivia, and a plateau zone that extends from the southern part of Peru, the northwestern and southern regions of Bolivia, the northern part of Chile and to the northwestern region of Argentina. The most important productive sector with reference to employment, income and food supply is agriculture with the predominance of potato crops, along with cereals, grains, vegetables and flowers combined with dairy cattle, sheep, minor animals, whose exploitation varies from country to country (Llambí 2002).

The mosaic of continental spaces contributes, in a natural way, to the first information of territorial zoning in Colombia, constituted by six of the nine continental spaces in South America[6], where we find the Colombian Andean Mass, corresponding to the northern and terminal parts of the Andes Cordillera. It goes from the Andean Pacific in the west, to Orinoquia in the east, and it occupies 323,000 km^2, which are equivalent to 28.3 % of the continental territory (Mendoza 2000, p. 44). The mountain and the high mountains, with the traditional farmers' production and with the major ethnic variety in Colombia, are the fundamental landscape.

This research develops in the context constituted by the farmers' communities of the Cundiboyacense High Plateau, which consists of two of the 32 states in which Colombia is divided territorially: Cundinamarca, with a surface 0f 24,210 km^2, which stands for 2.12 % of the national territory, with 15 provinces and 115 municipalities (Republic of Colombia 2011b), and Boyacá, with 23,189 km^2 equivalent to 2.03 % of the national territory, with 12 provinces and 123 municipalities (Republic of Colombia 2011a). The Cundiboyacense High Plateau, a territory that integrates the states synthetically described, is located in the Oriental Cordillera, in the high zones of the Andean system. It consists of mountain ecosystems and páramo regions which reach 3600 m above sea level, inhabited by a population descendent from the Cundiboyacense Chibcha culture, one of the most important ethnic groups in the country.

The socio-cultural scenario of the research study, where the Field Work is also done, is the potato-producing sub-region of the Cundiboyacense Plateau, characterized by a farming culture resulting from the influence and projection of the culture and mentality of the Chibcha ethnic group[7], where the man is narrowly attached to the surrounding environment from which he extracts his vital forces. The sun, the moon, the lakes, the mountains, rocks and physical phenomena for him "were bound to the spirits, a reason why they were considered their main deities" (Ocampo 1983, p. 29), which stimulate the care of nature. Paradoxically, the precepts inherited

[6] The Colombian continental spaces are as follows: Amazonia, Orinoquia, Marabina Basin, Andean Mass, Caribbean Space and Pacific Space (Mendoza 2000, p. 42).

[7] The Chibcha culture refers to the peoples existing in the Nueva Granada in the XVI century, at the arrival of Spaniards. The most important of those peoples were Chibcha-Carib and Chibcha; the latter settling what it is today Cundinamarca, Boyacá, Western Atrato, Cauca and Central-Oriental Nariño. The predominant language was the one distinguished by Spaniards as the Muisca Language or Mosca, with as many dialects as linguistic families (Ariza 1992, p. 75).

from the Green Revolution, predominate in the present agricultural exploitations, they promote the use of agricultural toxins, machinery and capital to ensure a high economic performance, without any environmental consideration and opposite to ancestral technology.

The present importance of the potato-growing sub-region lies in being not only the territory where the water flows furnishing the Bogota aqueduct and where other cities of the country are born, in the ample and varied farming, coal and hand-made production, but also in being the most important agricultural region of the country concerning potato crops. In effect, this Cundiboyacense High Plateau sub-region counts on more than 99,500 hectares cultivated which produce about 1,800,000 tons of potatoes— about 18 tons per hectare—out of a tally of 134,640 hectares cultivated in Colombia, which yield 2,833,795 tons. This means that 74 % of the Cundiboyacense High Plateau is cultivated and produces about 73 % of the total production in the country (Fedepapa 2010, pp. 10–13). It is important to highlight that from the 90,000 families linked to direct exploitation, about 70,000 are located in this sub-region, thus generating approximately 11 out of the 15 million wages a year; besides, it becomes the activity that most uses the terrestrial transportation services, with more than 2 million t a year. This is a cipher which increases with the mobilization of the required supplies (Fedepapa 2010, p. 9).

This sub-region characterizes by its difficult access for the information and communication technologies (TIC) due to the topographic and economic conditions already described. Its centers are among those defined by the Central Administration as of difficult access because, among others, "the access to telecommunications services is still deficient in those geographically distant rural places (National Planning Department 2009, p. 5).

The socio-cultural phenomenon, the comprehension object in the research study, consists of the young peoples, their families and physical spaces—farming and mining production units, governmental and communal educational and institutional facilities –, and their actions and interactions, among themselves and with the other social actors and with the rural space where they are located. The findings of this research study allow one to approach this reflection on the perception that these rural young peoples immersed in the potato-growing sub-region of the Colombian Andean high mountains have on the Rural Quality of Life. They also state the importance of the qualitative methodology approach to studies on the rural quality of life in the Colombian Andean high mountains.

9.3 Conceptual References that Support the Study

9.3.1 *Rural Quality of Life: From Social to Psychosocial Welfare*

The traditional concept of quality of life, initially assumed as an expression by the people in their daily life, refers to observable situations of reality recognized by people as highly positive, which strengthens itself from the 70s by the influence of great scientific debates[8] happening in North America and in Western Europe. These debates are added to the positive recognition of these situations of reality, the idea of value or collective, agglutinant and widely shared aspirations of social change with the perspective of a better situation.

As a matter of fact, according to Ferrán Casas, the social challenge consisting of obtaining better life conditions becomes the condition of being an objective and a process with concrete developments according to the sphere of actuation where it is adopted, but in which each sphere looks for forms of conciliation with previous developments, be they scientific, political or technical. Thus, the meaning of "quality" is noticeably different depending upon the sphere from where it is approached. For example, from the political and professional perspective, quality, assumed as an observable quality of the services rendered, relates to satisfaction measurements by the users and, from Organizational Psychology, Total Quality is a notion that includes the objective quality of services or products, related to the satisfaction by all users (Casas 1999).

Now, from the psychosocial perspective, the notion of "quality" contains a sense of "tendency towards", more than a "concrete objective". It refers to a utopian tendency, unreachable in its last consequences as it shows a concrete route to a last blurry target or goal. The achievement of happiness and satisfaction with life or with specific spheres of life, for example, seems to correspond to respectable aspirations and to values consensuable from moral rationality (psychosocial rationality, according to Weber), which opens the door to a critical psychosocial utopia, oriented by a psychosocial man model (Fernandez 1990, quoted by Casas 1999).

The quality of life, seen as an observable reality by the people or by the communities, has meanings that differ from the quality of life seen from the macro-social perspective. As an observable reality, it is given various meanings with reference to how to get many quality products, to live surrounded by a quality environment, to appreciate that there is quality in the various spheres of people's life and how to be able to satisfy one's own expectations of comfort or well-being (Blanco 1985; Casas 1989, 1996).From a macro-social perspective, the quality of life is understood as strongly pervaded with psycho-social components and, in this sense, it is a function both of the material environment (social well-being) and of the psycho-social environment (psychological well-being), although some authors recognize it with reference to other components (Casas 1999). These two concepts about the quality of life, such as social well-being and psychosocial well-being, have implications on the meaning of social and psychological well-being.

Social well-being corresponds to what in Anglo-Saxon literature is approached from its roots as well-fare, that is, how to go or journey along a good way; a positive

[8] The Rome Circle or Rome Club promotes in Europe the most specific philosophical-ideological debate about human quality through Peccei (1976), who defines the quintessential objective of humankind as "to perfect the quality of the human person"; thus approximating the idea of "quality" to the capacity of the population and to human renovation, presented as collective challenges or aspirations. For Peccei, the divulgation of the information concerning the improvement oflife conditions on Earth is one of the most essential topics, thus proposing a periodical publication to be entitled "Information to the citizens of the world" (Casas, 1999).

connotation related to external situations which are observable by the people. In this sense, "it is not a matter of subjective states of consciousness, but of conditions and objective circumstances" (Moix 1986, p. 23). It refers to the psycho-social order to promote the satisfaction of shared individual needs as well as pluri-personal needs (Casas 1999).

Psychological well-being corresponds, according to its English root, "well-being", to be or to feel fine. This is a positive connotation related to subjective states of consciousness, which indicate its psychological or psycho-social dimension and characterizes because: (a) it is based upon the individuals' own experiences and on their perceptions and evaluations of those experiences, (b) its physical and material context may influence their psychological well-being, but it is not always seen as an inherent and necessary part of well-being itself, (c) it includes positive measurements, not only negative ones or the lack of negative aspects and, (d) it includes some type of global evaluation about the person's whole life, commonly referred to as *vital satisfaction* (Casas 1999).

Recently the term "well-becoming" has been introduced in the Anglo-Saxon literature to emphasize the objectives and expectations to be achieved in the course of a process (Casas 1999).

A synthesis of conceptualizations about the quality of life constructed by North American and European researchers allows identifying their considerations as a joint function of the material and the psycho-social environments, as defined by Casas (1999), as the only proposal that makes it possible to approach reality in all its amplitude and complexity. It allows one to recognize people who are "objects of study" as "subjects" of a reality about which they also have valid knowledge which; at the same time, it allows them "to engage themselves in some social and political dynamics that want to be democratic, participative and promoters of a profound respect for human rights".

Nowadays, among the Latin American countries, Argentina sets the trend in the approach of research studies on the quality of life. The well-known researcher Graciela Tonon in her publication entitled *To investigate the quality of life in Argentina,* makes an emphasis on the possibility of a new theoretical look to the meaning of these studies. As a matter of fact, they are research studies that are approached from the potentialities, more than from the lacks and from the community anchoring, of the psycho-social type, that include the analysis of the socio-political context. Such studies start from the consideration of the material environment along with the social one, thus considering the person traditionally called "object" as "subject", as the protagonist of the acting. Accordingly, the new theoretical look on quality of life suggests a social and political reality based on the respect for human rights which generates the need to work in an integrated way (Tonon 2008). Likewise, it becomes a privileged look which, when trying to integrate the macro and micro dimensions, attempts to have the protagonists' visions be taken into account at the moment of making decisions about public policies, when becoming innovating information with reference to the traditional measurements of social well-being.

Specifically and with reference to *The studies on quality of life and the perspectives of positive psychology*, Tonon coincides with Kreitler and Niv (2007) when defining quality of life as a phenomenological construct which provides an image of the situation without explaining why or how it appeared. In this sense, she defines it as "experiential and evaluative as it presents a judgment with no intention to relate it with objective variables; it is dynamic, flexible and meaningful for every subject and it is multi-dimensional as it is not based only on a global measurement, but in specific domains identified as constitutive of the quality of life" (Tonon 2009, p. 78).

The importance of this theoretical look transcends the Argentine borders to be taken into account all over the Latin American region as the actions concerning the quality of life of members the traditionally poor and vulnerable. The communities are assumed, in these countries, from the State, through the political actions and decisions in which the point of view of the community is not generally taken into account, just the attributions of quality made by the public sector experts are admitted.

On the basis of what has been presented so far, "rural quality of life" is assumed, in this reflection, as a category constructed according to the following connotations: political, derived from the liberties the young peoples from the Colombian Andean high mountains have to participate actively and effectively in the decisions that affect or may affect what they consider a good rural life, for their families and the surrounding communities where they are immersed; economic, resulting from the opportunities to use the physical-material resources of the environment to execute actions they consider necessary to have a good rural life and; socio-cultural, resulting from the opportunities to access the fundamental rights that the State must provide. These considerations are framed in the traditional concept of social well-being, as elaborated by different authors (Bauer 1966; Duncan 1969; Smith 1973; Andrews and Withey 1976; Michalos 1980).

The concept of rural quality of life has also a psycho-social connotation resulting from the evaluation done, at a certain moment, by rural young peoples, about their future perspectives and their global visions of life in general. These considerations are stated in the solid conceptualization presented by contemporary authors (Evans et al. 1985; Casas 1989, 1999; Andrews and Withey 1976; Campbelll et al. 1976; Tonon 2008, 2009).

9.3.2 The Rural Matter

The space, in this case the rural space or "the rural matter", as a social construction, implies recognizing the affections deriving from the activities developed by the inhabitants in a certain time, which manifest themselves through life expressions influenced by their historicity. The space/time takes its form, in the globalized present world, of malleable and adjustable "recipients" or "containers" defined as "concrete but transitory units of human occupation" (Fals Borda 2000, p. 2). Contrary to its stillness and to resistance to change resulting from its physical or material consideration in the XX century, the space is an entity of relative, modifiable and changing dimensions resulting from its joining to expansions and to historical and demographic contractions related to collective needs; determined, then, by the point of view of the qualified observer.

The "recipients" in which the historical dimension is considered and its rigid and intangible conception of the linear block of spatial containers is put aside, and according to their physical or material consideration, are conceived as *bio-spaces,* "places" or "sites" defined as units predisposed to be adjusted or revised as a reflection of live realities. They configure themselves as a "response to local or regional processes of social, economic and political development which bind vital production and reproduction activities with the places where they are executed and from where elements of social continuity and cultural diversity are derived" (Fals Borda 2000, p. 9).

The social space thus perceived is an abstract representation that is the result from a specific construction work which provides a point of view about the set of points from where the common agents, in their current behaviors, "direct their looks towards the social world" (Bourdieu 1998, p. 169). In this sense, the biospaces[9] are fundamental because of the role they play in the formation of personality and culture, as they are the places where the inhabiting people use their collective memory permanently, with the aim to infer the present on the basis of their own stories and to presuppose the future based upon their personal goals.

Based upon these considerations, the "rural space" is recognized as the space/time determined by the point of view of rural young peoples who are considered highly-qualified current agents, to manifest themselves through expressions where the reality of the various rural processes of economic, social or cultural nature are taken into account. The Colombian Andean high mountains thus become a *bio-space* with a relatively homogeneous historical-cultural binding that makes its young observers valid elements to express their points of view and, consequently, trains them to act as key research informants. Taken into account that in these bio-spaces, collective life is expressed and felt in its ordinariness, the meanings that they construct on the space where they are immersed become an entangled network of meanings whose interpretation contributes, altogether, to the comprehension of the meaning they give to the "rural quality of life", "rural young people" and "the rural" environment.

9.3.3 Berger & Luckmann Phenomenological Constructivism

Berger and Luckmann (2001) propose an interpretation of the construction of society and of the configuration of social identity. Social identity is assumed as a part

[9] In "the rural matter", bio-spaces are formed by relatively homogeneous zones such as "ecosystems, uncultivated lands, hydrographic basins, historical-cultural regions, ethnic territories and indigenous reservations, farming reservation zones, natural parks, provinces, associated municipalities and neighborhoods- small villages", while in the city, neighborhoods, localities or zones, diverse circuits, districts and metropolitan and sub-urban areas are founded" (Fals Borda 2000, p. 9).

of a continuous and dialectical process consisting of three periods: externalization, where a social order constituted through social interaction processes is constructed; objectification, where the social order that has been constructed objectifies by hiding its human genesis in symbolic representations and becomes strange to new generations and; internalization, where the objectified social world projects itself again in consciousness through the process of socialization. In this sense, the habituation and institutionalization categories define the externalization moment, while those of primary and secondary socialization and re-socialization define the moment of internalization. The habituation process, which precedes any institutionalization, identifies itself with the actions that retain the meanings of the individuals, which embed themselves as routines in their "store of general knowledge", remain available and save energy which facilitates the development of activities with a minimal decision margin (Berger and Luckmann 2001, p. 74).

Institutionalization, on its part, emerges when habitualized actions typify reciprocally among types of actors, constructing themselves in the course of a shared history, but not in a determined moment, a situation that makes it impossible to understand what an institution is if we do not understand the historical process where it is produced. In young peoples, the typification of meanings constructed by themselves derives, first, from the possibility acquired to participate in the same events and in the same vital contents; that is, to belong to a same generation, and not the fact of being born chronologically at the same time or "to be young in the same period as others" (Mannheim 1993, p. 216). Second, the institutions, by the fact of existing, independent from any sanction mechanism created for their support, control human behavior when establishing guidelines previously defined which define a determined action, thus defining "social control" (Berger and Luckmann 2001, p. 76).

From this perspective, the traditional conception that identifies adolescence and young people as transition states to the future enjoyment of rights, when being in legal age, or as a preparation to assume responsibilities when in legal age, has been modified. Instead of this legal character, citizenship acquires a social and political character in the family, at school, at work, where primary and secondary socialization processes are implemented, and where children, adolescents and young peoples acquire behavior guidelines to construct social control, in this case, in the rural context of the Colombian Andean high mountains.

At the moment of internalization, the individual is trained to become a member of the society through the primary and secondary socialization and through the re-socialization processes (Berger and Luckmann 2001). Through primary socialization, the internalization process goes on in early childhood when the individuals come into contact with members of the family and close relatives with whom they have strong affection ties, they accept the roles and attitudes of those other signifiers, internalize them and takes them over when they identify with them in a generalized form; that is, with a generality of others, it is to say, with a society. In this sense, the formation within consciousness, of the generalized other marks a decisive stage in the socialization process. It implies, consequently, the internalization of society per se and by the objective reality established in itself and, at the same time, the subjective establishment of a coherent and continuous identity (Berger and Luckmann 2001, p. 16).

The secondary socialization induces the already socialized individuals to new sectors of the objective world of their society and imposes them a new social order as a regulatory framework of human action, without emotional burdens or great biographic impacts; an absence that complicates the destruction of the internalized entity in the primary socialization. This process advances after early childhood in spaces such as school, work or other places different from home or the family. Re-socialization, for its part, known as "alternation", makes possible the transformation of that internalized reality through the reinterpretation of the past according to the current reality. This process, which requires a plausibility structure, permits a rupture in the subjective biography of the individual, in the form of "before…" and "after…". Contrary to secondary socialization in which the ground of reality is in the past, the basis of re-socialization lies in the present (Berger and Luckmann 2001, p. 198).

This perspective sets out the role, which for the young peoples in the Colombian Andean high mountains, is provided by the family, the school, the work in its various modalities and by the State, by means of public management, in the construction and interpretation of "rural young peoples'" condition and in the construction and interpretation of the "rural quality of life". In this sense, we pretend to understand the way how the rural young peoples in the Colombian Andean high mountains are configured as social actors capable of transforming the rural environment where they are immersed, with the aim to reach a better rural quality of life for themselves, their families and for their surrounding community.

9.3.4 Alain Touraine's Social Actor and Subject Theses

Alain Touraine's theses have become the theoretical support which allows one to understand how rural young peoples, in the context of the study, configure themselves as "Subjects" and, subsequently, as "Social actors", thus facilitating a better interpretation of the findings.

As Subjects they configure themselves when they acquire the capacity to assume themselves as actors of their own lives, that is to say, when they are "able to have projects, to elect, to judge positively or negatively, and they are able also, more simply, to have social relations, be they cooperation, consensus or conflictive relations" (Touraine 1996, p. 41). The capacity to be the protagonists of their own history is of great importance as lacking such a capacity makes such forms to be lived "as an incoherent series of accidents" (Touraine 2000, p. 272). This configuration as "Subjects" is determined by the family which provides protection, security and initiative in childhood which, at the same time, offers the capacity to transform oneiric wishes in realistic projects; the school that provides, through language and the information supplied in the course of study, the capacity "to know the social field where action will take place", and the work which provides the social space where these capacities are exerted.

The condition of "Social actor" transcends that of the "Subject" when, besides being the protagonists of their own transformation, the individuals configure themselves as protagonists of the transformation of the environment where they are immersed, a case in which, besides having the conditionings which define them as Subjects, they also acquire the Citizen Consciousness. This consciousness is acquired only when the individuals recognize that their participation, besides being active is effective, that is, when the expression of their opinions are taken into account in the decisions and actions of those who have the power to decide and act. Effectively, only when the people perceive that their appreciations influence government decisions and actions, it is to say, that they are taken into account in "the decisions that affect their collective life, which is recognized and visibilized" (Touraine 1996, pp. 43–44), that is when citizen consciousness is acquired.

Research assumes the rural young peoples of the Colombian Andean high mountains as "Subjects" who are in the capacity to act, opine, contradict, argue, and construct life projects and to impose scopes to achieve their goals. They are also assumed to be "Social actors" or essential protagonists for the development of the rural community where they live and coexist every day, that is, as individuals who not only have personal projects but try to achieve objectives and personal projects in an environment constituted by other actors; an "environment which constitutes a collectivity to which they feel they belong to and whose culture and functioning rules become their rules, although just partially" (Touraine 1996, p. 43). From this theoretical perspective the young peoples from the Colombian Andean high mountains are assumed to be "Subjects" and "Social actors", that is to say, as people who are valid to be consulted and taken into account with respect to their perception about the "quality of life" and "life projects".

9.4 Methodological Design

Methodologically, the study is based upon a sound theory that makes it possible to widen the existing theory or to generate a new one, derived from the data systematically compiled and analyzed by means of a research process. It is a method where the data gathering, its analysis and the emerging categories have a straight relation among themselves and, where the analysis meets the requirement to be the interaction among researchers and the data, thus being, at the same time, science and art. It is science in the sense that it keeps a certain degree of rigor and is based upon data analysis and, it is art in the sense that creativity "manifests itself in the capacity of researchers to adequately denominate categories, ask stimulating questions, make comparisons and make an innovating, integrated and realistic outline of sets of disorganized data (Strauss and Corbin 2002, p. 14).

The Grounded Theory establishes the difference between description and theory. The first refers to what is happening, events, actions, scenes, emotions, moods and expectations, and it nourishes with the current vocabulary to express ideas about things, people and places; it also makes use of similes and metaphors, facilitates the communication among people. In short, "the descriptive details chosen by who is telling a story are usually consciously or unconsciously selective and are based upon what the teller saw or heard or thinks that it is important" (Strauss and Corbin 2002, p. 20). When making theory, on the contrary, events and happenings are not only described "but also the analysis is extended in a way to include interpretations to explain why, when, where, what and how events happen" (Strauss and Corbin 2002, p. 21).

From Grounded Theory, theories are classified as substantive and formal. A theory derived from a substantive area or theory is used to explain and to handle the problems of a social group, in a specific place, such as the one concerning rural young peoples in the Colombian Andean high mountains, whose results are secured in this reflection. It relates to the permanent interaction achieved by the researcher in the process of data gathering, from which new hypotheses to be verified emerge. In this sense, "it is the result of the systematic processing by means of coding and categorization of the field data" (Murcia and Jaramillo 2000, p. 73). Formal theories are less specific with reference to a group and a place, being this the reason why they are applied to a wider range of problems and disciplinary topics (Strauss and Corbin 2002); they are identified through the style of gathering and analysis of theoretical data, by which hypotheses are constructed and the substantive theory is constantly compared.

9.4.1 Type of Study

This research study is a qualitative one which, due to its interpretativist character accepts its reflexivity principle, the rationale of ethnographic research and, at the same time, makes emphasis on the social actors' "lived experiences"; in this case, the rural young peoples of the Colombian Andean high mountains in their daily lives, as the researcher's experience and knowledge, in the world of social sciences. We turn then to Martyn Hammersley and Paul Atkinson (1994), mainly to the first, who has been recognized and quoted as the "representative of interpretativists who pursue a synthesis between social realism and constructivism" (Valles 1999, p. 60).

To assume the material and social reality of the rural young peoples from the Colombian Andean high mountains as a representation built by everyone implies to unveil the meanings with which they, individually or collectively, intervene in this reality. In this sense, the researcher, with the intention to understand the meanings that rural young peoples give to "Rural Young people" and to " rural quality of life", gets into and becomes part of the socio-cultural system under study, interacts as one more element of the structure and reflects about one's own perception being elaborated (Hammersley and Atkinson 1994, pp. 15, 31). An emphasis is made on the experience lived by the rural young peoples, an experience that the researcher shares in the field work and that leads him to a permanent reflection about the incidence of his participation and his own experience and that of the "rural young peoples", subjects of this study. From this perspective, the role of ethnography is not to describe, but to "reflect on the perception that the researcher progressively constructs on that reality" (Murcia and Jaramillo 2000, p. 71).

The methodological "complementarity" in this research retakes all and every one of the elements of reflexive ethnography and similar perspectives and makes it possible to use a plurality of approaches and techniques, methodologies and theories aiming at the comprehension of behaviors and conducts that respond to the complexity of the problems under discussion, and not, on the contrary, that the problem be presented as a response to a certain approach and exclusive theory, a procedure that at present encounters a generalized refusal. In this sense, the inquiry is guided by an "emergent design" which is structured from the successive findings obtained during the full development of the research and is characterized by its "construction and reconstruction in the search for information (Briones 2002, p. 12).

The "emergent design", as the basis of *reflexive ethnography* and the method of Grounded theory to build a new theory, faces the problem by which the researcher cannot start a research with a list of preconceived concepts, a guiding theoretical framework or a well-defined design, because "the concepts and design must be allowed to emerge from the data" (Strauss and Corbin 2002, p. 38). Accordingly, a process through which the development of a research is designed, once started, finds a free way "through a slow process of gradual configuration, which would manifest itself in categories apparently unconnected and, which when being reflected would show a connection among themselves" (Murcia and Jaramillo 2000, p. 96). The problem lies, then, in that the initial data must give way to the design of a guide to focus on the gradual development of the research, and the initial data obtained at the very first moment of research.

Accordingly, *the initial exploration of reality* allows one to define relevant initial data that favor the extraction of hypotheses and questions to be demonstrated with methods, instruments and techniques used in the remaining moments where the research develops. The results from the application, analysis and interpretation of data are contrasted permanently with the formal theory referents, the research background and the information on the socio-cultural scenario, with the aim to permanently state the possible substantive categories and their relations whose final reflection, at the last moment, widens or modifies the existing theoretical and conceptual referents.

The methodological premises already presented allow one to elaborate, initially, a survey that will be administered to a representative sample of 544 rural young peoples, men and women, workers and students, with ages ranging from 16 to 29 years, from the potato-growing sub-region in the Cundiboyacense High Plateau, with the aim to complete its general characterization. Subsequently, detailed interviews will be administered to a significant sample of rural young peoples, from which the accounts can permit to reflect on their perceptions on the "rural quality of life" are extracted.

9.4.2 The Use of Triangulation

Research methods and techniques are defined by the object of research and taking into consideration that in the field of Sociology various objects are demarcated—society with its own dynamics, society as a product from man and the man as a product from society—the resulting explanation of social reality depends on which of these objects is put ahead (Cea 1999, p. 44). The object of study in this research has to deal, first, with the man being as a product of society, in this case, with the configuration of "rural young people" in the context of the Colombian Andean high mountains. It is also worth to consider the results from the guarantees offered by society to potentiate the corresponding capacities and to exert one's own rights and, second, with the society as a product of man, which refers to the "rural young people" as a psycho-social actor, trained to influence the development processes of the rural community, to exert the rights to become a guide or an example of life in the search of what is perceived as the "rural quality of life".

This pluralistic conception of the object of research leads to triangulation, which could be of different types: (a) triangulation of information sources, whose value consists of verifying the inferences extracted from an information source by means of another information source; (b) triangulation among researchers, generated by different observers who favor the formation of a constellation of complementary data and (c) triangulation of techniques that facilitates the comparison of information obtained from the application of different techniques (Hamersley and Atkinson 1994).

Through the triangulation of information sources, the information about the same phenomenon is compared, although obtained in different moments of the field work, at different points of the temporary cycles existing in that place or, as it happens in this research, by comparing the narrations from the various participants (the ethnographer included) involved in the field. In case diverse types of information lead to the same conclusion, it is possible to rely a little more on the conclusions. The triangulation of techniques, for its part, permits, from the perspective of reflexive ethnography, their combination, which makes it possible to prove the validity of the data from different and from each one of the techniques used (Hammersley and Atkinson 1994, pp. 216, 217). The triangulation of methods consists of their combination and the measurement of the same analysis unit (Cea 1999, p. 54). Triangulation in the interpretative presentation of data refers to the presentation of categories from the support of a formal theory that sustains its interpretation and comprehension, from the socio-cultural narrations and from the researcher's subjective interpretation. Finally, triangulation from the reviewing of formal theories consists of interpreting the category under study from various theoretical approaches (Murcia and Jaramillo 2000, p. 160).

Triangulation of information sources is used in this research study as it compares the information obtained by different actors according to their age ranges and gender, occupation and working activity they are devoted to. Equally, the triangulation among techniques is also used as it verifies the validity of statistical data from the initial administration of a survey, with the ethnographic data from the participating observation in the socio-cultural context, along with the data from the administration of in-depth interviews applied to rural young peoples in their own milieu. Obviously, triangulation is used in the interpretative presentation of data, as the categories are presented from the support of various theories, from the socio-cultural narrations by rural young peoples and from the researcher's subjective interpretation. Besides, triangulation is implemented from the reviewing of formal theories, which consists of reflecting about the categories of "the rural", "young people" and "quality of life", from different theoretical approaches.

9.4.3 Research Moments

First moment: exploration of reality

It refers to the complementary and parallel reviewing of documents, maps, texts and standards that permit, on the one hand, to define the research substantive or problem area, to structure a theoretical framework, to formulate hypotheses from formal theory and to review research antecedents and; on the other hand, to gradually discover the various parts that define the socio-cultural tangle of the Colombian Andean zone. Besides, an exploratory visit to the socio-cultural context is made, which facilitates its empirical knowledge and the delimitation of the adequate scenario for the development of the research field work. The findings from this *general exploration of reality* allow one to structure the research project and to design a possible guideline that will pave the road to the *pre-configuration of reality,* to take place in the second moment.

The exploratory visit to the socio-cultural context takes place in the course of four weeks, in three-day trips per week to the rural zone of the municipalities of Pasca and Villapinzón, in the state of Cundinamarca. These municipalities are selected taking into account their belonging to the Cundiboyacense Plateau, the settlement of high-mountain rural communities with the presence of both male and female young peoples, and their differentiating agricultural and cattle production. This visit aims at exploring the "rural young people's" reality through observations that range from non-participative ones to participative observations, apart from informal interviews to rural young peoples who are devoted to different occupations. This very first moment of the research is facilitated by the knowledge the researcher has of the zone where other research studies and field works have been done, and by the collaboration of assistant professionals, regional technicians, agricultural engineers and zootechnician veterinary doctors from the University of Cundinamarca, while being the Dean to the School of Agriculture and Livestock Sciences of the above mentioned institution, professionals to whom informal interviews are also administered.

This first exploration allows obtaining general data related to occupation, working performance, study, civil status, dependence and family of rural young peoples, besides it permits one to have information about land tenure and propriety of the crops. Once these data have been identified, which are considered as possible pre-categories or emergent subjective categories, it is necessary to deepen, at this precise moment, in the formal theory with reference to modernization and its influence on the design and formulation of young people policies, based upon the validity of the 1991 Constitution with all its antecedents.

The findings from the *general exploration of reality* allow one to elaborate, as a conclusion from this first moment, a thematic dimension entitled *Modernization and Young people in Latin America and in Colombia,* where socio-cultural categories from the modernization paradigm are identified (Parsons and Platt 1973; Parsons 1974, 1984; Almond and Powell 1972; Rostow 1973), and also possible substantive pre-categories are envisaged.

Guideline for the pre-configuration of reality.

Before the lack of reliable information, it is planned to carry out a second moment of the research: a general characterization of the young people population belonging to the selected socio-cultural scenario by means of the design, application and interpretation of a survey oriented to them. In this sense, the results from the *general exploration of reality* facilitate the design of a guideline to pre-configure reality in the following moment, which contains the following elements:

- Formulation of questions. Such questions orient the process at the second moment of the research. ¿How are the high-mountain young peoples and the traditional farming production in the Colombian Andean zone characterized? ¿How does the socio-cultural context have an impact on this characterization?
- Survey design. Its application, analysis and interpretation allow to characterize juvenile population and to identify relations among some of the emerging pre-categories, with the aim to confront them with formal theory and to define the second *thematic dimension* of the study. The surveys designed are submitted, at the same moment of the *general exploration of reality*, to a pilot test in the municipality of Pasca, where 30 of them are administered; errors in the formulation of questions are detected and, at the same time, they are adequately corrected.
- Definition of places where to administer the test. Provinces, municipalities and rural villages where to administer the tests are defined; the assignment of four months and of a team of four people, a main researcher and three assistant professionals for the application and analysis, as well as for the determination of a representative sample of the population to apply the test. Almeidas and Ubaté are selected as the high representativity provinces in the rural zone of the potato-growing sub-region at the Cundiboyacense High Plateau, in view of the presence of a rural population higher than 70 % of the total population, a high farming vocation that offers more than 80 % of jobs to the rural young peoples located 2700 m above sea level, and the possession of the biggest rural extension of all the other provinces lying in the socio-cultural scenario previously identified.
- A conglomerate sampling design is used as the object of a study population—as the rural young people of the Cundiboyacense High Plateau potato-growing sub-region is distributed in the villages of the municipalities belonging to the provinces selected. The conglomerates correspond to the influence geographic areas in which the Province of Almeidas and the Province of Ubaté are divided. In the

Province of Almeidas, the municipalities of Machetá, Manta, Sesquilé, Suesca and Tiribitá are selected, while in the Province of Ubaté are the municipalities of Carmen de Carupa, Cucunubá, Fúquene, Lenguazaque and Tausa, all of them with their corresponding rural villages.

- The selection of rural villages and the determination of their population are at random, as all of the villages of the municipalities have the same probability to be selected. Before the lack of the exact information about the population by age ranges in the villages, the population percentage between 14 and 29 years is determined in the rural zone of the state of Cundinamarca, on the basis of SISBEN[10] data. Given that 42 % of the rural population is in this age range, the population in each of the villages of the municipalities of the sample is estimated. Because of equal affixation for all of the villages of each municipality, the application of 554 surveys is determined, from which at the moment of cleaning the applied forms, eight (8) of them are discarded, for a total of 546.
- Determination of observation places and application of surveys. The populations where rural young peoples devote to study and to work, and the populations where farming, commercial, mining or home activities (exclusively by young women) are carried out, are taken into account. Likewise, the communicative manifestations of rural youngsters reflecting an attitude toward their daily practices, understood as observation elements to be carried out parallel to the administration of the surveys, are also taken into account. These practices must be consigned in the field diaries that each of the members of the survey team must fill out.
- Determination of software for the analysis of surveys. It has been stated to use the Statistical Package for the Social Sciences (SPSS), version 15.0, which permits to obtain descriptive statistics, contingency tables and correlation analyses, among others.

Second moment: Pre-configuration of reality

At this moment and for the first time, there is an access to the selected socio-cultural scenario, with the aim to do the referential field work represented in the application of surveys to rural young peoples within the ranges and the villages selected in the preceding moment. The characterization of young peoples in the socio-cultural scenario where the research takes place as a result from the surveys, the relations and correlations defined and the confrontation with formal theory with which the substantive area of the study is approached and with the theory that re-dimensions it, facilitate the elaboration of a second thematic dimension entitled *Rural young people and social integration in Colombia*, which becomes the socio-cultural pre-structure of reality. The "working young people" and the "studying young people" categories, which refer to the situation of young peoples in the Andean high

[10] SISBEN. Information system that permits one to identify, classify and select the people and the families who live in poverty, with the aim to let them have access to subsidies and other benefits provided by the Government. The data were supplied by the State Office of SISBEN, at the Office of Planning of the State of Cundinamarca, by its Coordinator Engineer José Delgado on August 1, 2007.

mountain context, the traditional farming production and the re-definition of "the rural matter" emerge from the above mentioned pre-structure.

From the substantive or problem area, the theoretical approaches from which it is dimensioned and re-dimensioned, the socio-cultural scenario and the thematic dimension constructed at the end of the first moment, as well as the characterization of young peoples in the study scenario, the relations and correlations established and the thematic dimension constructed in the second moment, envisage the design of the guideline for the configuration of reality; this configuration is developed in the third moment of the research.

Guideline for the configuration of reality. Reality is configured through the development of the following activities.

- Formulation of new questions. These result from the analyses of surveys and correlation studies. ¿What meanings do the young peoples from the Colombian Andean zone give to everything that influences their perception about their own reality and the reality of the Andean rural world where they are immersed? At the same time, other questions resulting from or turning around these questions appear: ¿What meanings do the young peoples from the Colombian Andean zone give to school, to work, to the State and to the incidence of these factors in their configuration as "rural young peoples"? ¿Do the young peoples from the Colombian Andean zone, who are students, configure in the same form as those of the same biological age and who already work? ¿What meanings do young peoples in this context give to the rural space where they are immersed?.
- Determination of the research scenario. The municipalities of Tausa and Cucunubá are defined as those where deep field work takes place, through the application of in-depth interviews, life histories and notes from field diaries.
- Design of a proof list. It permits one to guide the in-depth interviews in order to define an adequate control by the interviewer. They are open questions that are applied once the key social actors have been selected; it is the result from the analysis of the surveys applied, from the characterization and correlation studies that were developed in the second moment and the questions formulated in this guideline.

Third moment: Configuration of reality

In this moment, the in-depth field work represented by the application of in-depth interviews, the participating observation and the notes of the field diary, is advanced. The interviews are applied to the selected "key informants", initially, as the product from the analysis of results obtained in the second moment, and on the field, because of its consideration as necessary, at random, using the "snowball" technique, through which an interviewee leads another with the characteristics required by the research and according to the moment. They are guided holistic interviews, previously elaborated as a result from the questions arising from the surveys and in accordance with the object of the research study, constituted by the life, experiences, ideas, values and symbolic structure of rural young peoples, here and now, everything with the aim to unveil their emotions, feelings and subjectivities.

The interviews go after personalized information by treating the subjects in their exclusive originality, from the meanings that they themselves elaborate by means of what they call "common sense" (Sierra 1998 pp. 299, 301). The topics to be dealt with, stated in the *guideline of configuration of reality*, elaborated in the preceding moment, and their interpretation, make up the *socio-cultural structure* of reality and stands for the major approximation to the substantive theory intended to be elaborated at the end of the research process, re-dimensioned by the bio-space and territory theories (Fals Borda 2000) and by the political conception of the "Subject" (Touraine 2000). This socio-cultural structure is achieved through the first conceptualization about the essence of the actions and interactions that have been exhibited by reality, thus structuring a new thematic dimension with the title of "the rural young people: from Subject to social actor".

The in-depth interviews are administered to Cucunubá and Tausa rural young peoples, taking care that they be either workers or students. With reference to the first, those performing working activities such as farming, commerce, mining, public and home; the second ones, taking different degrees of formal or non-formal education. Men and women; single, married or even in free union; in age ranges from 14 to 18 years, from 19 to 24 years, and from 25 to 29 years, are selected.

The municipalities where the interviews are administered—Cucunubá and Tausa in the province of Ubaté—are selected due to the presence of both male and female young peoples and to the fact that the interviews detect a shared presence of young peoples, men and women, single, married and in free union, students, workers and unemployed, of different ages, who carried out the activities already described. Besides, they take into account the presence of young peoples that have constituted a family and have left the paternal home, of young peoples who, although having constituted their own home, they continue living in the paternal home, and of young peoples, "family children", who receive the protection from their parents, being these aspects identified in the analysis of the surveys administered. These conditions differentiate the selected municipalities as an adequate space for the administration of the in-depth interviews that allow the young peoples to answer, besides the initial questions of the research, those that arise in different moments. On the other side, the socio-economic and socio-political conditions of the selected municipalities are similar to the conditions of the municipalities in the Cundiboyacense High Plateau and, in general, of the Colombian Andean zone.

The participant observation gradually accompanies all the development of the research, that is, it goes from the passive participation of the first and second moments to the active and complete participation in this third moment of the research process. The researcher involves himself in these activities and deeply observes the situation through the selection of topics of interest, social situations, scenarios, groups and individuals (Valles 1999, p. 169). This observation is done in units of farming production, mainly in potato crops, and in mines, schools and other rural spaces where there are activities involving the young peoples.

The notes of field diaries become a fundamental instrument in the study. They literally register the "native" language used by rural young peoples which differs from that used by the researcher; when describing observations, the trend to use the language of social science is avoided. The notes are taken at the moment or immediately after an in-depth field work session and they include all types of notes about everything seen and heard by the observer, without being too detailed (Valles 1999, p. 170). They are *expanded*, that is, they are written from the preceding notes, some hours after field work has taken place, and they register experiences, affection, fear, anger, confusion and solution feelings, as well as other aspects that are useful not to put aside the researcher's biases. Everything that has been observed, the theoretical perspectives being used and the researcher's training are in the *analysis and interpretation notes*, which are located between the preceding notes and the final writing.

Guideline for the configuration of reality. The findings from the third moment of the research are fundamental for the design of the *guideline for the re-configuration of reality,* which takes place in the fourth and last moments. It is based on the reviewing, analysis and interpretation of the information gathered in each of the preceding moments, with the aim to widen and to modify the existing theoretical and conceptual referents, on the basis of the experiences shared by the researcher with the rural young peoples, the corresponding researching experience and the knowledge of the context.

The reconfiguration guideline formulates, as the result from the three moments already described, the question that finally tries to meet the objectives of the research study: ¿How to understand the meaning that the young peoples of the Colombian Andean zone give to their condition of protagonists of their own development and of protagonists of the development of the rural society where they are immersed? Other questions derive from these questions, which ask about ¿How to understand the meaning young peoples who are students give to their condition? ¿How to understand the meaning young people of the same biological age who work give to their condition? The answers to these questions allow one to interpret their perceptions about what they consider a good rural life and the way to get it, which is the rationale of the reflection in this chapter.

Fourth moment: Re-configuration of reality

It deals with the theoretical and conceptual condensation of the critical analysis of the socio-cultural structure resulting from the work developed in the preceding moments and its relation with each of the categories that make it; in other words, it is the synthesis of the whole process. It is formulated and supported in this sense, in the general conclusions, under the title of "*Rural young people: between the social present need and the social moratorium*", the thesis that states not only the existence of "rural young people" with its own characteristics but also states the existence of "different types of rural young people" in the Colombian Andean high mountain zone and in the traditional farming production.

It is precisely in this moment when the "rural quality of life" categories and the "rural subject", "rural social actor" and "rural psychosocial actor" sub-categories emerge, as a result from from the interpretations developed on the perceptions of the rural young peoples in the context of the research study. The purpose, then, of this work, is the comprehension of the meaning given to the "rural quality of life" and the way young peoples believe that it can be reached in the Colombian Andean high mountains.

9.5 The Way How the Category "Rural Quality of Life" Emerges

The life histories and the in-depth interviews administered to key informants, three workers and three students, selected from the 11 people who define the significant sample in the original research study, allow one to describe the way they construct their meanings about the rural quality of life. They orient themselves, in general terms, by the characteristics of the rural context where they act day by day and their meddling and determination in what they perceive as a good and satisfactory life style, the way how life passes in reality and the way how they assume themselves as trained to reach what they consider necessary to live satisfactorily or to reach, what 'Sen' calls, "valuable functioning" (Sen 1996, p. 56), that is, how to define scopes and how to construct life projects.

In this section, there is initially the description of the perceptions concerning the evaluation of the conditions that the rural contexts offer the young peoples in order to satisfy their material and physical, individual and collective needs, and to bet on new targets, short and medium term, that will let them "go ahead" in life. "To go ahead" is perceived as betting the targets defined by themselves where each target offers personal and community satisfactions that will give them the possibility to go on positively toward other targets whose accomplishment will be translated in the accumulation of great satisfactions. In this sense, "to go ahead" demands sacrifices that will be rewarded with great satisfactions which, at last, allow them to improve the living conditions.

Afterwards, the perceptions derived from the evaluation of their experiences, present situations and global visions of life, on their way to reach a last objective that is consolidated when they reach what they call to "be somebody" in life are described; as a process in which material and psychosocial connotations are also taken into account. To take into account these connotations comprehensively favors the emergence of the "quality of life" socio-cultural category, which derives, ultimately, from the interpretation of the Colombian Andean high mountain rural young peoples, workers and students' perceptions, as constructed by the researcher.

9.5.1 To "Go Ahead" in Life by the Young Workers

Rural young peoples who are devoted to work, be it in the mines, in farming activities or in commerce, perceive "the rural matter" as a means that meets the physical or material conditions to live one's life. In this sense, they relate with the hard effort they must make to reach the goals they define from an early age when they integrate themselves to society through work or they form new homes independent from their parents. It is the way it is perceived by three young workers of the Cundiboyacense High Plateau potato-growing sub-region who respond to the in-depth interviews:

The first is a young 26-year-old potato farmer, born in the Paramo Alto village of the municipality of Tausa, state of Cundinamarca, who starts working at the age of 11, thus accumulating a great experience at his age.

> I was born in the Paramo Alto village, Tausa […] We are four [referring to himself and to the number of siblings], two women and two men […] my sisters at home with my parents, my other brother is working there in the countryside […] With reference to study, I only completed the fifth grade of primary school, my sisters finished secondary school, and they are studying to be teachers, and when my brother will complete the fifth grade of primary school he will start working in the countryside […] My father is a farmer […] my mother is a housewife. (H/Ed:26/JoTa)[11].
> Now at present, here in this village, I have […] more or less 8 hectares (he refers to hectares cultivated in potatoes), because up there in Ladera Grande I have other 20 hectares […] and about 15 workers. (H/Ed:26JoTa).

The second is a young worker at one of the coal mines in the municipality of Tausa. He is 23 years old and was born in the village of Sabaneque, in this municipality. This is the way he describes his history:

> I studied until I was 12 and at that moment I started to work and when I was 15 I started living with a woman who is my wife nowadays […] I started working from that time on: I have three children and I work in the mine […] I'm a coachman […] there are 12 strikers, they go in and strike coal and I pick it up with a coach. I work at 90 m under the surface. (H/Ed:23/JoTm).

The third informant is a young lady with an age of 22, the owner of a small store in the Paramo Bajo village, in the municipality of Tausa, who hopes to continue her professional studies using her own resources:

> I took all my primary school here, from Kindergarden, here at the same high school [high school refers to the school at Paramo Bajo village], up to the eleventh grade in the same institution […] we have always worked to […] *go ahead*. (M//Ed:22/JoTc).
> With me, we are seven [with reference to the number of siblings], some of them work, others are studying and others are already married […] and the rest of them are farmers, they grow potatoes (M//Ed:22/JoTc).
> I have my small business [a grocery store in the village] and God willing, next year I will start studying in Ubaté (M//Ed:22/JoTc).

For these young workers, the rural zone is the space where they must work hard, far from the presence of the State, to reach the goals that will let them "go ahead" in life, as they say. In this sense, they are very critical about the scarce help from the State, both to guarantee the right to an education and to work in the farming zone, a situation which induces them, from an early age, to define short-term goals which

[11] **(H/Ed:26/JoTa)**. This is the coding used in this chapter which accompanies the narrations from now on. [H or M] refers to the informant's sex, thus, H: male, M: female; [Ed:26] is the age of the informant, in this case, 26 years; [Jo] means young and [T] means work or the informant's activity, thus: E: student, Ta: farm worker, Tc: commercial worker, Tm: mine worker, and Th: home worker.

contribute to abandoning school or to abandoning the early integration to society. This is how they express it:

> I live here in the countryside, what do I study for [...] it means we lose our motivation ¿What am I studying for, what for? If I will never become a professional, then ¿what do I spend money studying for? (H/ED:26/JoTa).

This very same perception, with reference to the support opportunities to study, is the same with reference to another young worker:

> One finishes the fifth grade of primary school and the first thing one has to do is to look for a job in a farm or in the mine, because there are no more options [...] Here in this town we never get any support (H/Ed:23/Jo/Tm).

The woman, for her part, expresses the critical situation with respect to the opportunities to work or study offered by the rural environment:

> There are no opportunities for the youngsters, this is why many times they say, for example, as a woman [...] what do we study for? If any way we will become housewives, as here there are no opportunities. (M/Ed:22/JoTc).

The perception they have about the incapacity of the State to guarantee the fundamental right to an education is the same as they have with reference to the State's incapacity to guarantee the right to rural work. As a matter of fact, they perceive the State's action as a timely and valid one for the big and technified agricultural production in the flat and in the medium-slope zones, but not valid for the farming production in the high mountains. In this sense, with reference to the affectations to agricultural production as a result from the climatic change, they express the following:

> One [...] has the same rights, but what happens is that the State, the administration, does not collaborate because we have nothing, for example, we will collaborate with this man who owns this farm, and to say something, because the dry period affected him, but as we do not have anything, we do not receive anything (H(Ed:26/JoTa).

The young person who does not work in farming, but in mining does not have a similar perception with reference to the State's actions concerning the support to rural lodging:

> Lodging, for example, we need it. Here in town, Col$300,000.oo are given to those of the urban sector, when somebody from the countryside comes and asks the Mayor: *Mayor I need a subsidy, there is nothing, there is nothing,* they simply support the people from the urban sector while they do not do it with the people from the countryside (H(Ed:23/Jo/Tm).

The young female worker, for her part, expresses the scarce interest of the State towards rural young peoples:

> Rural people, we are left at God's mercy, the State does not show any interest, I do not see whether they are interested in rural young peoples. (M/Ed:22/JoTc).

With reference to medium-term goals, young peoples express their desire to consolidate a major economic stability that will let them offer working possibilities to the members of the rural community where they are immersed. This is the way they perceive this situation:

> In my case my expectations [...] are to have my little farm and to employ people, as in this moment [He refers to having a property on the cropland; although the crops are ours or they are shared with other people, the land is rented (H/Ed:26/JoTa).

The medium-term goal for the young lady refers, basically, to getting married and afterwards to have access to a university career; she expresses herself as follows:

> My project is [...] first to get married, then to study a systems career and if it is not possible here, we would have to move to the city (M/Ed:22/JoTc).

In the long term, the working young peoples define coinciding goals dealing with the future of their children, when they manifest the interest they have in their children to study, to become professionals and not to follow their parents steps by working from an early age. In this sense, they express the following:

> In my case, my children, I want them to become professionals, not to be the same as I am, I will die here [...] I want them *to be somebody* in life, where they will not have to crop potatoes as we do, but that they will have a good level of education, that they will have their positions, something different from being exposed to the sun and to the rain. (H/Ed:26/JoTa).

In this sense, Alexander expresses:

> My project would be to have children, to have them study at the university and to become professionals [...] (H/Ed: 23/JoTm).

The young business woman also expresses herself with the same intention:

> My dream is to have my son *go ahead*, so that he will have a good future. (M/Ed:22/JoTc).

But at the same time the working young peoples identify "the rural" zone as a space of freedom, nature, peace and tranquility, of responsible and affective people where values, such as solidarity among the members of the community, are evidenced. A space that will offer them better opportunities to "be somebody" in life, that is, to reach an ultimate objective, superior to all goals previously defined. They express it as follows:

> Here, at least, we breathe pure air and we live with more tranquility, but in the city that is not possible, here we live well, that is well, for me, in the countryside. (H/Ed:26/JoTa).
> Here there is more freedom, more support within the family, everybody shares, everybody supports everybody else. (M/Ed:22/JoTc).

Up to now, we have the description of working young peoples' perceptions with reference to the conditions offered by the rural environment, to what they call to "go ahead" in life, the conditions that differ from the way the young peoples perceive the dedication to study.

9.5.2 To "Go Ahead" in Life by Young Students

The rural young students recognize "the urban" as the space where the State offers better possibilities, with reference to "the rural", to "go ahead" in life. This is an expression that they, as well as workers, understand as reaching the short, medium and long-term goals that have been defined in the course of life. Accordingly, the urban sector is the place where young peoples can consolidate their rights, the same rights rural young peoples have, but that in the countryside they cannot consolidate or consolidate just in a partial or deficient manner. This is evidenced by the affirmations by three young students, two women and a man:

One of the women is 16 years old, was born in La Florida village, in the municipality of Cucunubá, state of Cundinamarca, and proudly expresses her dedication to both study and work:

> I was born at the Ubaté Hospital, I completed kindergarden, I started when I was four and a half years old, and then I started studying at Policarpa Salavarrieta Public School, there I finished fifth grade and I have been studying at Divino Salvador high-school, from sixth grade on [Educational institutions in the municipality of Cucunubá], my father works as a mechanic and as a farmer…, or whatever there is to be done, my mother is a housewife […]. I started working about 15 days ago on weekends and I like it … I have been working in a bakery. (M/Ed:16/JoE).

The man is a young student, 17 years old, born in the municipality of Zipaquirá and is an inhabitant at the Paramo Bajo village in the municipality of Tausa, state of Cundinamarca, who highlights his condition of both student and worker. He describes the situation as follows:

> I completed my primary school at the high school here […], I had my secondary school there too, the name is Páramo Bajo Rural Basic High School […]. My father is a farmer, he crops potatoes, and my mother is a housewife, but she also has her cows and the like, to see them, to live from them, that is […] both completed the fifth grade of primary school. (H/Ed:17/JoE).

The third person who was interviewed was a young lady university student, 21 years old, born in Tausa and inhabitant in Paramo Bajo village, who studies Food Engineering at La Salle University in the city of Bogota:

> I was born 21 years ago in Tausa […] I took part of my primary school here at the Paramo Bajo Rural high school, and the other at the municipality of Tausa, downtown [She refers to the county town]. I completed my secondary school at La Presentación High School in Zipaquirá and then I entered La Salle University, where at present I am taking the ninth semester of Food Engineering […]. My father is a farmer and my mother is a housewife. (M/Ed:21/JoE).

The knowledge about the importance of the rural matter as a material and physical space in the satisfaction of needs is expressed by the recognition of the inequalities undergone with reference to the urban, with feelings of frustration before the incapacity to implement in the rural space the rights which in the urban zone are evidenced as consolidated. It is expressed as follows:

> If the rural young people were taken into account, it would not be the same kind of education we are being offered, but it would be the same as in the urban sector. In the rural sector […], for example, there is just one teacher for five courses, very different from the urban sector where, for example, there is a teacher for each classroom […]. We lack well-prepared teachers in English […], in the systems classrooms there is a lack of computers […] many laboratories are missing, such as the Chemistry one […] the objects existing there have been acquired by us, be it to meet some goals or as a donation situation, but the State's help is minimal. (M/Ed:16/JoE).

Similarly, the young university student expresses the following:

> The higher education level is highly neglected, then it is a situation that partially affects the quality of life of the people because they do not have the opportunity to have jobs yielding good incomes. (M/Ed:21/JoE).

As it can be easily observed, young students relate education with the opportunity to have better jobs, different from being simple farming or mining workers, and those with better income levels to achieve, according to their perceptions, a better quality of life. This perception, although it does not correspond to that of young workers, coincides with the expectations that the latter have for their children.

Now then, the goals students fix to "go ahead" in life are different from those of the workers, as they do not expect to integrate to society at an early moment, but to skill themselves by means of study for a future integration when they well be ready for it. In case to have a job, they assume it as something temporary, as a means to access some economic resources to be able to reach the goal consisting in finishing their studies. For the young students interviewed, these goals are only achieved with the obliging migration to the city. In this sense, they say the following:

> I finish this year [referring to finishing the secondary studies] and I think to go on with my studies for not staying here, to go to the city to *look for a better life*, in other words. I would like to be in the city, to study my electronics, *to go ahead.* (H/Ed:17/JoE).

The young female secondary student has short-term goals which are similar to those expressed by the man:

> Well, this year I am going to graduate with honors [...], next year I will go on studying, maybe to take a course [...] and then I will work and get some money to be able to register at a university [...] I expect to get out of here, because here the economy is poor [...] the dream I have is to become a Systems Engineer [...], that would be mainly in the Capital city. (M/Ed:16/JoE).

The university students about to finishing her professional studies talks about her future plans:

> To finish the career right now, maybe to take a specialization program [...]. (M/Ed:21/JoE).

With reference to further expectations to finish the studies, the students express their intention to return to the rural sector, to service it, to offer jobs and to create business to benefit the rural community where they are from. They express it as follows:

> One should study something [with reference to studying in the city] and to work here in the countryside to develop it, to stay here, in the countryside, to help the most needed rural people [...], for example, as an engineer or something similar, to help. (H/Ed:17/JoE).

In this very same sense, the young secondary student expresses her intention to come back and work in the rural sector:

> To set a business but with things related to the countryside. Let's say, with potatoes at an industrial level thus to foster industry here. (M/Ed:21/JoE).
> Rural development would be like allowing that the people have the opportunity to study, but that they apply their knowledge in the same rural sector, that they create business or things that benefit the rural sector in order to have development. (M/Ed:21/JoE).

In general terms, to "go ahead" in life is assumed by rural young peoples from the Colombian Andean High Mountains as the achievement of permanent short, medium and long-term goals imposed by daily life, which are fulfilled with sacrifice and dedication before the generalized perception on the State's absence in the rural communities in the Colombian Andean high mountains. But, ¿what makes the young workers do not want to migrate to the city, no matter the sacrifices they must undergo to "go ahead" in life, and what makes students desire to go back to the rural sector, once they have graduated, after having migrated to be able to finish their studies in the city?

The answer transcends the consideration of the rural sector as a space where the State does not provide the conditions necessary to meet the material needs that allow them to "go ahead". Young peoples cannot assume this sector as a bio-space that provides the possibility to reach a higher goal, an ultimate objective to which they get near only when they are recognized by the others and they acquire the capacity to recognize themselves as "somebody" in life; this is how these situations are evidenced in the narrations given below.

9.5.3 To "Be Somebody" in Life According to Rural Young People

The perceptions defined by young peoples, men and women, workers and students, allow them to identify how they construct knowledge on what they call "to be somebody" in life. This means simply to be recognized by the other members of the rural community in the Colombian Andean high mountain zone, and to be perceived, by themselves, as valuable, respectable and admirable people, as life models or examples to follow. They express it in the recognition they have about their parents:

> My father […] taught me how to work […] he was my teacher or he will go on being my teacher because any way I think I will never reach his height […] God willing someday I will be like him. (H/Ed:26/JoTa).

The recognition, admiration and respect that the young worker expresses about his father, whom he identifies as a life guide or model coincides with the recognition the young student makes for all his elderly:

> One guides oneself by following the more responsible people […] it is like a guide, like an example for one to *go ahead* and to redo one's life […]. Some people are already neat and tidy, more honest and they are a guide, one says that person is a good one, it is necessary to be honest, that is all. (H/Ed:17/JoE).

The interviewed young peoples perceive that a person "becomes somebody" in life when his behavior in the community becomes an example to be followed, a guide to be imitated because of honesty, neatness at work and good behavior as a member of the family and of the rural community. In this sense, the young student says:

> To be somebody in life for me would be to be nice with everybody; that at the moment I arrive in this town everybody would greet and say there goes such a person, and tell the children I would like you to be like him someday. (H/Ed:23/JoTm).

Now, to assume oneself as "somebody" in life and to be assumed as such by the rural community where the youngsters are immersed day by day allows them to be closer to happiness. This is expressed by rural young peoples without distinction because of occupation:

> To be somebody in life contributes to be happy, it is like being a good young person, I think, that is to be a good person, because being a bad person does not mean to be happy [...] to have a better friend no matter where you go, to be happy, to have friends that is all. (M/Ed:21/JoE).
>
> Happiness is to feel fine with oneself, with the surrounding environment, to be happy with the environment. (M/Ed: 21/JoE).
>
> Quality of life is to be happy, it is like being nice to people, to have friends and to be able to talk to them and to collaborate with people [...] to be responsible at home with everything that may be needed there. (H/Ed:26/JoTa).

9.6 Conclusions

The cultural practices of the rural young peoples of the Colombian Andean high mountain zone make an entangled network of meanings whose interpretation allows one to define, as a conclusion, a thematic dimension where perceptions, among others, are discerned with reference to the quality of life to be reached. The interpretation of these perceptions holds onto the considerations on the quality of life and other related categories that have been approached synthetically at the beginning of this chapter. These interpretations are as follows.

A theoretical look on the quality of life in conjunction with the material and psychosocial environment that allows one to recognize people as "subjects" of a reality about which they also have some knowledge that validates them to engage in social and political, democratic and participative dynamics as well as in activities that deeply promote the respect for human rights (Casas 1999), and, therefore, to be action protagonists (Tonon 2008), are evidenced practically in this research study. As a matter of fact, one of the most important aspects of this research study is the recognition of the young peoples in the Colombian Andean high mountain zone as people who are valid to be consulted, among other aspects, about their perceptions on the rural quality of life and on how to reach it, how to advance towards the achievement of personal and collective goals resulting in those satisfactions, so that they can reach what they consider the ultimate goal which provides them with the maximal satisfaction and moves them closer to happiness.

In this sense, when rural young peoples express critical arguments on the necessity of the presence of the State to guarantee the fulfillment of their rights, they behave as "rural subjects". And when they acquire their citizen consciousness in that their arguments are taken into account to implement actions and make decisions for the collective benefit by those who, from the State, have the power to make them in a certain moment, such young peoples behave as “rural social actors” who influence the betterment of their material environment to contribute to guaranteeing better life conditions or social well-being. Now, when they gradually reach the goals imposed that let them better their life conditions and those of the rural community, they pave the road to reach their ultimate goal, that is to be recognized as life examples to be followed by future generations. In this sense, when there is the subjective consciousness that their presence contributes to the psychosocial wellbeing of the members of the rural community, they are provided with satisfactions that move them closer to happiness, the ultimate goal of rural young peoples of the Colombian Andean high mountain zone.

The possible existence of two types of rural young peoples, derived from their occupation in rural work or education, that aim at reaching their ultimate goal in their lives and who consider it as the achievement to “be somebody” in life, it is simply their search for the recognition by the rural community where they are immersed and their own recognition as life examples or models to be followed by future generations. The reaching of this ultimate goal requires reaching other goals that could be short, medium or long-term ones, which gradually move them closer to this purpose. Accordingly, both the young worker and the young student aim at configuring themselves as “rural psychosocial actors” in their daily life. But this search is done through different ways: the worker, through the early integration to society in a kind of social pressing need that consolidates itself through their working bind or through the conformation of a new home; the student, with the postponement of that integration to society until acquiring the training or learning considered as indispensable, in a kind of rural social moratorium.

The attempt to argue, criticize or to propose options, according to their knowledge, to reach the goals aiming at the betterment of their life conditions, configures the rural young peoples of the Colombian Andean high mountain zone as “rural subjects” or people able to have projects, to judge something or somebody positively or negatively, and also to have social relations. These abilities ease the way to their configuration as “rural social actors” but not to their achievement. This happens given the lack of citizen consciousness, which is obtained only when the young peoples perceive they are recognized by the appropriate State authority to implement actions and make decisions taking into account their proposals, that is, when their participation becomes really effective.

Besides, when rural young peoples configure themselves as “rural social actors” or as agents who can contribute to the social wellbeing of their own community, they can go on the way to their configuration as “rural psychosocial actors” or agents able to contribute to the psychosocial wellbeing of their own community. But this configuration, which becomes their ultimate goal or life project, is not consolidated until, besides being perceived by the other members of the community, they perceive themselves as a life example or model to be followed by the members of the rural community where the young peoples coexist day by day, that is, until they acquire the subjective consciousness about this situation.

To move, then, positively along a route on which, short, medium and long-term goals are consolidated by young peoples, one configures them gradually as rural subjects and rural social subjects and ends with the goal which provides the most satisfaction and moves them closer to happiness: to be "rural psychosocial actors". This is a very fundamental goal, which without deciding and without having their actions propose it, their peers in the rural space where they coexist, including their children and the other young peoples' children, interiorize it, appropriate it and try to achieve it. In short, it is a collective, agglutinant and widely shared aspiration of psychosocial change aiming at consolidating a better situation. Accordingly, the rural young peoples' relation with the "others" is not a relation based upon the belonging to the same farm culture or to the same rural society, but an established one with the purpose to become "rural psychosocial actors" in rural life. It is a friendship relation that respects the distance, at the same time that generates communication, a relation that basically consists of considering the other as equal to oneself. It is a relation that, given the satisfactions generated, has positive implications in the community psychosocial wellbeing.

The solid purpose to recognize and to be recognized by the community as life examples and models to be followed by future generations motivates rural young peoples to reach their goals at work or at school. Besides, the desire that their children have "a good future" is not different from the intention to achieve that they also be recognized as life examples of models in their rural community. With this purpose, values such as solidarity, friendship, respect, admiration and care of nature, responsibility at work and at home are transmitted by parents from generation to generation. According to the workers and students' perception, the strong relation between the education level acquired by the parents and that acquired by the children is translated, towards the future, in a relation where the children's level of education is much higher than their parents' due to the desire that their children have a better rural quality of life.

Accordingly, psychosocial wellbeing is represented by the defense that rural young peoples make about their farming culture and about their rural space as a space of comprehension and solidarity. Consequently, when the informants manifest that they live calmly in the village because "we do not have problems with anybody, if we go somewhere we are everybody's friends" or because "the people here are very devoted to their work, they are very united", it reflects the defense of the farming culture which induces them to manifest their refusal to the intention of living elsewhere. This moral defense of the rural area that causes the working young peoples not to abandon the rural environment and that students want to go back home once they have finished their professional studies, is related to the perception that it is possible to enjoy a good rural life there, a satisfactory rural life that integrates social wellfare with psychological well-being.

Taking into account the interpretations constructed so far, the quality of young peoples' rural life in the Colombian Andean high mountain zone may be defined as a process through which they propose goals whose gradual achievements allow them to move along a positive way towards the obtaining of a higher or ultimate goal which will provide them with the maximal satisfaction that will move them nearer to happiness. The achievement of these goals, which are reached when the young peoples configure and exert as rural social subjects and actors, allows them to improve their life conditions, referred to as the satisfaction of needs and the consolidation of their fundamental rights that deal with the lack of property on the land on the part of young peoples, the inexistence of incentives for agricultural production, the need to improve the rural working conditions, access to rural education, lodging and health services. These conditions are considered precarious due to the traditional absence of the State and because they are really inferior with reference to those of young peoples in other contexts. The ultimate goal is reached when, at the moment of evaluating the goals reached in the course of life, there is a satisfaction that will permit these people to recognize themselves or to have the subjective consciousness to be life examples, models or guides to be followed by the new generations.

The rural quality of life is, then, a permanent construction process stimulated by the rural young peoples' aspiration to gain a collective recognition as good people in the Colombian Andean high mountain zone where they are immersed and to acquire the subjective consciousness of such recognition.

For quality of life studies and particularly for those concerning the rural quality of life, qualitative research is important as it presents its results in this chapter and it permits the approach of meaning interpretations that social actors in a determined context give to the daily practices with the aim to improve them. In Latin American countries characterized by social inequality and exclusion and, particularly in countries such as Colombia with the presence of social conflicts derived from this situation for more than 60 years, comprehensive studies on the quality of life that permit one to consolidate tolerance and to reduce discrimination on the basis of respect for differences become a need.

This study highlights the importance of qualitative research. As a matter of fact, the modification of the apathy *ethos* derived from the rural adolescents' formative ability to imitate the molds of the adults' apathy due to "rationalism in progress" that comes along with modernization, and which permits to recognize their unequal position in society, and how it worsens due to the strengthening of economic, commercial and financial globalization which, at the same time, intensifies social inequalities and the concentration of richness and opportunities in the hands of a few. Qualitative research allows one to identify, as in this case, the existence of an adequate sense of social injustice and to understand the just claim for the presence of the State which allows them to train themselves to encounter actions and decisions to reach what they perceive as a good quality of life, and how to consolidate their fundamental rights.

Only when those people who have the capacity and are empowered to make decisions and take actions with reference to the people's quality of life in a highly vulnerable contexts, when there is the want to recognize the inhabitants as valid subjects and actors to be consulted about those matters that they consider are affecting their lives, their families and the rural community's life, the results desired will be achieved. This will permit to reduce social conflicts as it will facilitate, in the possible Colombian post-conflict era, a look at the vulnerable populations such as the rural young people, rural subjects and social actors, who are to be recognized as valid, listened to and taken into account, by themselves, by the State and by the society.

From the methodological point of view, triangulation becomes a fundamental element in the research process done here. In this sense, the characterization required at the beginning of this study, as in the majority of studies on the quality of life, where reference to the socio-cultural context of the research study and the scenario where the field work takes place, requires the use of the qualitative method. It is also required the use of the quantitative method with its statistical support, given the existence of particular contexts where there is a lack, as in this case, of adequate information previously elaborated.

With reference to the triangulation of the information sources, information resulting from observation, which starts as non-participating information and ends as a participating one; the gathering of secondary information which, for example, from formal theory permits one to construct a theoretical framework that references the study and the primary information derived from the in-depth interviews, makes possible the emergence of the substantive theory represented in the definition of emergent categories such as the "rural quality of life", "rural subject" and "rural social actor", presented in this chapter.

It is also correct to emphasize on the importance of the theoretical triangulation used in this study, as it allows one to approach the theories which, from North America, Western Europe and Latin America, are constructed by contemporary researchers on the quality of life and to define the way to configure Touraine's subject and social actor. Such theories define the way in which the subject is configured and how it transcends to social actor. These approaches and interpretations resulting from the research findings make possible the emergence of categories such as rural quality of life and subcategories such as rural subject, rural social actor and rural psychosocial actor.

References

Almond, G., & Powell, B. (1972). *Política comparada. Una concepción evolutiva*. Buenos Aires: Editorial Paidos.

Andrews, F. M., & Withey, S. B. (1976). *Social indicators of Well-Being: Americans perceptions of life quality*. New York: Plenum Press.

Ariza, A. (1992). *Los dominicos en Colombia*. Tomo I. Bogotá: Ediciones Antropos.

Bango, J. (2000). *Políticas de juventud en América Latina en la antesala del 2000: logros, desafíos y oportunidades*. Madrid: Organización Iberoamericana de Juventud—Centro Internacional de Investigaciones para el Desarrollo. http://www.cinterfor.org.uy/public/spanish/region/ampro/cinterfor/temas/youngpeople/doc/not/libro237/libro237.pdf. Accessed 27 Oct 2007.

Bauer, R. (1966). *Social indicators*. Cambridge: M.I.T. Press.

Becerra, H. C. (2001). *Consideraciones sobre la juventud rural de América Latina y el Caribe* [Versión electrónica]. Documento preparado para el Primer Congreso Mundial de Jóvenes Empresarios y Pymes celebrado en Zaragoza, España, en 2002. http://www.rlc.fao.org/prior/desrural/juventud/considera.pdf. Accessed 27 Nov 2008.

Berger, P., & Luckmann, T. (2001). *La construcción social de la realidad*. Buenos Aires: Amorrortu Editores.

Blanco, A. (1985). La calidad de vida: supuestos psicosociales. In J. F. Morales, A. Blanco, C. Huici, & J. M. Fernández (Eds.), *Psicología social aplicada* (pp. 159–182). Bilbao: Desclée de Brouwer.

Bonilla, R., et al. (2004). *Situación actual y prospectiva de la niñez y la juventud en Colombia.* Bogotá: Universidad Nacional. http://www.colombiajoven.gov.co/documentos/generales/doc_siju.pdf. Accessed 16 Sept 2006.

Bourdieu, P. (1998). *La distinción. Criterio y bases sociales del gusto.* Santafé de Bogotá: Santillana.

Briones, G. (2002). Metodología de la investigación en las ciencias sociales y en el derecho. Seminario Internacional presentado en la Universidad Libre de Bogotá, Colombia, en octubre de 2002. http://www.redsociojuridica.org/documentos/metodologia_investigacion_ciencias_sociales.pdf. Accessed 19 July 2007.

Casas, F. (1989). *Técnicas de investigación social: Los indicadores sociales y psicosociales*. Barcelona: PPU.

Casas, F. (1996). *Bienestar social. Una introducción psicosociológica.* Barcelona: PPU.

Casas, F. (1999). Calidad de Vida y Calidad Humana. *Revista Papeles del Psicólogo 74* . Instituto de Investigación sobre calidad de vida. Girona (España). pp. 2–14. http://www.papelesdelpsicologo.es/vernumero.asp?id=812. Accessed 27 April 2014.

Campbell, A., Converse, P. E., y Rodgers, W. L. (1976). *The quality of American life: Perceptions, evaluations and satisfactions*. New York: Russell Sage Foundation.

Cea, D' Ancona. (1999). *Metodología cuantitativa. Estrategias y técnicas de investigación social.* Madrid: Editorial Síntesis.

CINEP. (2007). *90 falsos positivos denuncia el CINEP* [Versión electrónica]. Bogotá: Red de defensores no institucionalizados. http://www.dhcolombia.info/spip.php?article434. Accessed 29 Jan 2009.

CINEP. (2013). *Informe especial sobre la situación de derechos humanos y derecho internacional humanitario en Colombia durante 2012*. CINEP/ Programa por la Paz, mayo 2013. http://www.jesuitas.org.co/documentos/108.pdf. Accessed 3 April 2014.

Departamento Nacional de Planeación. (2009). *Lineamientos para implementar el proyecto satelital de comunicaciones de Colombia.* Documento CONPES 3579 del 25 de marzo de 2009. Bogotá: DNP.

Duncan, D. (1969). *Toward social reporting: Next steps*. New York: Russell Sage Foundation.

Durston, J. (2002). Juventud rural en Brasil y México. Reduciendo la invisibilidad. Ponencia presentada en el XX Congreso de la Asociación Latinoamericana de Sociología, ALAS, Brasil. http://www.eclac.cl/publicaciones/xml/6/4646/indice.html. Accessed 20 Dec 2005.

Escobar, R. et al. (2004). *Estado del arte del conocimiento producido sobre jóvenes en Colombia.* Bogotá: Colombia Joven—Presidencia de la República de Colombia. http://www.colombiajoven.gov-co/documentos/raes/informe_estado_arte.pdf. Accessed 5 Oct 2006.

Evans, D. R., Burns, J. E., Robinson, W. E., & Garrett, O. J. (1985). The quality of, life questionnaire: A multidimensional measure. *American Journal of Community Psychology, 13,* 305–322.

Fals Borda, O. (1961). *Campesinos de los Andes. Estudio sociológico de Saucio*. Bogotá: Universidad Nacional.

Fals Borda, O. (2000). *Acción y espacio. Autonomías en la nueva República.* Bogotá: Tercer Mundo.

Fedepapa. (2010). Acuerdo de competitividad de la cadena agroalimentaria de la papa en Colombia. http://www.fedepapa.com/wp-content/uploads/pdf/ACUERDO-COMPETITIVIDAD-CADENA-AGROALIMENTARIA-PAPA.pdf. Accessed 7 Oct 2008.

Feixa, C. & González, Y. (2006). Territorios baldíos: identidades juveniles indígenas y rurales en América Latina [Versión electrónica]. En: Papers, Revista de Sociología de la Universidad Autónoma de Barcelona, No. 79. (pp. 171–193). Accessed 18 August 2014. http://www.raco.cat/index.php/papers/article/viewFile/51828/57557.

Fernández Dols, J. M. (1990). *Patrones para el diseño de la psicología social*. Madrid: Morata.

González, Y. (2004). Óxidos de identidad: memoria y juventud rural en el sur de Chile (pp. 1935–2003) [Versión electrónica]. Tesis para optar el título de Doctorado en Antropología. L.

http://www.tdx.cat/bitstream/handle/10803/5508/ygc5de6.pdf;jsessionid=F1BFDB6B41DED357E43BD3DBB9F8F911.tdx2?sequence=5. Accessed 15 June 2014.

Hammersley, M., & Atkinson, P. (1994). *Etnografía. Métodos de investigación*. Buenos Aires: Paidos.

Hopenhayn, M., et al. (2004). *La juventud en Iberoamérica. Tendencias y urgencias*. Santiago de Chile: CEPAL. http://www.cepal.org/publicaciones/xml/6/20266/CEPAL_OIJ.pdf. Accessed 13 Nov 2008.

Kessler, G. (2005). *Estado del arte de la investigación sobre juventud rural en América Latina*. Buenos Aires: Secretaria de Agricultura, Ganadería, Pesca y Alimentos-Argentina. http://www.relajur.org/tema%20del%20mes/Tema%20del%20Mes%20Enero.pdf. Accessed 21 Aug 2013.

Kreitler, S., & Nive, D. (2007). Quality of life and coping in chronic pain patients. In S. Kreitler, D. Beltuti, A. Lamberto, & D. Niv (Eds.), *The handbook of chronic pain* (pp. 77–99). USA: Nova.

Llambí, L. (2002). El desarrollo rural sostenible de la ecorregión tropical andina. *Políticas Agrícolas. Revista de de la Red de Instituciones vinculadas a la capacitación en economía y políticas agrícolas en América Latina y El Caribe*. No 12, 9–15.

Mannheim, K. (1993). El Problema de las generaciones. *Revista Española de Investigaciones Sociológicas, 62,* 193–242.

Mendoza, A. (2000). *Colombia: Estado regional. Ordenamiento territorial*. Bogotá: Sociedad Geográfica de Colombia.

Michalos, A. C. (1980). *North American Social Report: A comparative Study of the Quality of Life in Canada and USA from 1964 to 1974*. Dordrecht: Reidel Publishing Company.

Moix, M. (1986). *Bienestar social*. Madrid: Trivium.

Murcia, N., & Jaramillo, L. (2000). *La complementariedad etnográfica. Investigación cualitativa*. Armenia: Kinesis.

Ocampo, L. (1983). *Historia del pueblo boyacense. De los orígenes paleo indígenas y míticos a la culminación de la independencia*. Tunja: Ediciones Instituto de Cultura y Bellas Artes de Boyacá.

Parsons, T. (1974). *El sistema de las sociedades modernas*. Ciudad de México: Editorial Trillas.

Parsons, T. (1984). *El sistema social*. Madrid: Alianza Editorial.

Parsons, T., & Platt, G. (1973). *The American University*. Cambridge: Harvard University Press.

Peccei, A. (1976). *La qualità humana*. Milano: Arnoldo Mondadori. (Trad.: *La calidad humana*. Informes al Club de Roma. Madrid: Taurus, 1977).

Quiroga, G. (2002). Las escuelas agrarias porteras adentro. Ponencia presentada en el IV Congreso de la Asociación Latinoamericana de Sociología Rural, ALASRU, Universidad Federal del Río Grande del Sur, Porto Alegre, Brasil, 25 al 29 de noviembre de 2002.

República de Colombia. (2011a). Gobernación de Boyacá—Fondo para el Financiamiento del Sector Agropecuario (FINAGRO)–Instituto Geográfico Agustín Codazzi (2012). Departamento de Boyacá Colombia. Ubicación, extensión, límites y actividades productivas. http://www.todacolombia.com/departamentos/boyaca.html. Accessed 14 June 2013.

República de Colombia. (2011b). Gobernación de Cundinamarca Colombia –Fondo para el Financiamiento del Sector Agropecuario (FINAGRO), Instituto Geográfico Agustín Codazzi, Departamento de Cundinamarca–. Ubicación y límites, División administrativa, Fisiografía, Hidrografía, Clima, Actividades económicas, Vías de comunicación, Turismo, Historia y Símbolos del departamento. Accessed 14 June 2013. http://www.todacolombia.com/departamentos/cundinamarca.html.

Rostow, W. W. (1973). *Las etapas del crecimiento económico. Un manifiesto no comunista*. Madrid: Ministerio del Trabajo y Seguridad Nacional.

Sarmiento, A. L. (2004). Política pública de juventud en Colombia. Logros, dificultades y perspectivas. In *Germán Muñoz* (Eds.), *Construcción de políticas de juventud. Análisis y perspectivas* (pp. 115–193) (Cap. III). Manizales: Colombia Joven-U. de Manizales-CINDE-GTZ–UNICEF.

Sen, A. (1996). Capacidad y bienestar. In M. Nussbaum, & A. Sen (Eds.), *La calidad de vida* (pp. 54–83). México, D. F.: Fondo de Cultura Económica.

Serrano, J. F., Bejarano L., Caicedo A., Hoyos D., Quintero F. (2002). Estado del arte de la investigación sobre juventud para la formulación de la política. Presidencia de la República–Programa

presidencial Colombia Joven. http://www.colombiajoven.gov.co/documentos_normatividad.htm. Accessed 9 June 2007.
Sierra, F. (1998). Función y sentido de la entrevista cualitativa en investigación social. In J. Galindo (Eds.), *Técnicas de investigación en sociedad, cultura y comunicación* (pp. 277–341). México: PEARSON.
Smith, D. (1973). *The geography of social well-being in the United States*. New York: McGraw-Hill.
Strauss A., & Corbin, J. (2002). *Bases de la investigación cualitativa. Técnicas y procedimientos para desarrollar la teoría fundamentada*. Medellín: Universidad de Antioquia.
Tonon, G. (2008). Investigar la calidad de vida en Argentina. *Revista Psicodebate 8. Psicología, Cultura y Sociedad*.Facultad de Ciencias Sociales. Universidad de Palermo. Bs. As. Marzo 2008. pp. 141–151.
Tonon, G. (2009). *Los estudios sobre calidad de vida y la perspectiva de la psicología positiva. Revista Psicodebate 10. Psicología, Cultura y Sociedad Facultad de Ciencias Sociales* (pp. 73–81). Buenos Aires: Universidad de Palermo.
Touraine, A. (1996). Juventud y democracia en Chile. En, *Revista Iberoamericana de Juventud No 1*, 36–48. Madrid: UNESCO.
Touraine, A. (2000). *¿Podremos vivir juntos? La discusión pendiente: el destino del hombre en la aldea global*. Ciudad de México: Fondo de Cultura Económica.
Valles, M. (1999). *Técnicas cualitativas de investigación social. Reflexión metodológica y práctica profesional*. Madrid: SÍNTESIS.

Chapter 10
A Qualitative Study on Yoga Practice in Quality of Labor Life

Lia Rodriguez de la Vega

10.1 Quality of Life

Although the interest in quality of life goes a long way back in time, its conception and systematic and scientific assessment are relatively recent; it became a popular idea in the 1960s and is, nowadays, a widely used concept in different spheres.

Tonon (2007) considers that the study of quality of life refers to the material and psychosocial environment, thus acknowledging two spheres of wellbeing: social and psychological, the latter corresponding with people's experience and the assessment they make of their own situations; this includes positive and/or negative outlooks and a global visión of their lives i.e. vital satisfaction. The social agents make general assessments of their lives, taking different aspects of them into consideration.

Dennis et al. (1994) sustain that the research focuses on quality of life may be classified into two types: a) quantitative focal points, which seek to operationalize quality of life through the study of different indicators and b) the qualitative ones, which adopt the attitude of listening to the subjects (Gómez Vela 2000). According to Veenhoven (1994), quality of life involves two meanings: (1) the presence of conditions considered indispensable to a good life and (2) the actual practice of good living, the latter being the one which submits the consideration of factors which largely depend on the subjects' actions and perceptions of their own lives.

García Martín (2002) points out that this objective-subjective dimensional differentiation has brought about an intensification of individual analysis as opposed

L. Rodriguez de la Vega (✉)
UNICOM, Faculty of Social Sciences, Universidad Nacional de Lomas de Zamora, Lomas de Zamora, Argentina

CICS, Faculty of Social Sciences, Universidad de Palermo, Ciuadad Autónoma de Buenos Aires, Argentina
e-mail: liadelavega@yahoo.com

G. Tonon (ed.), *Qualitative Studies in Quality of Life*,
Social Indicators Research Series 55, DOI 10.1007/978-3-319-13779-7_10

to the social or structural ones, thus allowing an approach on the subjective dimension of of human welfare by laying emphasis on internal components.

According to Diener and Diener (1995), we may assert that the concepts of welfare may be grouped into three categories: (1) which describes welfare as the individuals' appraisal of their own lives in positive terms ("satisfaction with life"), (2) which has a bearing on the superiority of positive feelings or affection over negative ones, and (3) the closest to philosofical-religious questions, which considers happiness as a virtue or grace—definitions derived from this perspective may be considered normative (García Martín 2002). Petito and Cummins (2000) uphold a perspective centered in the individuals, thus considering welfare in terms of individual assessment on their quality of life, which has two components: satisfaction with life—implying a cognitive assessment—, and a component of affection, which involves feelings and moods.

10.2 Work and Quality of Labor Life

León Palacios (2003) expounds that the combination of capitalist restructuring and information technologies have direct effects on the international división of labor, the circulation of financial capital, and industry, thus implying changes in the social order. This is occuring in an asiymetrically inter-dependent world, revolving round Europe, the United States, and Asia, polarized by an axis that divides wealthy regions with high information rates, from indigent regions—socially empoverished and with devaluated economies. In such a setting regarding Latin-America, Rendón and Salas (2000) have established the following tendencies in the labor market: (a) plain unemployment, loss of warranties derived from seniority and empyrical knowledge, flexibilization, increase in the number of employed family members, feminization, reduction of the state and employers' contributions to social security, increasingly precarious labor conditions, decentralization of collective bargaining, etc.

Castel (1995), on the other hand, adopts a posture regarding the individuals' constitution through the emergence and transformation of problem fields and devices which define the base of the modern man's individuality. His view is directed to that increasingly fragile base, i.e., to the loss of affiliation processes and their vulnerable zones. He focuses on a contemporary social process with which most post-industrial societies are faced: the growth of unemployment together with a general weakening of labor conditions and protection of the laborers, underlining its effect on the construction of the individuals' social support.

In this context, he considers centralizing the analysis of the existence or non-existence of a relationship between individuals and their work, for he does not conceive work as a technical relationship involving production, but as a privileged support which allows a subscription to the social structure. He considers the existence of a profound correlation between the position occupied by individuals in the social division of labor—as well as their participation in socialization networks, and the protection systems to safeguard them, when faced with existencial contingencies. According to this author, the individuals' protective layers may be metaphorically considered as social cohesion zones. Thus, a solid insertion in the labor networks, where they may enjoy relative security in terms of salary and health insurance, among other aspects, implies situating the individuals in an integration zone while, an insertion in weak labor networks would, on the contrary, derive in a process of social vulnerability.

He claims that individuals need to occupy a certain space in society in order to develop their capacity to become individuals (Castel and Haroche 2003) which is directly linked to the processes of cohesion and social vulnerability, but also to the social instances that allow the creation of spaces for the individuals' support.

Proceeding with Castel's considerations, we coincide with Martuccelli (2002), who believes that, though there is no denying the need for different resources, social rights and the access to certain protective institutions, the construction of modern individuals must contemplate that "their possibility to create themselves from the sphere of sense production should not be overlooked for one moment, by considering it, inevitably, anchored to a supportive base" (p. 96).

As to the Quality of Labor Life, Duro Martín (2002) points out that the workers' psychological labor welfare and their mental health at work are personal consequences of their work, of their subjective experience, and that they affect the workers' own organization and family life. Moreover, his writings have allowed us to verify the following: (a) the existence of a mixture of both types of consequents, as shown in various studies on the different aspects of the workers' psychological welfare and labor mental health, for instance: professional self-esteem and stress and/or burnout (Gil-Monte and Peiró 1997); on labor satisfaction, and anxiety, depression and irritability (Hackman and Oldham 1980); on excessive work and labor satisfaction, etc; (b) awareness of the existence of a certain amount of concealment and confusion among labor syndrome and psychological conditions, for instance: depression and burnout (Leiter and Durup 1994; Schaufeli and Enzmann 1998), stress and burnout (Mearns and Cain 2003), etc., and (c) that the workers' psychological welfare and labor mental health have a common background (for example, an adequate amount of work offers a psychological sense of wellbeing while excessive work may begin by deteriorating that sense of wellbeing and, eventually, damage the workers' labor mental health).

10.3 Yoga

Yoga is considered to be what is popularly called Complementary or Alterative Medicine. Bowling (2010) points out that in the field of complementary and alternative medicine (CAM, English acronym/MCA, Spanish acronym) different terms are used. A broader one is "non-conventional medicine", alluding to therapies which are not normally taught in medical school, or not available in hospitals. The terms "complementary" and "alternative" refer to the way in which the therapies are applied: complementary therapies are applied together with conventional medicine; while alternative therapies actually replace conventional medicine.

These medical practices are defined, in connection with conventional medicine. An example of this is the fact that they are defined by the U.S. National Health Institutes as: "*healing practices* […] *which differ from the politically predominant health system in a particular society* […] *within a certain historical period*". (p. 4). These techniques are diversely found in countries all over the world (OMS/WHO 2002). On the other hand, within that denomination (MCA/CAM, also generally associated to Traditional Medicine, according to OMS/WHO 2002) numerous practices are included: non-medicated therapies (yoga, accupuncture, manual therapies, Gigong, Tai ji, thermal therapy, and other physical and mental therapies), or therapies requiring medication (using medicines obtained from herbs, animal and/or mineral parts) (OMS/WHO 2002).

The root of the word "yoga" is "juj" (to bind, oppress, yoke, etc.). The actual term Yoga is used to designate "all ascetic techniques and any other method of meditation" (Eliade 1998, p. 18), though classical Yoga exists; a philosophical system ("darsana", a system of coherent assertions extended to human experience, which it endeavours to interpret as a whole, with the intention of delivering men from ignorance) expounded by Patanjali in his treatise Yoga-Sutra, and other innumerable popular forms. Yoga is one of the six orthodox Indian philosophical systems, and the best known in the Western World, by its formulation of Patanjali.

One of the features of Yoga, apart from its practical aspect, is its initiation structure, since it is not only learnt from a teacher (guru). In India, all philosophical systems are taught by teachers, which confers them such character, for initiations are transmitted orally, "from mouth to ear". Nevertheless, Yoga further adds the fact that the yogi begins by abandoning the profane world (family, society) and devoting himself to successively overcoming the conduct and values inherent to human conduct, through their guru. Thus, it may be said to impy a form of death (of a manner), and the rebirth (of another being: liberation) (Eliade 1988).

Yoga, the philosophical system, is very similar to another Indian philosophical system, actually considered by Zimmer (1979) as two aspects of the same discipline. While Samkhya upholds a theoretical exposition of human nature—including an enumeration and definition of its elements, analyzing the way in which they collaborate in the binding state (Bandha) and describing its state of liberation (moksha), Yoga concretely approaches the dynamics of the sepatation process and points out the liberation practices. Although it is believed that the fundamentals of Samkhya and Yoga are extremely ancient, they were not found in orthodox Indian texts until a relatively late date (Upanishads and Bhagavad Gita), in which they are found harmonized with Vedic philosophy (Zimmer 1979).

In the aforementioned texts of Yoga Sutra –which date is controversial, given the fact that the first three books might date back to the second century B.C., the fourth one seems to have appeared later, probably in the fifth century, according to Zimmer (1979)-, Patanjali, the autor refers to the eight step path of Yoga (or "Ashtanga Yoga", in Sanskrit), namely: (1) Yama (Sanskrit term which alludes to moral restrictions, abstention and self-restriction), (2) Niyama (Sanskrit term for observances, values and precepts), (3) Asana (Sanskrit term to designate postures) (4) Pranayama (Sanskrit term which refers to breathing/energy regulation), (5) Pratyahara (Sanskrit term which alludes to the retraction of the senses), (6) Dharana (Sanskrit term refered to concentration), (7) Dhyana (Sanskrit term alluding to meditation, to contemplation) y (8) Samadhaya (Sanskrit term which alludes to the absorption of conscience within the self, deep meditation, super conscience) (Iyengar 2002, pp. 31–32, pp. 140–142).

Finally, it is worth mentioning that Hatha Yoga (Hathayoga, in Sanskrit) is one of the major Yoga systems and the most widely spread in Western practices, its best known text being Hatha Yoga Pradipika (Svatmarama 2002). The practice of Hatha Yoga is considered to bring equilibrium and balance on solar and lunar energies –Ha means "sun" and Tha means "moon", in Sanskrit- (Maheshwarananda 2009).

10.4 Disquiet and Self-Care/Self-Practice

Foucault (1987) points out the precept that looking after oneself is imperative to different doctrines, that it has impregnated ways of living, and developed in the procedures and practices which are being developed and taught; "it has, thus, constituted a social practice, giving way to inter-individual relations, exchange and communication, and even to institutions; it has, finally, generated a certain mode of learning and the elaboration of a certain knowledge" (p. 43).

In his view, self-care is understood as a set of pracrices through which a subject establishes a certain relationship with him/herself and, thus, becomes subject of his/her own actions (Chirolla 2007). This self-care implies self knowledge (Robbins 2007, quoted in Garcés Giraldo and Giraldo Zuluaga 2013), is directed to the soul, but it involves the body in its infinite details, and constitutes a preparation for a complete fulfilment in life (Giraldo 2008).

Lanz (2012) points out that, according to Foucault, self-care comprises three fundamental aspects: (1) an attitude of respect for oneself, for others, and for the world, (2) a particular attention, a view from the outside to the inside, focused on one's thoughts. It is an outlook of the practice of subjectivity, (3) it names a series of actions, actions which are carried out by oneself, through which one takes charge of oneself and is transformed. Self-care also requires a reflective movement about oneself, a permanent review of the ways in which one has sought to orient one's conduct, examining it in order to improve it. Thus, the techniques which allow us such procedure are known as technologies of the "self":

> They allow individuals to carry out (on their own accord, or with the help of others), a certain number of operations on their bodies and souls, thoughts, behavior, or any other aspect of their being, thus achieving a transformation within themselves in order to reach a state of happiness, purity, wisdom, or immortality (Foucault 1990, p. 48).

He proposes four principal types among these technologies and points out that each one represents a matrix of practical reasoning: (1) technologies of production, which allow us to produce and transform things, (2) technologies of sign systems, which allow us to use signs or significations; (3) technologies of power, which determine the individuals' behavior, submitting them to certain ends and (4) technologies of the Self, that allow subjects to do a certain number of operations on their bodies and souls, or any other aspect of their being, thus achieving a transformation within themselves in order to reach a state of happiness, wisdom, or immortality (Foucault 1990).

Sáenz Obregón (s./f.- no date) points out that these practices stem from the individuals'dissatisfaction with their present state and their quest for transformation, with an underlying knowledge-power relation, at the point of relating to their own knowledge and that of others. Britos (2005) claims that these self practices delimit self knowledge within a series of practices and physical, behavioral, and meditation exercises aimed at the construction of a better existence and the pursuit of happiness. Along with that, Sossa Rojas (2010) adds that such instruction on living techniques will allow, or contribute to finding the truth, the personal truth, and the transformation of subjectivity. Thus, resorting to Yoga, as a practice itself, is a way of considering it a voluntary practice through which those who practice it act upon themselves in order to achieve a transformation.

Whether individual or collective, the practices in question are social practices (Foucault 1994) and they, therefore, have varied according to the historical contexts in which they were carried out, from ancient times up to the present. Considering the present time, Ravettino (2008) believes that there is an obsession with the body, which has surpassed bodily superficiality, since not only is it a quest for adequate weight and appearance but also for body welfare, through the advent of health prevention practices. Bauman (2006, quoted in Ravettino 2008) adds that, in consumerist societies, the subjects' obsession with health and personal care becomes increasingly outstanding, "being fit". Thus, this state of "feeling better" is reflected, not only in eating habits but also in physical training and leisure activities. Moreover, in this context, physical activity is raging among major organizations, seeking to reduce absenteeism and boosting the emplyees' performance; several Argentine firms are offering their staff a variety of physical activities during labor time (or out of schedule, on the premises). This is the echo of a phenomenon originated in the United States, following directions emanated from the main offices.

Regarding choices, interests, and motivations, Lewin (1939), considers, from the view-point of Psychology, that the subjects' aims and needs are dynamizing elements in their behavior while, according to Nuttin (1985), there is the so-called "tendency towards self-fulfilment", an inner force that urges the subjects to fulfil their potentialities and carry out their projects, in a process of unity and differentiation between what they wish to become and the image they have of the environment. In this respect, D'angelo (2013), point out the existence of an orientation towards self-fulfillment which urges the subjects to develop their essential potentialities, values and interests, in the context of their social activities.

10.5 The Body as a Semantic Vector

According to Le Breton (2002), the body is the semantic vector through which the evidence of the actors' social relationship with the world is constructed, and is responsible for the generation and propagation of "the significations that constitute the basis of an individual and collective existence. It is the axis of their relationship with the world, the place and the time in which existence becomes part of the actors' flesh as a result of their singular outlook on it" (pp. 7–8). It is through their corporeal condition that the subjects transform the world into a familiar and coherent fabric, available both for action and comprehension. "Both by emitting and receiving, the body produces continuous sense, thus, men are actively inserted in a given social and cultural space." (p. 8). Social order filters through their body, through the education they have received, identifications of the subject, cultural transformations in their life-styles, etc.

The representations of the body are a function of the representation of people and both are inserted in the world's vision of the community/group they belong to. The modern conception of the body regards men as being separate from the cosmos, from other men, and from themselves. Yet, there are societies in which such separation does not exist, and the body is inscribed in a complex network of correspondence—between body and cosmos—i.e. the body and its representations, knowledge systems it is referred to, etc., alter from one society to another. It is important to highlight that, in our societies, there are various body models associated to different medical practices (biomedical formal and dominant cognizance, parallel or popular medical practices, etc.). "In the foundations of all social practices, as a privileged mediator and pivot of human presence, the body is situated at the crossroads of all cultural instances; it is the supreme imputation point in the symbolic field". (p. 32). Thus, it is essential to consider the fact that the body does not exist in its natural shape, it is always inserted in a web of sense i.e., the body is construed as a base of values. "The body is a metaphor of the social aspect, and the latter is a metaphor of the body". (p. 73).

10.6 Yoga and Quality of Life

The studies on quality of life are numerous and embrace different aspects. Quality of life studies and alternative or complementary techniques are, generally, approached from a medical perspective (Taylor 2012; Wells et al. 2007; Matthees et al. 2001; Astin 1998).

As to the quality of labor life, Duro Martín (2002) considers that the workers' psychological labor welfare and their mental health in the same context are the personal consequences of work; they constitute its subjective experience, and have certain effects on the actual organization (effects on productivity, direct and indirect costs) and on the workers' families (break-ups, other conflicts, etc.). He further adds that the different approaches on workers' psychological welfare are, basically, made in the field of study on quality of labor life, considering different aspects, such as: labor satisfaction (Bravo et al. 1996); labor satisfaction, welfare and quality of life (Requena 2000), absenteeism (Burton et al. 2002; Harrison and Martocchio 1998); person-environment adjustment (Kahn and Boysiere 1992); task contents (Karasek et al. 1998), etc. Parallel to this, the approaches on workers' psychological welfare, in broader terms, and the themes of labor mental health, have mostly been dealt with in studies on social psychlogy applied to labor health; for instance, in studies on stress (Spielberger et al. 2003), burnout or syndrome of being burnt out by work (Bakker et al. 2002), labor harassment or mobbing (González de Rivera 2002), sexual harassment at work (Harned et al. 2002), and other more general psychological disorders, and a diversity of symptoms, namely, studies on: depression, anxiety, alcohol consumption, somehow, associated to work.

Among the studies on the use of alternative and/or complementary techniques in the work place, Smith (2005) concluded that the employees of very small firms are more open to the use of those techniques, in connection with labor induced stress and fatigue. Halpern (2011); Kellner et al. (2002); Coulter and Willis (2004), among others, consider that the use of "alternative techniques" has become common in the Western World, Yoga being one of the best known and more widely used, including a diversity of physical practices (postures or asanas, breathing exercises, relaxation and meditation) as well as philosophical formulations on reality and the life styles derived from it.

There are several studies on the effect of the different meditation techniques which, though close to the yoga practice are not classified as forming part of it, such as Transcendental Meditation (MT)™ (Ospina et al. 2007), Budhist Zeb Meditation (Chiesa 2009; Chiesa and Serretti 2010; Ospina et al. 2007), Vipassana meditation (Chiesa and Serretti 2010; Chiesa and Serretti 2009), and several other contemporary forms of meditation (Ospina et al. 2007; Chiesa and Serretti 2009). There are also studies on the effects of non-yoga contemporary relaxation techniques, which share certain similarities with Yoga techniques (Carlson and Hoyle 1993), on "stretching" (Thacker et al. 2004; Herbert and Gabriel 2002; Andersen 2005; Shrier 2004), and on isometric training techniques (Millar et al. 2007; Peters et al. 2006; Taylor et al. 2003).

There are also numerous studies on the effects of Yoga practice, though varying in quality, method, and population. Most of them apply protocols which incorporate, at least, two elements of Yoga practice (such as, e.g. asana and relaxation, or pranayama and meditation), while a few have settled on the effects of a single Yoga practice (asana, pranayama, relaxation or meditation).

Different research papers have demonstrated the beneficial effects of Yoga practice on sleep disorders and insomnia (Shannahoff-Khalsa 2004, 2006; Manjunath and Telles 2005; Cohen et al. 2004; Halpern 2011, Chen et al. 2008, 2009, 2010; Patra and Telles 2009, 2010; Telles et al. 2000, etc.). There are also studies on the offect of Yoga practice on depression—which are said to have obtained seemingly positive results—though further research is required, considering the heterogeneity of the protocols used and the quality of the methodology (Pilkington et al. 2005-idea shared by Uebelacker et al. 2010). On the other hand, few studies have been made on the effect of those practices on anxiety and anxiety disorders, though they have been proved effective, while requiring more research on the topic. (Kirkwood et al. 2005).

A research on practices of the Iyengar Yoga method to reduce stress showed significant improvements over the measuring of self-perceived stress and indicators of physical welfare (Michalsen et al. 2005). On the other hand, the studies on the effects of Yoga practices on muscular-skeletal pain, proved that the achievement of pain reduction and general physical improvement (Raub 2002; Sherman et al. 2005; John et al. 2007; Garfinkel et al. 1994; Kolasinski et al. 2005, etc.) moreover, Yoga practice has been shown to reduce factors of risk in connection to chronic diseases, including blood pressure, cholesterol, trigliceric acid, oxidative stress, glucose and clotting factors (Yang 2007; Innes et al. 2005; Innes and Vincent 2007, etc).

The approach on the effects of Yoga on the cardio-respiratory function offers several relevant studies that show significant improvement in different parameters which include the lung function, improvement in the work average, and in physical exercise as well as a reduction in oxygen consumption. Some studies even suggest that these practices may cause significant improvement in chronic asthma symptoms and in bronchitis. (Raub 2002). In this connection, the research on the scope of Pranayama practice makes reference to its beneficial effects in the reduction of anxiety, stress, and depression; it further shows improvements in the use of oxygen and in immune system markers, reduction of blood pressure, etc. (Brown and Gerbarg 2005a, b; Janakiramaiah et al. 2000; Shannahoff-Khalsa 1993; Kjellgren et al. 2007; Sharma et al. 2008; Raju et al. 1994; Pramanik et al. 2009, etc.)

Other studies focus on the effects of non-yoga stretching, and to the effect of the cycles of sometric effort and rest periods which, owing to their similarities with Asana practices, may be considered to have equivalent results (Herbert and Gabriel 2002; Thacker et al. 2004; Andersen 2005, etc.). The aforementioned studies indicate that stretching does not necessarily reduce the risk of wounds, but may contribute to shorten their period of recovery, reduce blood pressure, etc.

Regarding the scope of meditation practices, Yoga Nidra (Yoga dream) has been instrumental in the studies thaat were carried out, and it has been attributed improvements in psychological and physiological level measuring including stress, anxiety, and self-assessed welfare, among others. (Pritchard et al. 2010; Kamakhya 2004; Vempati and Telles 2002; Lou et al. 1999; Amita et al. 2009, etc.).

There are further studies which consider the effects of Yoga practice on the needs of senior adults (Krucoff et al. 2010; Manjunath and Telles 2005; SAY 2010, etc.), while a few other works have compared the effects of Yoga practice to that of non-Yoga practices (Streeter et al. 2010; Ross and Thomas 2010).

In the same field of work, a group of researchers from Ohio University, authors of an abridged versión of Yoga practice, applied it to a study made on participant members of weekly group gatherings held in the lunch hour at work, during which meditation and Yoga practice were carried out on the premises and, after six weeks' practice, they (among other things) were able to report an increased awareness of the participants regarding external stress factors; a sense of relief of the stress caused by events in their lives; and a reduction in sleeping disorders, as compared to the members of the control group that did not take part in the experiment (Klatt et al. 2009).

The Supervising Office of Traditional Medicine and Intercultural Development, Secretary of Health, Mexico 2007, (In Spanish: Dirección de Medicina Tradicional y Desarrollo Intercultural, Dirección General de Planeación y Desarrollo en Salud, Secretaría de Salud de México 2007) highlights the contributions of Yoga to its diagnosis made by the different clinical therapeutic models for diabetes mellitus. While in Brazil, Dantas de Carvalho and da Silva Correia (2011) studied the beneficial effects of Yoga in women undergoing the process of counteracting the habituation effects of Diazepam, certifying that the Yoga practices allowed a more accurate self-perception in the women included in their study by producing awareness of their dependence on that medicine; furthermore, they observed a significant reduction, and even total abstention, in the use of the aforementioned tranquilizer.

Fajardo Pulido (2009) considers that Yoga practice in Bogotá (Colombia) conceives a particular vision of the body which promotes a holistic mode of existence whithin the logics of a spiritual experience, materialized in individual bodies. He claims that oriental spirituality entails "new forms" of experiencing, both of health and illness, which is having a comercial repercussion among complementary health service institutions and in urban Bogotá. Moreover, he believes that, to those who embrace the promise of a better life, the time devoted to weekly Yoga practice is no longer a mere corporeal experience but rather a lifestyle, through a body in permanent construction in different strata, thus transforming their vision of the world. Also in Colombia, Ramírez Suárez (2011) focuses on Yoga as a practice of the self and according to his study the people who practice it belong to the high and high middle class from the city, which possesses the economic and socio-cultural means to gain access to the aforementioned practice. The reasons alleged for the practice of Yoga are: emotional crises, physical disquiet produced by illness; or sheer interest in leading a healthy life, the quest for a treatment to combat the stress and anxiety caused by the hustle and bustle of city life. On the other hand, the incorporation of Yoga practice as a life style varies according to the degree of involvement in the practice, the institutional commitment with the practice centers, and the aims of those who practise it.

Araiza Díaz (2009), focuses on "learning" and "being" through Yoga practice, highlighting the teacher-disciple relationship in Yoga and recovering, among other things, through Foucault (2004), the other kind of teacher who once existed in the Western World, committed to cultivating the self, and the technologies of "being" i.e. not only implying self-knowledge but also self-care.

On the other hand, Ravettino (2008) relates the practice of certain disciplines, such as Yoga, with a "light" life-style, and points out that physical activity in the workplace is becoming increasingly popular among major organizations. This is reflected in the offer of gym and relaxation activities made to employees by several Argentine firms, in labor hours, in the hope of reducing absenteeism and stimulating higher performance. He further adds that, around 2003, Argentine firms began to develop these programs, following the tendency of the United States.

Different authors analyze the arrival and development of Yoga practice in Argentina, such as Saizar (2006, 2007, 2009a, 2009b, 2011); Sarudiansky and Saizar (2007); Giménez y Saizar (2011); D'angelo (2012, 2013) and Viotti (2010).

To conclude, we agree with Chakraborty (1986) who believes that the path towards the "will-to-yoga" constitutes a desirable choice in the enhancement of quality of labor life.

10.7 Yoga and its Significance to Quality of Life, in our Study

The study in question was developed from a qualitative perspective, and was carried out through semistructured interviews of 20 people, females and males between 21 and 65 years old, who practice Yoga, and reside in Ciudad Autónoma de Buenos Aires, República Argentina, analized with Thematic Analysis (Braun and Clarke 2006).

Regarding the motives which have led the interviewed subjects to practice Yoga are, in some cases, stimulated by someone close (their couple, for instance). Such is the case of one of the interviewed subjects, a 40 year old woman: "(Yoga) wouldn't have entered my life if it hadn't been for C. her husband [due to his health problem]" (female, 40 years old).

Self disquiet is also reflected in the fact that it attracts others who are in a personal pursuit, as expressed by another interviewed subject (female, 41 years old):

> Look, it was an inner search. I really needed something for my soul. I got pregnant with S. and, at that moment, my head began to spin, maybe due to the responsibility it represented, because it was something I couldn't control, because we can't control Nature, and then, well, I was really afraid and felt insecure, though we had really wanted this baby. I began to perceive a lot of things that I must have had bottled up inside, and I needed peace and a reconnection with myself and then, well, a lady I happened to know, who practiced Reiki, said, " Why don't you come and give it a try?", and that's how I started with G. [Yoga instructor]...

In some cases, disquiet of the self, may be rooted it health issues, leading to the development of the Yoga practice by medical prescription, or recommendations made by family or friends. Such is the case of another interviewed subject (male, 55 years old), who comments:

> On June 29, 2009 I had a heart attack, followed by heart failure, on that same night,; in September of that same year they, well, they tried to do something but, well, they couldn't because my heart was too weak, in fact only 60% is functioning properly, to this day. In Septemnber they inserted three stents, but this wasn't enough and, in February 2010, I was operated on. The operation lasted eight hours, my heart was artificially stopped, and I've got five by-pass operations; I'm technically disabled, but there was nothing else they could do and, thankfully, I'm perfect now. When I returned home, a friend of mine (without asking for my opinión), introduced me to a Yoga teacher called G., he himself paid the fees for the first month's clases, and here I am.

Another interviewed subject (male, 44 years old) suffering from ankylosing spondilitis, begins a quest for different activities, which he carries out with his couple.

Regarding the personal outlook on Yoga (exclusively as a technique, or as a phylosophical-practical system), it may be pointed out that Foucault, upholds that self care may be understood as set of practices through which an individual establishes a certain relationship with himself and, in that relationship, he becomes the subject of his own actions (Chirolla 2007). Foucault states that one can not take care of oneself if one does not know oneself enough. Britos (2005) adds that self care implies self knowledge, but also the knowledge of rules of behaviour or principles embodying truths and prescriptions. Thus, by taking care of oneself would involve being equipped with those truths.

In this connection, an interviewed 46 year old male, points out:

> Of course, this impact from the point of view of values and all that, somehow, comes later; one's first perception is the impact on the body, isn't it? From the physical or mental points of view, depending on one's interests, what one feels should be deepened in order to reach those values; I do it from both points of view, don't I? But [,..] from both, yes from both, I also practice meditation, I then do something for my spirit, to put it some way, I'm interested and I try to go deeper, yes, yes.,

According to Robbins, the care of the self involves knowledge of the self, the inevitable relationship between practice and learning, for there is a strong bond between knowledge and action, whether as a principle to regulate action, as an aim to be achieved through it, or as a process through which it is made manifest (Robbins 2007, quoted in Garcés Giraldo and Giraldo Zuluaga 2013). Giraldo, on the other hand, adds that self care aims at the soul and it is a way of preparing oneself for a complete fulfilment of life (Giraldo 2008). In that sense, in some cases, this self care reflects the different practices developed by the subject. Such is the case of 42 year old interviewed male, who explains that he seizes the practical aspect of Yoga and the values transmitted by his instructor, G. and, in general lines, anything that may complement his own Budhist practice.

The body appears as a vector which produces a sense that enhances the subject's active social and cultural insertion; and, in this regard, a 42 year old female points out:

> Yes…I don't know, whether to consider it as a phylolophy, let's say, to which I strictly respond as a religión; I simply put into practice some of the principles, some of the values of Yoga which I agree on, er, yes, I believe it spreads, not as a sports practice, it isn't a mere sports practice, but something, I insist, that began as something for the body, to be able to relax, to sleep better, but I'm beginning to find, somehow in spite of myself, I'm beginning to find a lot of things which involve a closenes to spiritual life […] For instance, unattachment, working on the notion of unattachment, beginning to work on the idea of non-violence, starting by the person itself, that is, starting by oneself, by us; beginnging to enjoy and concentrate on "here and now",er, well, on joy, that state of joy or samadio…isn't it? Erm, being somehow conscious and active because one is sometimes prejudiced into believing that it's only a relaxation practice, while it really involves great consciousness of our bodies or of the state we're in, don't you think? We must respect all that […] Yes, yes, I believe that it's like a whole exercise, I mean, like beginning to work on certain things such as unattachment, for instance. Life catches hold of you, it makes you grasping, so to speak. Er, I believe it's all about working, it requires work, not hard labor, but pleasant work, a process that is gradually incorporated.

Regarding quality of life in general and quality of labor life, previous to the practice of Yoga, and on its initiation, it should be remembered that Foucault hightlights that self care comprises three basic aspects: firstly, that it is an attitude of self respect, of respect for others, and for the world in general; secondly, that it is a certain manner of attention, an outlook; and thirdly, that the notion of self care designates a series of actions which are exercised over oneself, actions which lead to taking charge of one's self and transforming it.

Care for others, explicit in actions, presumes ethical care of oneself. The body, as a vector which connects material practice to the other scopes of Yoga, also expresses an interrelation with others (made evident in stress, pressure, etc.), as inferred from the following interview with a 37 year old woman:

> Well, er, before I began to practise Yoga, my physical body and my mental body, were ravaged by stress, you see? They were my own pressures, let's say, because I can't very well say that they were external issues related to labor achievement, and it was a kind of mandate imposed by reality, a mandate that I had received, and I think that what Yoga did was help me break with all that, just that really, it changed my approach to labor, I now work fewer hours…

Another woman we interviewed highlights that Yoga practice elicits order:

> I think it has a lot to do with temperaments and the extent of the effects of these practices. I experience great serenity but…it's difficult, you see…how, how…to express what really transmits so much serenity but, well, I'm a highly strung person, therefore, very hyperactive, very anxious, and with a perfectionist streak, so er…there are moments, when I feel it's doing me good, I complete the practice, but later on, if this is projected to calm me down a second time, no, I don't think it's possible, ha, ha […]I think that what is useful to me—I'm a devoted student and, more so in my "nest" within my structure—but what I've noticed is that I need daily practice, discipline, but I'm not disciplined myself. I notice that I've maybe become more organized; it seems that the practice has brought order into certain aspects one doesn't always have an eye on, such as complying with college, with work, with doing things right, and showing this to the people involved. That are things which are personal so, in those aspects that are my own, like this question of discipline, though I find it hard, I've noticed small changes such as—since I like doing things properly—I've become more orderly.

A 52 year old woman we interviewed, on the other hand, talks about Yoga practice as evidence of self care, regarding oneself, regarding others, and the world in general:

> Well, I should say that, after going through the Yoga experience, one becomes conscious not only of the body but also of the thought of where one's quest is oriented,; through it I have incorporated something that I cannot learn from a book because it's a personal experience, there is enegy in the group and this often helps, when one is lazy or whatever, there is interactive energy with the other members of the group; this also happens when I'm working in a team, but it doesn't when I'm working on my own, in my workshop, they're different things.[…]my interest was focused in incorporating that [group energy].

A 63 year old woman we interviewed, comments on Yoga practice as a source of embetterment, made evident in specific values:

> They're two different worlds, you go in as one kind of person and end up being completely different […]at least, you become acquainted with the reasoning of a spiritual person, with being a better person each day, with being proper, pleasant and, above all, a kind person.

Regarding the scope of Yoga practice in labor life, in the relation with the above mentioned, it should be remembered that the care for others, implicit in actions,

reflects ethical care of oneself. Britos (2005) acknowledges that self-care requires self-reflection, and questioning oneself to examine behavior in order to polish up its forms and procedures.
A 42 year old woman we interviewed points out the following:

> What I can tell you is that, now I work on my own, I have clients who entrust me with their businesses, with their communications […] All I can say, right now, is that I'm happy with my clients, happy because they're human and, by having that kind of clients, I have slowly ruled out others, you see?, the lazy, aggressive guys, competitive people. I said to myself, "As from today, I'm only working with people who make me happy!"[…] The others fell away and that's great, you see? […] We all ended up hugging and kissing each other, they say I'm fantastic, but I know the clients I now have are amazing […] They're the people I want to do business with, and if any of them tells me, "Look, Silvina, let's review the fees", still it's people I feel happy to work with […] It's wonderful, because it's a job I love, it's something I want to go on doing and, apart from everything else, they're wholesome people.

In a further interview with a 41 year old woman, she says:

> Yes, yes, I try to create an atmosphere; I've been working here for nine years, almost ten, and I try to have a wholesome atmosphere for everyone, so that we can live in harmony, have fun—since we have to spend ten hours cooped up in here –, at least, I try, I don't know. What is more, two of the girls who come here are also taking Yoga classes with G. [the instructor] […]Yes, one of them is my boss and, what I mean is I try to show them that there are others.

It would be advisable to consider the development of self care relating others. It is necessary to take care of oneselves by taking care of others. Thus, the so-called technologies of the self enable subjects to carry out (on their own or with the help of others) operations on their bodies and souls and behavior, in a process of transformation resulting in a state of happiness, wisdom, etc. (Foucault 1990). Thus, a 46 year old male expresses during an interview:

> Yes. No, I'd say no to that[some element in Yoga practice in particular I use at work], basically in this question of achieving harmony, taking one's distance from certain things […] give relative importance to things, you see?, but no, I don't practise breathing […]I might, if my muscles are stiff at work, I try to divert my attention away from the muscle in question, or from the affected zone, and I attempt to practice breathing, visualization and […] [it's a kind of attitude towards life that begins to show …] yes, yes, yes.

In coincidence with Daros (2007, quoted in Garcés Giraldo and Giraldo Zuluaga 2013), we say that the self develops thechnologies in its construction which do not exclude discipline, a rational use of pleasure, and the breeding of practices through which subjects preserve themselves. In connection with this, a 50 year old woman we interviewed points out:

> I think it's a whole, but I also think that the beneficial effects one experiences in the long-run are, all in all, this single benefit, a certain emotional stability. Of course, in my case, it is complemented by meditation which also helps, doesn't it? Anyway, before starting with meditation your begin to feel the positive effects because that's the way Yoga works, from the physical point of view, I mean, posture, for asana is the physical part, but the result is gradually felt inside the body, through a better health state, higher spirits, er, intellectually perhaps even more; your mind becomes slightly more alert, more open, and then you begin to experience overall results, at all levels, you see? I believe that to be the greatest asset

> of this practice, more than anything else [...including the question of work]. Yes, exactly, exactly, it offers you a lot and, I don't know, that's why I like it and that's why I do it.

Further, a 55 year old prosecuting attorney expresses in the interview:

> Breathing.That's very useful to me at work; I practice deep breathing. Breathing is very useful to me and, er, when I'm anguished at having to rush from one place to another, I practice breathing, trying to take, to walk with, to keep my mind a blank and breathe, and that helps me a lot...

Inherent in self care, specific ethics underlie in coherence with caring for others. Thus, a 63 year old woman expresses in the interview:

> The element Yoga gives you is, above all, "a sense of balance", so you're never going to have impulsive reactions, you're always going to have a smile on your lips or in your eyes, and that's going to help you interrelate with people and, besides, whoever wants to listen may do so when you say, "Hey! I'm practising Yoga". Don't miss it, because when you're doing something you want to share it with those around you, you want them to live it, to feel it...

10.8 To Conclude

In coincidence with Lewin (1939), the subjects' aims and needs make their behavior more dynamic. Thus, self care, expressed through Yoga practice, appears as a temporal space marker for those who indulge in it, and as a route which leads from a state of being un-well/organized/balanced to the contrary, with the addition of related values and consequent changes in relation to others, and to the world in general.

Among the reasons leading to the practice of Yoga—practice of the self, we may mention disquiet related to health problems, the stimulus of another signifier, a personal quest on the part of the interviewed subjects, and it may even be attributed to chance. Most of the subjects interviewed relate Yoga to something that exceeds the mere practice (restricted to the physical plane) thus, the body comes across as a full semantic vector, expressing values, changes in the relationships with others, and with the world in general. Those changes are reflected in quality of life, in general, and in quality of labor life in particular, and are explicitly acknowledged, in some cases, as being the source of improvement in productivity.

As aforementioned, the globalization context produces a pronounced circulation of people, goods, cultural elements, etc., related to improvements in means of transport and communications. The circulation of cultural elements of diverse origins is an ancient phenomenon, product of a convergence of cultures, thus generating not only circulation but also resemantization of the them, sometimes related to the development of the self; in other words, to quality of life itself, both general or explicit, particularly in the work place. Such is the case of Yoga, a system applied nowadays in different spheres including business organizations which offer it to their employees as an added benefit in their workplace. In any case, Yoga, as a practice of the self, entails inner changes, changes in relation to others and to the world in general.

References

Amita, S., Prabhakar, S., Manoj, I., Harminder, S., & Pavan, T. (2009). Effect of yoga-Nidra on blood glucose level in diabetic patients. *Indian Journal of Physiology and Pharmacology, 53* (1), 97–101.

Andersen, J. C. (2005). Stretching before and after exercise: Effect on muscle soreness and injury risk. *Journal of Athlete Training, 40*(3), 218–220.

Araiza Díaz, A. (2009). Conocer y Ser a través de la práctica del Yoga: una propuesta feminista de investigación performativa. (Tesis de Doctorado/PhD Thesis, Universitat Autònoma de Barcelona). http://www.tdx.cat/bitstream/handle/10803/5474/aad1de1.pdf;jsessionid=D2682BFBC06C9F499F36CC7A4FA0099F.tdx2?sequence=1.

Astin, J. (1998). Why patients use alternative medicine: Results of a national study. *JAMA, 279,* 1548–1553.

Bakker, A. B., Demerouti, E., & Schaufeli, W. B. (2002). Validation of the Maslach Burnout inventory—general survey: An internet study. Anxiety, stress and coping. *An International Journal, 15*(3), 245–260.

Bauman, Z. (2006). *Modernidad líquida*. México: FCE.

Bowling, A. (2010). Medicina complementaria y alternativa: Un tema de EM importante en todo el mundo. *MS in focus, 15,* 4–6.

Braun, V., & Clarke, V. (2006). Using thematic analysis in psychology. *Qualitative research in Psychology, 3,* 77–101.

Bravo, M. J., Peiró, J. M., & Rodriguez, I. (1996). Satisfacción Laboral. In J. M. Peiró & F. Prieto (Eds.), *Tratado de Psicología del Trabajo*, (Vol. 2, pp. 343–397). Madrid: Síntesis.

Britos, M. del P. (2005). La problematización de la relación con la verdad. Interrogantes a partir de la lectura de Foucault. *Tópicos, 13,* 29–43. http://www.scielo.org.ar/scielo.php?script=sci_arttext&pid=S1666485X2005000100002&lng=pt&nrm=iso.

Brown, R. P., & Gerbarg, P. L. (2005a). Sudarshan Kriya yogic breathing in the treatment of stress, anxiety, and depression: Part I—neurophysiologic model. *Journal of Alternative and Complementary Medicine, 11*(1), 189–201.

Brown, R. P., & Gerbarg, P. L. (2005b). Sudarshan kriya yogic breathing in the treatment of stress, anxiety, and depression. Part II—clinical applications and guidelines. *Journal of Alternative and Complementary Medicine, 11*(4), 711–717.

Burton, J. P., Lee, T. H. L., & Holtom, B. C. (2002). The influence of motivation to attend, ability to attend, and organizational commitment on different types of absence behaviors. *Journal of Managerial Issues, XIV*(2), 181–197.

Carlson, C. R., & Hoyle, R. H. (1993). Efficacy of abbreviated progressive muscle relaxation training: A quantitative review of behavioral medicine research. *Journal of Consulting and Clinical Psychology, 61*(6), 1059–1067.

Castel, R. (1995). *Les métamorphoses de la question sociale*. París: Gallimard.

Castel, R., & Haroche, C. (2003). *Propiedad privada, propiedad social, propiedad de sí mismo.* Buenos Aires: Homo Sapiens.

Chakraborty, S. K. (1986). The will-to-yoga: Key to better quality of work life. *Vikalpa, 11*(2), 113–124.

Chaufeli, W. B., & Enzmann, D. (1998). *The burnout companion to study and practice: A critical analysis*. Washington, DC: Taylor & Francis.

Chen, K. M., Chen, M. H., Hong, S. M., Chao, H. C., Lin, H. S., & Li, C. H. (2008). Physical fitness of older adults in senior activity centres after 24-week silver yoga exercises. *Journal of Clinical Nursing, 17*(19), 2634–2646.

Chen, K. M., Chen, M. H., Chao, H. C., Hung, H. M., Lin, H. S., & Li, C. H. (2009). Sleep quality, depression state, and health status of older adults after silver yoga exercises: cluster randomized trial. *International Journal of Nursing Studies, 46,* 154–163.

Chen, K. M., Chen, M. H., Lin, M. H., Fan, J. T., Lin, H. S., Li, C. H. (2010). Effects of yoga on sleep quality and depression in elders in assisted living facilities. *Journal of Nursing Research, 18,* 53–61.

Chiesa, A. (2009). Zen meditation: An integration of current evidence. *Journal of Alternative and Complementary Medicine, 15*(5), 585–592.

Chiesa, A., & Serretti, A. (2009). Mindfulness-based stress reduction for stress management in healthy people: A review and meta-analysis. *Journal of Alternative and Complementary Medicine, 15*(5), 593–600.

Chiesa, A., & Serretti, A. (2010). A systematic review of neurobiological and clinical features of mindfulness meditations. *Psychological Medicine, 40*(8), 1239–1252.

Chirolla, G. (2007). Reseña de Foucault y el sujeto político. Ética del cuidado de sí, de Humberto Cubides Cipagauta. *Nómadas, 26*, 241–243.

Cohen, L., Warneke, C., Fouladi, R. T., Rodriguez, M. A., & Chaoul-Reich, A. (2004). Psychological adjustment and sleep quality in a randomized trial of the effects of a Tibetan yoga intervention in patients with lymphoma. *Cancer, 100*(10), 2253–2260.

Coulter, I. D., & Willis, E. M. (2004). The rise and rise of complementary and alternative medicine: A sociological perspective. *Medical Jornal of Australia, 180*(11), 587–589. https://www.mja.com.au/journal/2004/180/11/rise-and-rise-complementary-and-alternative-medicine-sociological-perspective. Accessed 28 Jan 2014.

D'angelo, A. (2013). Tendiendo puentes: La apropiación terapéutica del yoga ante la dimensión emocional de los padecimientos. *RBSE – Revista Brasileira de Sociologia da Emoção, 12*(34), 321–360.

D'angelo, A. (2012). Difusión mediática de discursos bio-psi y técnicas corporales de origen oriental. Transformaciones en los procesos de salud-enfermedad-atención. VII Jornadas de Sociología de la UNLP. Memoria Académica. http://www.memoria.fahce.unlp.edu.ar/trab_eventos/ev.1814/ev.1814.pdf.

Dantas de Carvalho, C., & Da Silva Correia, N. (2011). Aplicabilidad del yoga como recurso terapéutico, junto a las mujeres en el proceso de deshabituación del diazepam. *Revista Chilena De Terapia Ocupacional, 11*(1). http://www.revistaterapiaocupacional.uchile.cl/index.php/RTO/article/viewArticle/17079/17816.

Daros, W. (2007). La identidad del "yo" como descubrimiento por el otro (M. burber) y como cuidado de sí mismo (M. Foucault). *Espíritu: Cuadernos del Instituto Filosófico de Balmesiana*, Año 56, N·136, 293–306.

Dennis, R., Williams, W., & Giangreco, MyC. (1994). Calidad de vida como contexto para la planificación y evaluación de servicios para personas con discapacidad. *Siglo Cero, 25*(155), 5–18.

Diener, E., & Diener, M. (1995). Cross-cultural correlates of life satisfaction and self-esteem. *Journal of Personality and Social Psychology, 68*, 653–663.

Dirección de Medicina Tradicional y Desarrollo Intercultural, Dirección General de Planeación y Desarrollo en Salud, Secretaría de Salud de México. (2007). Diagnóstico de los aportes de diferentes modelos clínico terapéuticos para la diabetes mellitus. http://www.dgplades.salud.gob.mx/descargas/dmtdi/carpeta4/Diagnostico_Aportes_Diabetes.pdf.

Duro Martín, A. (2002). Calidad de Vida Laboral y Psicología Social de la Salud en el Trabajo: hacia un modelo de componentes comunes para explicar el bienestar laboral psicológico y la salud mental laboral de origen psicosocial. Resultados preliminares. *Revista del Ministerio de Trabajo y Asuntos Sociales, 56*, 57–98. www.empleo.gob.es/es/publica/pub_electronicas/…/56/Inf02.pdf. Accessed 23 Jan 2014.

Eliade, M. (1988). *Yoga, inmortalidad y libertad*. Buenos Aires: La Pléyade.

Fajardo Pulido, J. A. (2009). Yoga, cuerpo e imagen: espiritualidad y bienestar, de la terapia a la publicidad. *Universitas Humanística, 68*, 33–47.

Foucault, M. (1987). *Historia de la Sexualidad*. México: Siglo XXI Editores.

Foucault, M. (1990). *Tecnologías del yo*. Barcelona: Paidós.

Foucault, M. (1994). *La ética del cuidado de sí como práctica de la libertad*. París: Gallimard.

Foucault, M. (2004). *Historia de la sexualidad*, vol. 3, *La inquietud de sí*. México: Siglo XXI Editores.

Garcés Giraldo, L. F., & Giraldo Zuluaga, C. (2013). El cuidado de sí y de los otros en Foucault, principio orientador para la construcción de una bioética del cuidado. *Discusiones Filosóficas, 14*(22), 187–201.

García Martín, M. A. (2002). El Bienestar Subjetivo. Subjective well-being. *Escritos de Psicología, 6,* 18–39.
Garfinkel, M. S., Schumacher, H. R., Husain, A., Levy, M., & Reshetar, R. A. (1994). Evaluation of a yoga based regimen for treatment of osteoarthritis of the hands. *The Journal of Rheumatology, 21*(2), 2341–2343.
Gil-Monte, P., & Peiró, J. M. (1997). *Desgaste psíquico en el trabajo: El síndrome de quemarse.* Madrid: Síntesis.
Giménez, A., & Saizar, M. M. (2011). Reeducando la mirada. Reflexiones sobre la refiguración de nociones católicas entre practicantes de terapias alternativas en Buenos Aires (Argentina). *Revista da FAEEBA–Educação e Contemporaneidade, Salvador, 20*(35), 151–161.
Giraldo R. (2008). La resistencia y la estética de la existencia en Michel Foucault. *Entramado, 4* (2), 90–100.
Gómez Vela, M., & Sabeh, E. (2000). *Calidad de vida. Evolución del concepto y su influencia en la investigación y la práctica.* Instituto Universitario de Integración en la Comunidad, Facultad de Psicología, Universidad de Salamanca. http://campus.usal.es/~inico/investigacion/invesinico/calidad.htm. Accessed 16 Dec 2013.
González de Rivera, J. L. (2002). *El maltrato psicológico: Cómo defenderse del mobbing y otras formas de acoso.* Madrid: Espasa Calpe.
Hackman, J. R., & Oldham, G. R. (1980). *Work redesign.* Reading: Addison-Wesley.
Halpern, J. S. (2011). Yoga for improving sleep qualty and quality of life in older adults in a Western cultural setting. Tesis de grado. Escuela de Ciencias de la Salud, Colegio de Ciencia, Ingeniería y Salud, Universidad R. M. I. T, Victoria, Australia.
Harned, M. S., Ormerod, A. J., Palmieri, P. A., Collinsworth, L. L., & Reed, M. (2002). Sexual assault and other types of sexual harassment by workplace personnel: A comparison of antecedents and consequences. *Journal of Occupational Health Psychology, 7,* 174–188.
Harrison, D. A., & Martocchio, J. J. (1998). Time for absenteeism: A 20-year review or origins, offshoots, and outcomes. *Journal of Management, 24*(3), 305–350.
Herbert, R. D., & Gabriel, M. (2002). Effects of stretching before and after exercising on muscle soreness and risk of injury: Systematic review. *BMJ* (*Clinical research ed.*), *325*(7362), 468.
Innes, K. E., & Vincent, H. K. (2007). The influence of yoga-based programs on risk profiles in adults with type 2 diabetes mellitus: a systematic review. *Evidence Based Complementary and Alternative Medicine, 4*(4), 469–486.
Innes, K. E., Bourguignon, C., & Taylor, A. G. (2005). Risk indices associated with the insulin resistance syndrome, cardiovascular disease, and possible protection with yoga: A systematic review. *The Journal of the American Board of Family Practice, 18,* 491–519.
Iyengar, B. K. S. (2002). *Light on the sutras of Patanjali.* London: Thornsons/Harper Collins.
Janakiramaiah, N., Gangadhar, B. N., Naga, V., Murthy, P. J., Harish, M. G., & Subbakrishna, D. K., et al. (2000). Antidepressant efficacy of Sudarshan Kriya Yoga (SKY) in melancholia: A randomized comparison with electroconvulsive therapy (ECT) and imipramine. *J Affect Disord, 57*(1–3), 255–259.
John, P. J., Sharma, N., Sharma, C. M., & Kankane, A. (2007). Effectiveness of yoga therapy in the treatment of migraine without aura: a randomized controlled trial. *Headache*, *47*(5), 654–661.
Kahn, R. L., & Boysiere, P. (1992). Stress in organizations. In E. M. D. Dunnette & L. M. Hough (Eds.), *Handbook of industrial and organizational psychology* (Vol. 3, pp. 571–650). Palo Alto: Consulting Psychologist Press.
Kamakhya, K. (2004). Yoga nidra and its impact on students' well-being. *Yoga Mimamsa, 36*(1), 71–76.
Karasek, R., Brisson, C. H., Kawakami, N., Houtman, I., & Bongers, P. (1998). The Job Content Questionnaire (JCQ): An instrument for internationally comparative assessments of psychosocial job characteristics. *Journal of Occupational Health Psychology, 3*(4), 322–355.
Kellner, M. J., Boon, H., & Wellman, ByW. (2002). Complementary and alternative groups contemplate the need for effectiveness, safety and cost-effectiveness research. *Complementary Therapies in Medicine, 10,* 235–239.

Kirkwood, G., Rampes, H., Tuffrey, V., Richardson, J., & Pilkington, K. (2005). Yoga for anxiety: A systematic review of the research evidence. *British Journal of Sports Medicine, 39*(12), 884–891.

Kjellgren, A., Bood, S. A., Axelsson, K., Norlander, T., & Saatcioglu, F. (2007). Wellness through a comprehensive yogic breathing program - a controlled pilot trial. *BMC Complementary and Alternative Medicine, 19*(7), 43. doi:10.1186/1472-6882-7-43.

Klatt, M., Buckworth, J., & Malarkey, W. (2009). Effects of low-dose Mindfulness-Based Stress Reduction (MBSR-ld) on working adults. *Health Education Behaviour, 36*(3), 601–614.

Kolasinski, S. L., Garfinkel, M., Tsa, A. G., Matz W., Van-Dyke, A., & Schumacher, H. R. (2005). Iyengar yoga for treating symptoms of osteoarthritis of the knees: A pilot study. *Journal of Alternative and Complementary Medicine, 11*(4), 689–693.

Krucoff, C., Carson, K., Peterson, M., Shipp, K., & Krucoff, M. (2010). Teaching yoga to seniors: essential considerations to enhance safety and reduce risk in a uniquely vulnerable age group. *The Journal of Alternative and Complementary Medicine, 16*(8), 899–905.

Lanz, C. (2012). El cuidado de sí y del otro en lo educativo. *Utopía y Praxis Latinoamericana, 17* (56), 39–46.

Le Breton, D. (2002). *La sociología del cuerpo*. Buenos Aires: Nueva Visión.

Leiter, M. P., & Durup, J. (1994). The discriminant validity of burnout and depression: A confirmatory factor analytic study. *Anxiety, Stress and Coping, 7,* 357–373.

León Palacios, P. C. (2003). Globalización y reestructuración capitalistas: cambios en el mundo y América Latina. *INNOVAR. Revista de Ciencias Administrativas y Sociales, 21,* 47–70.

Lewin, K. (1939). Field theory and experiment in social psychology: concepts and methods. *The American Journal of Sociology, 44,* 868–897.

Lou, H. C., Kjaer, T. W., Friberg, L., Wildschiodtz, G., Holm, S., & Nowak, M. (1999). A 15O-H2O PET study of meditation and the resting state of normal consciousness. *Human Brain Mapping, 7*(2), 98–105.

Maheshwarananda, P. S. (2009). The meaning of "Hatha Yoga". http://swamiji. Accessed 4 Dec 2013.

Manjunath, N. K., & Telles, S. (2005). Influence of yoga and ayurveda on self-rated sleep in a geriatric population. *The Indian Journal of Medical Research, 121*(5), 683–690.

Martuccelli, D. (2002). *Grammaires de l'individu*. París: Gallimard.

Matthees, B. J., Nantachoti, P., Kreitzer, M. J., Savik, K., Hertz, M. I., & Gross C. R. (2001). Use of complementary therapies, adherence and quality of life in lung transplant recipients. *Heart Lung, 30*, 4, 258–268.

Mearns, J., & Cain, J. E. (2003). Relationships between teachers' occupational stress and their burnout and distress: Roles of coping and negative mood regulation expectancies. *Anxiety,-Stress-and-Coping:-An-International-Journal, 16*(1), 71–82.

Michalsen, A., Grossman, P., Acil, A., Langhorst, J., Lüdtke, R., & Esch, T., et al. (2005). Rapid stress reduction and anxiolysis among distressed women as a consequence of a three-month intensive yoga program. *Medical Science Monitor: International Medical Journal of Experimental and Clinical Research, 11*(12), CR555–561.

Millar, P. J., Bray, S. R., McGowan, C. L., MacDonald, M. J., & McCartney, N. (2007). Effects of isometric handgrip training among people medicated for hypertension: A multilevel analysis. *Blood Pressure Monitoring, 12*(5), 307–314.

Nuttin, J., & Lens, W. (1985). *Future time perspective and motivation. Theory and research method.* Hillsdale, New Jersey: Erlbaum.

Organización, Mundial de la Salud –OMS-. (2002). *Estrategia de la OMS sobre Medicina Tradicional.* Ginebra: OMS. http://www.sld.cu/galerias/pdf/sitios/mednat/estrategia_de_la_oms_sobre_medicina_tradicional.pdf. Accessed 23 Nov 2013.

Ospina, M. B., Bond, K., Karkhaneh, M., Tjosvold, L., Vandermeer, B., & Liang, Y., et al. (2007). Meditation practices for health: State of the research. *Evidence Report Technology Assessment, 155,* 1–263. (http://www.ncbi.nlm.nih.gov/bookshelf/br.fcgi?book=erta155. Accessed 3 Nov 2013).

Patra, S., & Telles, S. (2009). Positive impact of cyclic meditation on subsequent sleep. *Medical Science Monitor, 15*(7), 375–381.

Patra S., & Telles, S. (2010). Heart rate variability during sleep following the practice of cyclic meditation and supine rest. *Applied Psychophysiology and Biofeedback, 35*(2), 135–140.

Peters, P. G., Alessio, H. M., Hagerman, A. E., Ashton, T., Nagy, S., & Wiley, R. L. (2006). Short-term isometric exercise reduces systolic blood pressure in hypertensive adults: Possible role of reactive oxygen species. *International Journal of Cardiology, 110*(2), 199–205.

Petito, F., & Cummins, R. A. (2000). Quality of life in adolescence: The role of perceived control, parenting style and social support. *Behaviour Change, 17*(3), 196–207.

Pilkington, K., Kirkwood, G., Rampes, H., & Richardsona, J. (2005). Yoga for depression: The research evidence. *Journal of Affective Disorders, 89*(1), 13–24.

Pramanik, T., Sharma, H. O., Mishra, S., Mishra, A., Prajapati, R., & Singh, S. (2009). Immediate effect of slow pace bhastrika pranayama on blood pressure and heart rate. *The Journal of Alternative and Complementary Medicine, 15*(3), 293–295.

Pritchard, M., Elison-Bowers, P., & Birdsall, B. (2010). Impact of Integrative Restoration (iRest) meditation on perceived stress levels in multiple sclerosis and cancer outpatients. *Stress and Health, 26*(3), 233–237.

Raju, P. S., Madhavi, S., Prasad, K. V., Reddy, M. V., Reddy, M. E., Sahay, B. K., et al. (1994). Comparison of effects of yoga & physical exercise in athletes. *The Indian Journal of Medical Research, 100,* 81–86.

Ramirez Suárez, Y. C. (2011). Subjetividades contemporáneas: el Yoga como práctica de sí. (Tesis de Maestría/Master Thesis, Universidad Nacional de Colombia). http://www.bdigital.unal.*edu.*co/4445/1/428270.2011.pdf.

Ravettino, A. J. (2008). El estilo de vida light. Hábitos y patrones de consumo. *Revista Científica de UCES, XII*(1), 103–117.

Raub, J. A. (2002). Psychophysiologic effects of hatha yoga on musculoskeletal and cardiopulmonary function: A literature review. *The Journal of Alternative and Complementary Medicine, 8*(6), 797–812.

Rendón, T., & Salas, C. (2000). El cambio en la estructura de la fuerza de trabajo en América Latina. En E. De la Garza (coord.). *Tratado latinoamericana de sociología del trabajo* (pp. 540–565). México: COLMEX/FLACSO/UAM/FCE.

Requena, F. (2000). Satisfacción, Bienestar y Calidad de Vida en el Trabajo. *REIS. Revista Española de Investigaciones Sociológicas, 92,* 11–44.

Robbins, S. (2007). *El cuidado de sí. La inversión del platonismo desde la mirada de Michel Foucault. Seminario de Pensamiento crítico. Chile*: Universidad Diego Portales.

Ross, A., & Thomas, S. (2010). The health benefits of yoga and exercise: a rev*iew* of comparison studies. *The Journal of Alternative and Complementary Medicine, 16*(1), 3–12.

Saizar, M. (2006). Reflexiones en torno de la complementariedad terapéutica entre ususarios del Yoga en el Área Metropolitana de Buenos Aires (Argentina). *Mitológicas, XXI,* 23–46.

Saizar, M. (2007). El yoga como terapia complementaria en pacientes con estrés en Buenos Aires (Argentina). *Mitológicas, XXII,* 69–83.

Saizar, M. (2008). Todo el mundo sabe. Difusión y apropiación de las técnicas del yoga en Buenos Aires (Argentina). *Sociedade e Cultura, 11*(1), 112–122.

Saizar, M. (2009a). Reflexiones acerca del ritual y la terapia en las prácticas del Yoga en el área Metropolitana (Argentina). *Espectáculo. Revista de Estudios Literarios,* 42. http://pendientedemigracion.ucm.es/info/especulo/numero42/rityoga.html.

Saizar, M. (2009b). La etiología de la enfermedad y el fluir de la energía. Relatos de ususarios y especialistas del Yoga en Buenos Aires (Argentina). *Mitológicas, XXIV,* 9–27.

Saizar, M. (2011). The Ideas of God, Good and Evil in the Refigured Yoga Practices in Metropolitan area of Buenos Aires city (Argentina). *Antrocom Online Journal of Anthropology, 7*(2), 251–262. http://www.antrocom.net/upload/sub/antrocom/070211/09-Antrocom.pdf.

Sarudiansky, M., & Saizar, M. (2007). El yoga como terapia complementaria en pacientes con estrés en Buenos Aires (Argentina). *Mitológicas, XXII,* 69–83.

SAY (2010). Silver Age Yoga. http://www.silverageyoga.org/.

Shannahoff-Khalsa, D. S. (2004). An Introduction to kundalini yoga meditation techniques that are specific for the treatment of psychiatric disorders. *The Journal of Alternative and Complementary Medicine, 10*(1), 91–101.

Shannahoff-Khalsa, D. S. (1993). The effects of unilateral forced nostril breathing on the heart. *International Journal of Neuroscience, 73*(1–2), 47–60.

Shannahoff-Khalsa, D. (2006). *Kundalini yoga meditation: Techniques specific for psychiatric disorders, couples therapy, and personal growth.* New York: W. W. Norton & Company.

Sharma, H., Datta, P., Singh, A., Sen, S., Bhardwaj, N. K., Kochupillai, V., et al. (2008). Gene expression profiling in practitioners of Sudarshan Kriya. *Journal of Psychosomatic Research, 64*(2), 213–218.

Sherman, K. J., Cherkin, D. C., Erro, J., Miglioretti, D. L., & Deyo, R. A. (2005). Comparing Yoga, Exercise, and a Self-Care Book for Chronic Low Back Pain. A Randomized, Controlled Trial. *Annals of Internal Medicine, 143*(12), 849–856.

Shrier, I. (2004). Does stretching improve performance? A systematic and critical review of the literature. *Clinical Journal of Sport Medicine: officia Journal of the Canadian Academy of Sport Medicine, 14*(5), 267–273.

Smith, C. J. (2005). *The use of complementary and alternative medical therapies among employees in small and very small businesses.* Phd Dissertation (Doctor of Philosophy in Social Ecology). University of California, Irvine.

Sossa Rojas, A. (2010). Michel Foucault y el cuidado de sí. *CONHISREMI, Revista Universitaria Arbitrada de Investigación y Diálogo Académico, 6*(2), 34–45. http://conhisremi.iuttol.edu.ve/pdf/ARTI000094.pdf. Accessed 3 Jan 2014.

Spielberger, CH. D., Vagg, P. R., & Wasal, C. F. (2003). Occupational stress: Job pressures and lack of support. In J. C. Quick & L. E. Tetrick (Eds.), *Handbook of occupational health psychology* (pp. 185–200). Washington, DC: APA.

Streeter, C. C., Whitfield, T. H., Owen, L., Rein, T., Karri, S. K., Yakhkind, A., et al. (2010). Effects of Yoga Versus Walking on Mood, Anxiety, and Brain GABA Levels: A Randomized Controlled MRS Study. *The Journal of Alternative and Complementary Medicine, 16*(11), 1145–1152.

Svatmarama. (2002). *The hatha yoga pradipika* (B. D. Akers, Trans.). Woodstock: YogaVidya.

Taylor, M. (2012). Complementary and alternative medicine preparations used to treat symptoms of menopause. *Menopausal Medicine, 20*(1), 1–8.

Taylor, A. C., McCartney, N., Kamath, M. V., & Wiley, R. L. (2003). Isometric training lowers resting blood pressure and modulates autonomic control. *Medicine and Science in Sports and Exercise, 35*(2), 251–256.

Telles, S., Reddy, S. K., & Nagendra, H. R. (2000). Oxygen consumption and respiration following two yoga relaxation techniques. *Applied Psychophysiology and Biofeedback, 25*(4), 221–227.

Thacker, S. B., Gilchrist, J., Stroup, D. F., & Kimsey, C. D. J. (2004). The impact of stretching on sports injury risk: A systematic review of the literature. *Medicine and Science in Sports and Exercise, 36*(3), 371–378.

Tonon, G. (2007). La propuesta teórica de la calidad de vida como escenario facilitador de construcción de redes de investigación. *HOLOGRAMÁTICA*, IV, 7, V1, pp. 15–21. http://www.hologramatica.com.ar/. Accessed 25 Oct 2013.

Uebelacker, L. A., Epstein-Lubow, G., Gaudiano, B. A., Tremont, G., Battle, C. L., & Miller, I. W. (2010). Hatha yoga for depression: critical review of the evidence for efficacy, plausible mechanisms of action, and directions for future research. *Journal of Psychiatric Practice, 16* (1), 22–33.

Veenhoven, R. (1994). Is happiness a trait? *Social Indicators Research, 32,* 101–160.

Vempati, R. P., & Telles, S. (2002). Yoga-based guided relaxation reduces sympathetic activity judged from baseline levels. *Psychological Reports, 90*(2), 487–494.

Viotti, N. (2010). El lugar de la creencia y la transformación religiosa en las clases medias de Buenos Aires. *Apuntes de Investigación del CECYP 18*, 39–68.

Wells, M., Sama, L., Cooley, M. E., Brown, J. K., Chernecky, C., Williams, R. D., Padilla, G., & Danao, L. L. (2007). Use of complementary and alternative medicine therapies to control symptoms in women living with lung cancer. *Cancer Nursing, 30*(1), 45–55.

Yang, K. (2007). A review of yoga programs for four leading risk factors of chronic diseases. *Evidence Based Complementary Alternative Medicine, 4*(4), 487–491.

Zimmer, H. (1979). *Filosofías de la India*. Buenos Aires: Editorial Universitaria de Buenos Aires.

Index

A
Acquired Immunodeficiency Syndrome *See* AIDS, 104
AIDS, 103, 106, 110
  diagnosis of, 101
  psychosocial effects of, 104
  research on, 118
  role of therapies in, 106
  symptoms of, 103

C
Children, 57, 89, 125, 127, 138, 205, 211
  quality of life in, 121
  sexuality of, 116
  social sciences research in, 125
Community,
  technique, 65
Context, 135, 144, 154, 159, 175, 180, 184, 195, 199
  cultural, 65
  heterogeneity of, 73
  historical, 89
Culture, 24, 67, 78, 126, 153

G
Geography, 63, 64, 66, 67, 82
  critical, 68
  evolution of theoretical thinking in, 65
  of the French tradition, 71

I
Impact in the researcher, 25
Integration, 29
  in quality of life research, 59
  in the research field, 53

L
Life satisfaction, 150
  assessment of, 79

M
Mixed-methods, 53

N
New methodological strategy, 53

P
Participation, 24, 58, 124, 132, 144, 159
  and research, 128, 130
  effective, 183
  political, 141
Personal dimension, 26
  concept of, 26
Political dimension, 26
  concept of, 29
Population, 64, 73, 78, 83, 89, 105, 181, 198
  agglomerated, 155
  child, 143
  study of, 110
  welfare, 125
Professional dimension, 26, 28

Q
Qualitative methodologies, 65, 72
Qualitative methods, 25, 35, 57, 109
Qualitative researcher, 23, 24, 35
  role of, 26
Qualitative techniques, 58, 64
Quality of life, 31, 73, 100, 128, 137, 138, 142, 165, 187, 207, 209, 212
  concept of, 76, 80, 185
  main components of, 152

G. Tonon (ed.), *Qualitative Studies in Quality of Life*,
Social Indicators Research Series 55, DOI 10.1007/978-3-319-13779-7

perceptions of, 58
research on, 54, 59, 125

R
Relationship culture-quality of life, 30
Rural,
community, 152, 154, 169
life, 171
matter, 188
quality of life, 180, 185, 202, 210
villages, 198
Rural young people, 154, 169, 181, 188, 193, 196, 209, 213

S
Semi-structured interviews, 25, 107, 108
Socio-cultural context, 196, 213
Space, 125, 142, 165, 188

T
Triangulation, 53, 54
Denzin's definition of, 53
uses of, 195, 213

U
Urban, 68, 175, 183
community, 152

W
Well-being, 80, 117, 170
psychological, 211
social, 186

Y
Young people, 31, 105, 112, 115, 152, 156, 163, 164, 166, 169, 171, 175, 179, 180, 182, 193, 198, 200, 208, 209, 212
with HIV/AIDS, 110

MIX
Papier aus verantwortungsvollen Quellen
Paper from responsible sources
FSC® C105338

If you have any concerns about our products,
you can contact us on
ProductSafety@springernature.com

In case Publisher is established outside the EU,
the EU authorized representative is:
Springer Nature Customer Service Center GmbH
Europaplatz 3, 69115 Heidelberg, Germany

Printed by Libri Plureos GmbH
in Hamburg, Germany